PRENATAL DIAGNOSIS – MORPHOLOGY SCAN AND INVASIVE METHODS

Edited by **Richard Kwong Wai Choy** and
Tak Yeung Leung

Prenatal Diagnosis – Morphology Scan and Invasive Methods
Edited by Richard Kwong Wai Choy and Tak Yeung Leung

Published by InTech
Janeza Trdine 9, 51000 Rijeka, Croatia

Publishing Process Manager Bojan Rafaj

Technical Editor Teodora Smiljanic

Cover Designer InTech Design Team

Additional hard copies can be obtained from orders@intechopen.com

Prenatal Diagnosis – Morphology Scan and Invasive Methods, Edited by Richard Kwong Wai Choy and Tak Yeung Leung
p. cm.
ISBN 978-953-51-0614-2

For EU product safety concerns:
IN TECH d.o.o., Prolaz Marije Krucifikse Kozulić 3, 51000 Rijeka, Croatia,
info@intechopen.com or visit our website at intechopen.com.

Meet the editors

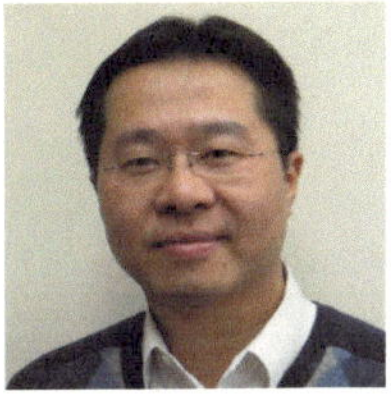

Dr Richard K. W. Choy obtained his BSc degree in Biomedical Sciences from the University of Bradford and M(Med)Sc in Immunology at University of Birmingham, UK. He received postgraduate training in research and was awarded Doctor of Philosophy by The Chinese University of Hong Kong in 1999. Dr Choy's main research interests include the development of novel molecular diagnostic strategies and innovative applications of molecular analysis tools in prenatal diagnosis. His current research focuses on the development of the microarray based Comparative Genomic Hybridization (array CGH) and massive parallel sequencing for prenatal diagnosis. In terms of professional service, Dr Choy is an Honorary Scientific Officer (medical) at the New Territories East Cluster of Hospitals, Hong Kong, where he is involved in the delivery of the laboratory diagnostic service. He is also the board member of the Hong Kong Society of Medical Genetics since 2009.

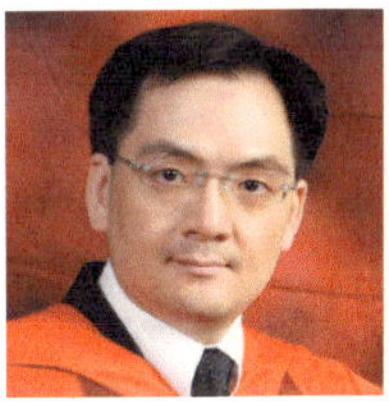

Tak Yeung Leung is Professor in the Maternal Fetal Medicine unit in the Department of Obstetrics and Gynaecology of The Chinese University of Hong Kong. His special interest is in perinatal medicine, prenatal screening and diagnosis of fetal abnormalities, with advanced genetic and ultrasound technology, including the non-invasive prenatal diagnosis using maternal cell-free fetal DNA and array comparative genomic hybirdisation. He has published more than 150 papers in international peer reviewed journals. He is also invited into the editorial board of international journals suchas American Journal of Perinatology and Pediatric Research (Fetus & Pregnancy Section). Besides, Professor Leung has strong international and Asian-Pacific connection with appointments in several international professional bodies including: Chairman of the Prenatal Maternal Screening Special Interest Group of International Society for Prenatal Diagnosis, Foundation Broad member of Global Obstetric Network (GONet), Foundation Secretary of The Chinese Fetal Medicine Foundation. He is also the Vice-president of Obstetrical and Gynaecolgical Society of Hong Kong, and co-opt council member of Hong Kong College of Obstetricians and Gynaecologists. Professor Leung is enthusiastic in teaching and training and is the organizer as well as trainer in many traning courses such as first trimester ultrasound, ALSO and PROMPT.

Contents

Preface

As new technological innovations arise, clinical medicine must also adapt and assimilate these advances into clinical practice. Prenatal diagnosis is no exception. When amniocentesis was introduced into practice, study of the unbanded chromosomes was the standard. With the introduction of G-banded analysis, duplications, deletions, and gross chromosomal translocations were detectable. By comparing the phenotypic to the genotypic findings, most of the detected chromosomal aberrations were quickly found to be clinically relevant. Integrating this new information into patient care and counseling required years of data gathering and analysis. As clinical and molecular technologies continued to evolve, similar questions concerning the appropriate clinical use of these technologies in prenatal diagnosis have also arisen.

Prenatal Diagnosis: Morphology Scan and Invasive Methods brings together distinguished contributors with extensive experience in the fetal ultrasound and prenatal diagnosis fields. Emphasis has been paid to the inclusion of molecular and sonographic techniques used in fetal medicine that are relevant to obstetricians and scientists performing prenatal diagnosis. These include how to diagnose iodine deficiency, skeletal dysplasisa; methods for molecular diagnosis of fetal diseases and treatment by fetal therapy. We hope that this book will be an invaluable reference for obstetricians and scientists in the process of prenatal diagnosis.

Richard Kwong Wai Choy and Tak Yeung Leung
The Chinese University of Hong Kong,
Prince of Wales Hospital,
Hong Kong, China

1

Invasive Prenatal Diagnosis

Sonja Pop-Trajković[1], Vladimir Antić[1] and Vesna Kopitović[2]
[1]Clinic for Gynecology and Obstetrics, Clinical center of Niš
[2]Clinic for Gynecology and Obstetrics, Clinical Center of Vojvodina
Serbia

1. Introduction

Prenatal diagnosis, traditionally used as a synonymous for invasive fetal testing and evaluation of chromosomal constellation, presently encompasses many other issues like pedigree analyses, fetal risk assessment, population screening, genetic counseling and fetal diagnostic testing as well. Ultrasound guided chorionic villus samling (CVS), amniocentesis and, to a lesser extent, fetal blood sampling are used routinely in fetal medicine units. Other fetal tissue biopsies such as skin, liver and muscle biopsy are used only rarely. In this chapter we discuss the invasive diagnostic procedures in maternal fetal medicine with specific interest of showing the list of indications basic principles used for choosing the particular invasive technique, linkage of non invasive with invasive diagnostic procedures, precise description of techniques, list of complications and their prevention and management, all of these based on the recent scientific results and clinical experiences publicized in the available literature.

2. Chorionic villus sampling

The ability to sample and analyse villus tissue was demonstrated in China, in 1975 (Department of Obstetrics and Gynecology THoAIaSCA, 1975). Trying to develop a technique for fetal sex determination, Chinese inserted a thin catheter into the uterus guided only by the tactile sensation and small pieces of villi were aspirated. By today's standards of ultrasonically guided invasive procedures this approach seems crude, but their diagnostic accuracy and low miscarriage rate demonstrated the feasibility of first-trimester sampling. Major advancements have occurred since that time in instrumentation, techniques for direct kariotyping, faster culturing of cells and in the molecular and biochemical assay of chorionic villi. Today in experienced centers, chorionic villus sampling (CVS) as a method of obtaining chorionic villi using transcervical or transabdominal approach, can be utilized as a primary prenatal diagnostic tool. Although CVS has the advantage of being carried out very early in pregnancy to the widespread amniocentesis, due to, more likely, the more technically demanding aspects of sampling, CVS has still not replaced amniocentesis in many centers.

2.1 Timing and technique

CVS is usually performed between 10 and 12 weeks of pregnancy. The risk and severity of limb deficiency appear to be associated with the timing of CVS: the risk before the end of 10 weeks gestation is higher than the risk from CVS done before that time. The upper limit for transcervical sampling has been suggested to be 12–13 weeks. Indeed, by the end of the first trimester, the gestational sac becomes attached to the decidual wall. Thereafter, any attempt to insert either a catheter or a biopsy forceps entails a higher risk of indenting and damaging the membranes .There are two paths for approaching placenta: through the maternal abdomen using a needle or through the cervical canal by catheter or biopsy forceps. For transcervical CVS, after ultrasound examination and determination of placental location, position of uterus and cervix is determined and a catheter path is mapped. (Vaughan & Rodeck,2001). The distal 3 to 5 cm of the sampling catheter is molded into a slightly curved shape and the catheter gently passed under ultrasound guidance through the cervix to the distal edge of the placenta under the ulatrasound visualization. The stylet is removed and a syringe with nutrient medium is attached. After obtaining negative pressure by a syringe the catheter is gently removed. In most cases chorionic villi are seen with naked eye in the syring (Dadelszen et al.,2005). For transabdominal approach the skin surface is treated with antiseptic solution. Trajectory of the needle should be chosen as much as parallel to the long axis of the trophoblast. The 20-gauge needle is inserted into chorionic villi (single needle technique). In some centers double needle technique is used. With this technique, 18-gauge needle is inserted into chorionic villi and the stylet is removed, then a smaller, 20-gauge needle with the aspirating syringe is inserted through this needle. Therefore if the sample is not adequate, sampling procedure with this smaller needle through 18-gauge needle can be repeated as necessary. Each technique (single or double needle) can be either free-hand or with needle-guide (alfirevic et al.,2003).

2.2 Counseling before CVS

Individualized counseling, by the obstetrician or an expert in genetics should always precede the procedure and support the couple in coming to a decision. Adequate time and personnel should be available to conduct a high-quality informed consent process in order to enhance the woman's decision making about prenatal testing. Counseling patients before CVS should emphasize some issues. First, the indication for invasive diagnosis in general and for CVS in particular. CVS is recommended for patients with very high risk of single gene disorder or chromosomal translocations in offspring. Although CVS should be also available to lower risk patients who wish karyotyping, the amniocentesis as an alternative should be offered. Second, specific data should be given to parents about failure, false-negative and false-positive results of the procedure and the need of amniocentesis in cases with confined placental mosaicism which occurs in approximately 1-2%. At the end, the risks of CVS should be discussed, especially the risk of fetal loss. The risk of other complications is low and should not be discussed routinely, unless the patient asks. Written material about CVS might also be given to the couple. It is good clinical practice to obtain formal written consent for CVS before the procedure and it is mandatory in most centers.

2.3 Indications

Prenatal diagnosis in the first trimester has advantages over midtrimester diagnosis for a number of reasons. The first one is the advantage of an earlier procedure which brings relief to the patient when the results are normal and on the other hand allows an easier and more private pregnancy termination when necessary. Earliest time for having the chromosome results is the 14th week with CVS and the 19th week with amniocentesis. First trimester abortion is followed by significantly lower rate of clinical complications. Speaking of emotional effect on patient, it is less stressful than labor induction and delivery at about 20 weeks. Also, by that time maternal-fetal bonding is not clearly established and the pregnancy is generally not visible to the environment. Additionally, early diagnosis is essential when there is a need for in utero gene or stem cell therapy for the correction a genetic defect. The earliest applications of CVS were fetal sex determination and prenatal diagnosis of hemoglobinonopathies by DNA analysis (Monni et al.,1993) Since then, advances in cytogenetic and DNA analysis techniques have remarkably expanded the number and types of genetic conditions detectable in the prenatal period. Currently, CVS is primarily indicated for chromosomal studies, DNA analysis of genetic disorders and prenatal diagnosis of inborn errors of metabolism. For chromosomal studies, the main indications for CVS are: maternal age over 35 years, previous pregnancy with a chromosomal abnormality or multiple anomalies, parents with proved chromosome translocations, inversions and aneuploidies, X-linked diseases, history of recurrent miscarriage, abnormal ultrasound scan and decrease or the absence of amniotic fluid in the first trimester. The development of first-trimester screening methods for the detection of fetal chromosomal anomalies has increased the demand for CVS. In fact, although maternal-related risk for fetal aneuploidy remains a common indication for CVS, the indication for CVS has evolved to become one of quick confirmation of an abnormal karyotype whenever chromosomal abnormality is suspected based on ultrasound scan or biochemical screening in the first trimester. Less common indications for fetal karyotyping are multiple miscarriages and pregnancies after assisted reproductive techniques. First trimester ultrasound screening for Down syndrome can occasionally bring to light a number of fetal abnormalities. Holoprosencephaly, omphalocele, cystic hygroma, diaphragmatic hernia and megacystis are well known features of either aneuploidies or other genetic syndromes. When they are detected in the first trimester, CVS is indicated for fetal karyotyping or molecular studies. DNA-based diagnoses of single-gene disorders, such as cystic fibrosis, hemophilia, muscular dystrophy and hemoglobinopathies, continue to expand with advancing technologies and the discovery of the additional disease-causing genes. Single gene disorders, which affect about 1% of livebirths, carry a high risk of recurrence and have unsatisfactory treatment so that prenatal diagnosis with termination of affected pregnancies is an important option for at-risk couples. Prenatal diagnosis of genetic disorders is based on the carrier detection procedures and genetic counseling of the couples at risk. Inborn errors of metabolism represent a vast group of disorders that are individually rare but together are a significant cause of human disease. Chorionic villi provide large amounts of metabolically active cytoplasm, therefore for many inherited metabolic diseases direct assay is possible, yielding diagnostic results within hours or a few days. Moreover, the amount of DNA obtained from a conventional sampling allows reliable analysis by recombinant DNA technologies. This is not the case with amniotic fluid cells, which provide too little DNA, which is frequently fragmented. Majority of these disease are very rare and new detection methods for specific disorders are constantly being reported so it is advisable to check with a specialists referral center on the current availability and preferred method for prenatal diagnosis. Some congenital infections such as rubella, toxoplasmosis, cytomegalovirus and parvovirus can also be detected by CVS.

CVS in multiple pregnancies require more experience, ability and an accurate planning of the procedure. The procedure is not complicated in cases with clearly separated placentas but it becomes a challenge in cases of fused or joined placentas, because in contrast to amniocentesis when one amniotic cavity can be marked with a dye, with CVS there is no technique to ensure that each sample has been obtained from a distinct placenta. To be sure to sample all fetuses one by one, and to reduce the risk of contamination, separate forceps and needles are inserted in succession and different samples are collected in close proximity to each cord insertion. A high level of expertise in technique of CVS is crucial. However, CVS can generally offer several technical advantages over midtrimester amniocentesis (Antsaklis et al.,2002). The easy evaluation of the membranes by ultrasound makes both the prediction of chorionicity and amnionicity and the identification of the affected twin(s) more reliable, the use of rapid analytical methods makes substantial changes in the uterine topography very unlikely, and if same-sex dichorionic twins are diagnosed, DNA polymorphism markers may be easily checked to assure retrieval of villi from the individual placentas. In the hands of experienced operators, CVS has the same efficacy as mid-trimester amniocentesis for genetic diagnosis of multiple gestations: diagnostic error, probably due to incorrect sampling, is between 0,3% and 1,5%. Speaking of safety, carried out by expert physician, CVS appears at least as safe as amniocentesis (Brambati et al.,2001). Postprocedural loss rate after CVS in multiple pregnancies is somewhat higher than in singleton pregnancies but comparable to midtrimester amniocentesis. In cases where selective reduction is indicated the advantages of the first-trimester approach include a significantly lower emotional impact and a lower risk of clinical complications (Brambati et al.,2004)

2.4 Laboratory considerations for chorionic villus sampling

In the early development of CVS there was a high rate of incorrect results due to maternal cell contamination and misinterpretation due to placental mosaicism. In the early 1990s the laboratory failure rate was 2,3%, which was significantly higher compared to amniocentesis. Nowadays CVS is considered to be a reliable method of prenatal diagnosis with a high rate of sucess and accuracy. Most centers report near 99% CVS sucess rate with only 1 % of the patients requiring a second diagnostic test (amniocenteses or cordocenetsis) to clarify the results (Brun et al., 2003). Maternal cell contamination is the first cause of potential diagnostic errors which can occur after CVS.Obtained samples after CVS typically contain two cell lines: fetal i.e.placental villi and maternal i.e. decidua. It is posible that maternal cell line completely overgrow the culture and lead to incorect sex determination ans potentially to false- negative diagnosis. However, today, maternal cell contamination occurs in less then 1% of cases and usually does not limit the possibilities of accurate diagnosis. Contamination of samples with significant amounts of maternal decidual tissue is almost always due to small sampling size. In experienced centers in which adequate quantities of villi are avilable, this problem has disappeared. The second major cause of potential diagnostic error associated with CVS is placental mosaicism (Kalousek et al.,2000). The rate of placental mosaicism in the frst trimester CVS is 1-2%. Although the fetus and placenta have a common ancestry, chorionic villus tissue will not always reflect fetal genotype. While initially placental mosaicism was considered as the main disadvantige of CVS in prenatal diagnosis, today it is an important marker for pregnancies at increased risk for growth retardation or genetic abnormalities. Two mechanisms can explain the occurance of placental mosaicism: mitotic error originally confined to the placenta and trisomic conceptus loosing of chromososme in the embryonic cell line. The most significant complication of placental mosaicism is uniparental disomy which is the case when both chromosomes originate from the same parent (Kotzot et al.,2001). The clinical concequence of uniparental disomy occurs when the involved chromososme carries an imprinted gene in which expression is dependent on the patern of origin. For example, Prader-Willi syndrome may result from uniparental maternal disomy for chromosome 15. Because of this, all cases in which trisomy 15 is confined to the placenta should be evaluated for uniparental disomyy by amniotic fluid analysis. There is also evidence that placental mosaicism might alter placental function leading to the fetal growth restriction. This is especially relevant to chromosome 16 where placental trisomy affects growth of both uniparental and biparental disomy fetuses in a similar manner. A decision of termination of pregnancy should not be done on the basis of mosaicism found on CVS. In such cases an amniocentesis should be offer to elucidate the extent of fetal involvement. Amniocentesis correlates perfectly with fetal genotype when mosaicism is limited to the direct preparation. When a mosaicism is observed in tissue culture, amniocentesis is associated with a false negative rate of about 6% and mosaic fetuses were reported to be born after normal amniotic fluid analysis (Los et al.,2001). Follow-up may include fetal blood sampling or fetal skin biopsy. However, the predictive accuracy of these additional tests is still uncertain.

2.5 Transcervical versus transabdominal chorionic villus sampling

In most cases, operator or patient choice will determine the sampling route, but the choice of the route is usually decided on a case-by-case depending on placental site. Anterior and fundal placentas are usually easily accessed transabdominally while lower, posterior located placentas are more accessible transcervically. However, operators must be skilled in both methods. Both techniques appear to be comparably efficient between 8 and 12 weeks, when the overall success rate after two sampling device insertions is considered to be very near to 100% (Philip et al.,2004).This efficiency has been confirmed in three national randomized trials of transabdominal vs.transcervical CVS (Brambati et al.,1991; Jackson et al.,1992; Smidt-Jensen et al.,1992). Although the data appear to confirm that the two techniques are equally effective in obtaining adequate amounts of chorionic tissue, transabdominal needling entailed a significantly smaller proportion of repeated device insertions (3.3 vs. 10.3%) and of low weight specimens (3.2 vs. 4.9%). Moreover, the complications due to undetected vaginal or cervical infection were much higher in the transcervical group. Additionally, speaking of safety, the Cochrane review showed that the transcervical CVS is more technically demanding than transabdominal CVS with more failures to obtain sample and more multiple insertions (Alfirevic et al.,2003). There are no differences in birth weight , gestational age at delivery, or congenital malformations with either method (Cederholm et al.,2003). Because of the specificity of the sampling route, transabdominal and transcervical sampling techniques are expected to have different types of contraindications. Vaginismus and stenotic or tortuous cervical canal, as well as myomas of the lower uterine segment, may severely hamper the introduction of either catheter or forceps. Active vaginal infection may also be an absolute contraindication to the cervical route. In the latter condition, vaginal and cervical culture and specific treatment do not seem sufficient to remove any risk of ascending infection. Transabdominal sampling may be relatively or absolutely contraindicated when obstacles such as intestines, large myomas or the gestational sac cannot be avoided. If olygohydramnios is present, transabdominal CVS may be the only approach available.

Transabdominal sampling, in our experience, has definitely become the method of choice, and our preference for this approach is based on the shorter learning time, the lower rate of immediate complications, the higher practicality and success rates at the first device insertion, the lower hazard of intrauterine infection, the opportunity to extend sampling beyond the first trimester, and the wider range of diagnostic indications.

2.6 Complications

The benefits of earlier diagnosis of fetal genetic abnormalities by chorionic villus sampling (CVS) or early amniocentesis must be set against higher risks of pregnancy loss and possibly diagnostic inaccuracies of these tests when compared with second trimester amniocentesis. The overall pregnancy loss rate following CVS has been reported in a number of relatively large clinical studies, and the values range from 2.2% to 5.4% (Odibo et al.,2008). The date used for determining the associated risks of fetal loss due to CVS are presented in the literature as case series with detailed outcome and comparative studies of CVS group versus amniocentesis and transabdominal versus transcervical CVS. Data evaluating the safety of CVS compares amniocentesis comes primarily from three collaborative reports (Canadian Collaborative group, 1989; Medical Research Council, 1977; Rhoads et al.,1989). The results of Canadian Collaborative group demonstrated equivalent safety of CVS compared to midtrimester amniocentesis There was a 7,6% loss rate in the CVS group and a 7% loss rate in the amniocentesis group. A multicentric U.S. (Rhoads et al.,1989) study found slightly higher fetal loss rate following CVS (7,2%) compared to the one following midtrimester amniocentesis (5,7%). A prospective, randomized, collaborative comparison of more than 3200 pregnancies, sponsored by the European Medical Council reported CVS having a 4,6% greater pregnancy loss rate than amniocenetesis.Based on the presented data, CVS is associated with a slightly increased risk of fetal loss when compared to amniocentesis. Noteworthy, that excluding the results of the MRC study, CVS is associated with no more then 1 % extra risk of fetal loss when compared to midtrimester amniocentesis. Also, the risks of fetal loss rate should not be compared between the studies since each study had its own criteria for total fetal loss (although most have described fetal loss before 28 weeks gestation). Moreover, while some have included only cytogenetically normal fetuses, others have evaluated a mixed population. The risk of fetal loss after CVS can also be obtained from the studies comparing CVS with early amniocentesis (Caughey et al.,2006). Most of these studies point to a relatively small risk of fetal loss (2-3%) associated with CVS on the one hand and a significantly increased risk of fetal loss in the early amniocentesis gropu on the other hand. Logistic regression analysis of the procedure-related variables showed a significant association between fetal loss rate and maternal age, the lowest rates occurring in the youngest women (1.22%) and the highest in the women of 40 years and over, while gestational age affected the abortion rate only at 8 weeks (3.78%), no differences in the odds ratio being present at 9 to 12 weeks. Moreover, procedure related risk remained low later in pregnancy, and total fetal loss rates for CVS cases performed at 13–14 weeks and at least 15 weeks compared favorably with early and midtrimester amniocentesis respectively. Single-operator experience presents an estimated fetal loss after CVS of about 2-3%. Although, single operator experience shows that the results (fetal loss rate) of early procedures are better in the hands of skilled operators, this remains controversial. Transabdominal CVS is considered by many to be safer than the transcervical approach.However, this observation is heavily influenced by the data from the Danish study (Smidt-Jansen,1992).Moreover no significant difference found between those two approaches from two of three randomized trials comparing techniques.Based on these studies, as well as myny single center reports, we believe that the poor results from the Danish study (where the Portex cannula was used) would not be repeated if the operators were equally good at the techniques being compared. Unfortunately, no study has randomly evaluated CVS versus non-sampled (with same risk) patients.

Among early post-procedural complications, spotting within a few hours has been more frequently observed in patients undergoing transcervical rather than transabdominal CVS (Brambati et al.1991). Other sequelae due to injury to the placental circulation include retro-placental hematomas and subchorionic hemorrhage. Significant amniotic fluid leakage after CVS is about 2-4 times less frequent when compared to early amniocentesis.

Localized peritonitis immediately after sampling occurs in very few cases, and only after transabdominal sampling, with an overall rate of 0.04%. Intrauterine infection (acute chorionamnionitis) should be considered a potential, although very rare, complication of transcervical CVS, having been reported in 0.1–0.5% of cases, and in some large series no cases at all were observed (Paz et al.,2001). However, there is some concern about the role of less serious infection in women who experience fetal loss after transcervical CVS. Because transcervical CVS involves passage of a cannula or forceps through the cervical canal from the perineum and vagina, microbial colonization and infection, with consequent morbidity for both mother and fetus, may result (Cederholm et al.,2003).

Feto-maternal hemorrhage following CVS has been demonstrated by a significant increase in maternal serum a-fetoprotein in 40–72% of cases, and in 6–18% of these the amount of blood transfused was calculated to exceed 0.1ml. Fetal hemorrhage should therefore be capable of initiating an immune response in RhD-negative women bearing an RhD-positive fetus. Moreover, an association between maternal serum a-fetoprotein increase and frequency of spontaneous fetal death has been suggested for the cases with the highest maternal serum a-fetoprotein levels (Mariona et al.,1986).

In general, the rate of fetal abnormalities after CVS is not different than in general population. Several case reports and cohort studies in the early 1990s have suggested a possible association between CVS and a cluster of limb defects and oromandibular hypogenesis. However, these findings were not repeated in other studies. The background risk of limb reduction defects (LRD) in the general population is low and varies between 1.6 and 4/10000. In an evaluation of CVS safety presented by WHO, LRD cases were observed in 5.3/10000. The possible mechanisms of LRD following CVS are unknown. However, there are three principal theories:

1. Vascular disruption caused by hemodynamic disturbances, vasoactive peptides or embolism
2. Amnion puncture with subsequent compression and entanglement of the fetus.
3. Immunological mechanisms causing increased apoptotic cell death

It is speculated that technical aspects of the procedure may have a bearing on the amount of placental trauma associated with the sampling procedure and the risk of limb deficiency. However, the rarity of limb deficiency following CVS means that none of the existing trials have the power to clarify the effect of technical factors on the risk. It also remains unresolved whether the risk of limb deficiency differs for transabbominal versus transcervical sampling (

Froster et al., 1996). Given the weight of current evidence supporting an association between early sampling and limb deficiency, it would be unethical to conduct a trial to investigate this prospectively.

No increased frequency of perinatal complications, i.e. preterm birth, small-for-dates neonates, perinatal mortality and congenital malformations, have been observed both in randomized and clinical control studies (MRC Working Party, 1992).

3. Amniocentesis

Amniocentesis is the invasive diagnostic procedure by which amniotic fluid is aspirated from pregnant uterus using transabdominal approach. This method was first performed as therapeutic procedure more than 100 years ago for decompression of polyhydramnios. Amniocentesis became a diagnostic procedure in 1950s when Bevis first used amniotic fluid for measurement of bilirubin concetration and prediction of the severity of Rhesus immunisation. Today amniocentesis is a significant diagnostic tool for prenatal detection of chromosomal as well as metabolic disorder. Tests performed on fetal cells found in the sample can reveal the presence of many types of genetic disorders, thus allowing doctors and prospective parents to make important decisions about early treatment and intervention (Wilson, 2005).

3.1 Timing and technique

For karyotyping amniocentesis is generally performed between 15 and 18 weeks of gestation with results usually available within three weeks. At this time, the amount of fluid is adequate (approximately 150ml), and the ratio of viable to nonviable cells is greatest. With the current technology amniocentesis is technically possible from 8 weeks of gestation but this is not usually recommended because there appears to be an increased risk of miscarriage when done at this time (Allen & Wilson,2006). The advantage of early amniocentesis and speedy results lies in the extra time for decision making if a problem is detected. Potential treatment of the fetus can begin earlier. Important, also, is the fact that elective abortions are safer and less controversial the earlier they are performed. For assessment of the fetal lung maturity the amniocentesis can be used until term (Hanson et al.,1990). Before the procedure, genetic couceling is mandatory and a detailed family history should be obtained. The parents should be informed about the complications and limitations of the procedure same as for CVS. After genetic counseling, a "level two" ultrasound is then done to check for any signs of fetal abnormalities, to check the fetal viability, to determine the position of the fetus and of the placenta, to examine closely the main fetal structures, and to double check the gestational age (Hanson et al.,1990). Ultrasound is used also to determine the best location for placing the needle-a pocket of substantial amniotic fluid well away from the baby and umbilical cord. When amniocentesis first came into use, they were done "blind" (without continuous ultrasound guidance during the procedure), and this resulted in a number of disastrous outcomes, including occasional cases of horrifying fetal damage and death(Gratacos et al.,2000) .Modern amniocentesis is done with continuous ultrasound and is much less dangerous. For the amniocentesis, the mother lies flat on her back on a table. Iodine solution is swabbed onto her belly in order to cleanse the area thoroughly, and sterile drapes are placed around the area. After an appropriate sampling path has been chosen , a 20 to 22-gauge needle is introduced into a pocket of amniotic fluid free of fetal parts and a umbilical cord. The pocket should be large enough to allow advancement of the needle tip through the free-floating amniotic membrane that may occasionally obstruct the flow of fluid. The first 2ml of amniotic fluid are discarded to reduce the risk of contamination of the sample with maternal cells which could occasionally lead to false-negative diagnosis. The amount of withdrawn amniotic fluid should not exceed 20 to 30ml (Blessed et al.,2001).There is confirmed relationship between higher fetal loss and aspiration of 40ml of amniotic fluid and more. Continuous ultrasound during an amniocentesis allows the doctor to see a constant view of the needle's path, the location of fetus and to identify uterine contractions that occasionally retract the needle tip back into the myometrium. If the fetus moves near the needle's path at any point, the doctor can then reposition the needle, or if necessary, withdraw the needle and try again in a different location. Continuous ultrasound has eliminated a great deal of the risk formerly associated with amniocentesis (Johnson al.,1999). The procedure should be performed either free-hand or with the needle guide. The free-hand technique allows easier manipulation of the needle if the position of the target is altered by a fetal movement or uterine contraction. Alternatively, a needle guide allows more certain ascertainment of the needle entry point and a more precise entry determination of the sampling path. A needle guide technique is helpful for obese patients, in cases of oligohydramnios and for relatively inexperienced sonographer (Welch et al.,2006). After the fluid sample is taken, the doctor immediately checks the viability of the fetus. Both uterine and maternal abdominal wall puncture sites should be observed for bleeding and anti-D should be given to Rh negative women. In experienced hands and after 11 completed weeks of gestation the pure amniotic fluid aspiration has a success rate of 100%. If the initial attempt to obtain fluid is unsuccessful, a second attempt in another location should be performed after reevaluation of the fetal and placental positions. If unsuccessful after two attempts, the patient should be rescheduled in several days. The technique of early amniocentesis is similar to amniocentesis performed at later gestational ages. However, in the first trimester there are two sacs, the amniotic cavity and the extra-embryonic coelome. The incomplete fusion of the amnion and chorion in early gestation may result in tenting of the membranes, which may necessitate more needle insertions. It is important to distinguish the two sacs ultrasonographically at the time of the amniocentesis, as the fluid in the extraembryonic coelome is jelly-like, difficult to aspirate, and has a different alpha-fetoprotein concentration than amniotic fluid. Retrieval of fluid from this sac should be avoided, as it will only rarely produce enough cells to allow a cytogenetic diagnosis (Sundberg et al.,1991). In order to assess whether amniotic fluid has been retrieved from both sacs in twin pregnancies, a marker (a dye or a biochemical substance) may be injected into the first sac. When the second sac is punctured, the absence of the marker in the amniotic fluid indicates that both sacs have been sampled. However, real-time ultrasound allows visually guided amniotic fluid sampling from both sacs, thus making dye-injection obsolete (Pijpers et al.,1988). Whether amniocentesis in twin pregnancies should be performed by using one or two needle insertions remains to be shown. A single needle insertion could reduce the abortion risk, but may on the other hand create the problems of amniotic band syndrome or a mono-amniotic twin pregnancy, or give rise to cytogenetic problems (Millaire et al.,2006).

3.2 Indications

Since the mid-1970s, amniocentesis has been used routinely to test for Down syndrome by far the most common, nonhereditary, genetic birth defect, affecting about one in every 1,000 babies. By 1997, approximately 800 different diagnostic tests were available, most of them for hereditary genetic disorders such as Tay-Sachs disease, sickle cell anemia, hemophilia, muscular dystrophy and cystic fibrosis (Summers et al.,2007).

Amniocentesis is recommended for women who will be older than 35 on their due-date. It is also recommended for women who have already borne children with birth defects, or when either of the parents has a family history of a birth defect for which a diagnostic test is available. Another reason for the procedure is to confirm indications of Down syndrome and certain other defects which may have shown up previously during routine maternal blood screening (Fergal et al.,2005). The risk of bearing a child with a nonhereditary genetic defect such as Down syndrome is directly related to a woman's age—the older the woman, the greater the risk. Thirty-five is the recommended age to begin amniocentesis testing because that is the age at which the risk of carrying a fetus with such a defect roughly equals the risk of miscarriage caused by the procedure-about one in 200. At age 25, the risk of giving birth to a child with this type of defect is about one in 1,400; by age 45 it increases to about one in 20. Nearly half of all pregnant women over 35 in the United States undergo amniocentesis and many younger women also decide to have the procedure. Notably, some 75% of all Down syndrome infants born in the United States each year are to women younger than 35 (Jacobson et al.,2004).

One of the most common reasons for performing amniocentesis is an abnormal alpha-fetoprotein (AFP) test. Because this test has a high false-positive rate, another test such as amniocentesis is recommended whenever the AFP levels fall outside the normal range (Sepulveda et al.,1995).

3.3 Laboratory considerations for amniocentesis

The cells within the amniotic fluid arise from fetal skin, respiratory tract, urinary tract, gastrointestinal tract and placenta. After obtained fetal cells, they are put into tissue culture, either in flasks or more often on coverslips. After 3 to 7 days of growth, sufficient mitoses are present for staining and karyotype analysis. Viable cells in the amniotic fluid are cultured and used for karyotyping, and investigation of metabolic and biochemical disorders. Uncultured cells may now be used to detect specific chromosome aberrations by using chromosome specific probes and fluorescent in situ hybridization (FISH) on interphase cells, but complete karyotyping is not yet possible on uncultured cells (Pergament,2000). Amniocyte culture is quite reliable, with failure occurring in less than 1% of cases. The culture failure rate increase with falling gestational age and it seems to occur more often in fetal aneuploidy. Chromosomal mosaicism most frequently results from postzygotic nondisjunction but can also occur from meiotic errors with trisomic rescue. The most common etiology is pseudomosaicism where the abnormality is evident in only one of several flasks or confined to a single colony on a coverslip. In this case the abnormal cells have arisen in vitro, are not present in the fetus, and are not clinically important. Alternatively, true fetal mosaicism is rare, occurring in 0,25% of amniocentesis but can be clinically important, leading to phenotypic or developmental abnormalities. Maternal cell contamination may cause misdiagnosis, if only maternal cells are examined or mosaicism is suspected. The rate of maternal cell contamination is 1-3 per 1000 cases, but this figure should probably be doubled as maternal cell contamination is only detected when the fetus is male (Tepperberg et al.,2001). A large study (Welch et al.,2006) sought to relate the frequency of maternal cell contamination in amniotic fluid samples that were submitted to a single laboratory for cytogenetic analysis to the experience and training of the physician who performed the amniocentesis.

Fluorescence in situ hybridization (FISH) probes are relatively short fluorescently labeled DNA sequences that are hybridized to a known location on a specific chromosome and allow for determination of the number and location of specific DNA sequences. Presently, it is suggested that FISH analysis not be used as a primary screening test on all genetic amniocenteses because of its inability to detect structural rearrangements, mosaicism, markers, and uncommon trisomies. Because all abnormalities would be detectable by tissue culture, FISH analysis is not cost effective. Presently, most laboratories use FISH to offer quick reassurance to patients with an unusually high degree of anxiety or to test fetuses at the highest risk, such as those with ultrasound anomalies. It is also beneficial in cases where rapid results are crucial to subsequent management, such as advanced gestational age (Sawa et al., 2001).

3.4 Complications

Amniocentesis is not without maternal and fetal complications and should be undertaken with due regard to the risks involved.

3.4.1 Maternal

The risk of intervention for the mother is minimal. The risk of an amnionitis after amniocentesis is less than 0,1% and the risk of a severe maternal infection reaches 0.03%-0.09% (Wurster et al.,1982). In a retrospective survey of 358 consecutive amniocentesis (Pergament, 2000) there were two patients who developed amniotic fluid peritonism and one with minor intraperitoneal bleeding. Amniocentesis is not associated with severe pregnancy complications such as placental abruption or placenta praevia. On the other hand after amniocentesis there is an increased risk of complications related to amniotic cavity, membranes and hypotonic uterine dysfunction (Cederholm et al.,2003).Feto-maternal hemorrhage occurs during amniocentesis in one out of six women, and may therefore theoretically give rise to subsequent isoimmunisation. In a prospective cohort study (Tabor et al.,1987) the immunization rate was 1.4%. The observed 1.4% immunization rate is not different from the spontaneous immunization rate. In spite of these findings, and since Rh-immune serum globulin is apparently harmless to the fetus and mother, its use is recommended in nonsensitized Rh-negative mothers after amniocentesis Practice differs between countries regarding whether this recommendation is followed or not. In American controlled study anxiety and depression varied similarly in women having amniocentesis and in control women. However, among women having amniocentesis due to advanced maternal age, the anxiety level was increased while awaiting the results of the test (Phipps et al.,2005).

3.4.2 Fetal

The major risk of mid-trimester amniocentesis is fetal loss. Two types of loss should be considered: (1) total pregnancy loss rate postprocedure, which includes both background pregnancy loss for that gestational age and procedure-related loss, and (2) procedure related pregnancy loss. The total post-amniocentesis loss rates are derived from studies of populations of pregnant women who underwent amniocentesis, with a control group consisting of populations of pregnant women who had another procedure. The amniocentesis-related pregnancy loss rates are derived from studies of pregnant women who had amniocentesis compared with a "no procedure" control group. A study published by Eddleman et al. suggests that the procedural loss rate of amniocentesis may be much smaller than previously reported, further challenging the indications for invasive testing in the context of a traditional "risk-benefit" ratio (Eddleman et al.,2006). Although the committee agrees that it is timely to re-evaluate this issue, it is believed Eddleman's conclusion that the rate of miscarriage due to amniocentesis of 0.06% (1/1600) is misleading and should be interpreted with caution. The study is based on a secondary analysis of data from the "First and Second Trimester Evaluation of Risk for Aneuploidy" (FASTER) trial, the primary goal of which was to compare first and second trimester noninvasive prenatal genetic screening methods. Among the 35 003 women enrolled the rate of spontaneous fetal loss prior to 24 weeks' gestation in the study group was 1%, not statistically different from the control group rate of 0.94%. The risk of miscarriage due to amniocentesis was reported to be the difference between these two rates, which was 0.06%. Letters to the editor have criticized the FASTER conclusion. Nadel (Nadel,2007) concluded that the likelihood of amniocentesis resulting in the loss of a euploid fetus is less than 0.5% .Smith (Smith,2007) commented that the methods used to include or exclude pregnancy termination patients resulted in the paradox of a statistically significant increase in spontaneous abortion for women not having amniocentesis with a positive screen and women who were aged 35 years or over. The lowest rate of risk for genetic amniocentesis derived from the literature is about 1 in 300 (Wilson,2007). In counseling patients prior to amniocentesis, it is important to convey to patients that at their stage of pregnancy there is still a background pregnancy loss rate, and that amniocentesis will contribute an additional procedure related loss rate. The notion of background population or individual loss rate is important, as the patient will not be able to determine whether her pregnancy loss was "background" or "procedural."Counselling should provide a woman with the total pregnancy loss rate to enable her to fully understand the possible sequelae of her decision. Individual procedural risks may be required for counseling because of the real variables that contribute to the population or individual background risk.

A. Patient factors

1. Maternal age/ paternal age (Kleinhaus et al.,2006)
2. Past reproductive history
3. Pre-existing maternal conditions (diabetes, hypertension, infertility, autoimmune)
4. Pregnancy/uterine (assisted reproductive techniques, vaginal bleeding, uterine fibroids, placental location, amniotic fluid loss, oligohydramnios, retro chorionic hematoma, single vs. multiple gestations)
5. Screening methodology
   i. timing (first trimester, second trimester, first and second trimester)
   ii. technique (ultrasound alone, biochemistry, biochemistry and ultrasound, nuchal translucency +/- biochemistry, single or multiple soft markers or congenital anomalies)

B. Procedure factors

1. Amniocentesis needle size variation
2. Operator experience
3. Ultrasound guided (freehand; needle guide)
4. Uterine/placental location
5. Maternal BMI

C. Postprocedure factors

1. Rest for 24 hours or normal activity (no evidence-based comparisons available)
2. Complications (ruptured membranes, infection)

Increasing maternal and paternal age are significantly associated with spontaneous abortion, independent of amniocentesis and multiple other factors (Kleinhaus et al.,2006). Also pre-existing maternal conditions, as well as assisted reproductive techniques and multiple gestations are "per se" risk factors for increase fetal loss (Bianco et al.,2006). Amniocentesis before 14 weeks gestation has an adverse effect on fetal loss (Alfirević et al.,2007). Rupture of membranes is an uncommon complication of genetic amniocentesis. Theoretically, a thin needle may have both advantages and disadvantages for fetal loss. One would expect a thin needle to cause a smaller hole in the membranes and to be less traumatic, thereby decreasing the risk of amniotic fluid leakage and feto-maternal hemorrhage. On the other hand, a thin needle increases the procedure time, and increased sampling time might be associated with an increased risk of chorio-amnionitis and fetal loss (Weiner,1991). It seems reasonable to assume the fetal loss to be lower if the operator has performed a large number of invasive procedures than if he/she is inexperienced. (Milunsky,2010). The number of annual procedures needed for amniocentesis to be safe is not known, and the recommendation of at least 150 amniocenteses per year is not based on scientific evidence. There is indirect evidence from nonrandomized studies that ultrasound guided amniocentesis is safer than blind amniocentesis, because feto-maternal hemorrhage occurs less often if the procedure is performed under ultrasound guidance than if it is done blindly and feto-maternal hemorrhage may be associated with an increased risk of fetal loss (Papantoniou et al.,2001). In the study by Weiner and colleagues, there was some evidence that the rate of fetal loss after amniocentesis increased with the number of needle insertions. On the other hand they did not find increased fetal loss after transplacental passage of the amniocentesis needle than after non-transplacental passage. Possibly, the most important thing is to perform the procedure as atraumatically as possible. Therefore, the puncture site that gives easiest access to a pocket of free fluid should be chosen. If the placenta can be easily avoided, it is probably wise to avoid it. Whether the amount of amniotic fluid removed has any effect on fetal loss rates is not known, but it is probably wise to remove as little as possible (usually 15-20 ml is enough to obtain a diagnosis). Spontaneous reseal of ruptured membranes after genetic amniocentesis can occur with conservative management and end with a favorable pregnancy outcome (Phupong & Ultchaswadi,2006).

The Table 1 summarizes the recent published reports (randomized controlled trials and cohort studies with or without a control group; the control group may have no procedure or an alternative procedure), showing a range of post mid-trimester amniocentesis losses of 0.75 to 2,1% .The FASTER study pregnancy loss difference (amniocentesis; no amniocentesis) is a clear outlier within these controlled study groups and reflects that this study's method of analysis underestimated the procedure-related pregnancy loss rate following mid-trimester amniocentesis by excluding the terminated pregnancies in the amniocentesis group, resulting in a lower intrinsic rate of pregnancy loss for this group than for the control group.

In conclusion there is *no* single percentage (or odds ratio) that can be quoted as the risk of pregnancy loss following midtrimester amniocentesis in singleton pregnancies. The risks unique to the individual and is based on multiple variables, as summarized in this opinion. The best estimate range to consider for the increased rate of pregnancy loss attributable to amniocentesis is 0.6% to 1.0% but may be as low as 0.19% or as high as 1.53% on the basis of the confidence intervals seen in the various studies.

The fetal loss rate in multiple gestations has not been estimated in a controlled trial and is difficult to determine due to the increased miscarriage rate per se in twin pregnancies. An increased post-amniocentesis abortion rate in multiple gestations may be expected, since most operators use more than one needle insertion, a variable associated with an increased fetal loss rate (Toth-Pal et al., 2004). In the largest Israel study fetal loss among bichorionic twin gestations undergoing genetic amniocentesis was compare with singletons undergoing the procedure and untested twins. Fetal loss was 2,73% in the first group, compared to 0,6% and 0,63% in the other two groups. It may thus be concluded that the risk of early fetal loss is apparently higher in twins undergoing amniocentesis than in untested twins or tested singletons. These data can be of value in counseling parents of twins because of the increased number of gestations resulting from fertility programs and the elevated risk of chromosomal abnormalities in twin pregnancies (Yukobowich et al.,2001). Whether amniocentesis in twin pregnancies should be performed by using one or two needle insertions remains to be shown. A single needle insertion could reduce the abortion risk, but may on the other hand create the problems of amniotic band syndrome or a mono-amniotic twin pregnancy, or give rise to cytogenetic problems (Wapner et al.,1993).

Considering perinatal mortality et morbidity, amniocentesis does not affect the preterm birth rate, the stillbirth rate or the perinatal mortality rate. This procedure does not affect neither the mean birth weight. In early experience with amniocentesis, needle puncture of the fetus was reported in 0,1% to 0,3% of cases (Karp & Hayden, 1977) and was associated with fetal exsanguinations (Young et al., 1977), intestinal atresia (Swift et al., 1979), uniocular blindess, porencephalic cysts, peripheral nerve damage and intestinal atresia (Karp & Hayden,1977) Continuous use of ultrasound to guide the needle minimizes needle puncture of the fetus and in the hands of experienced operators those are extremely rare complications. The British study (Medical Research Study, 1978) also found an increase in postural deformities such as talipes and congenital dislocation of the hip. The possible mechanism of this deformity is compression due to olygohydramnios or tissue injury from the amniocentesis needle. This study was criticized for biases in the selection of the control patients who were younger, had less parity, entered later in the gestation in the study and some of the matched controls were replaced with other controls.No long-term adverse effects have been demonstrated in children undergoing amniocentesis. Finegan and colleagues (Baird et al.,1994) showed that the offspring of women who had had amniocentesis were no more likely than controls to have a registrable disability (such as hearing disabilities, learning difficulties, visual problems, and limb anomalies) during childhood and adolescence. At the ages of 4 and 7 years, there was no difference between the two groups regarding child social competence, behaviour, growth and health. The results suggest that the wide range of developmental and behavioural variables studied is not influenced by removal of amniotic fluid in the mid-trimester.

A. Total pregnancy loss rates post amniocentesis

Study	Type	Mid-trimester amniocentesis	Control	Post-amniocentesis loss rate	Significance
Reid (1999)	C	3953	-	0,7%	_
Antsaklis (2000)	C	3910	EA 5324	2,1%/1,5%	P=0,01
Horger (2001)	RCT	4600	_	0,95%	_
Caughey (2006)	C	30893	CVS9886	0,83%/0,46%	_

B. Procedure-related pregnancy loss rate

Study	Type	Mid-trimester amniocentesis	Control (no procedure)	Procedure -related Loss rate (loss rate amnio group: loss rate no procedure group)	Significance
Muller (2002)	C	3472	47004	0,7%(1,12%;0,42%)	95%CI 0,39-1,13
Kong (2006)	C	3468	1125	0,86%(corrected for Background loss rate)	95%CI 0,19-1,53)
FASTER(2006)	C	3096	31907	0,06%(1%;0,94%)	95%CI0,26-0,49
Seeds (2004)	Review	11372	12097	0,6%(1,68%;1,08%)	95%CI 0,31-0,9

RCT: Randomized controlled trial; C: cohort/case–control study; CVS: chorionic villus sampling (TA: transabdominal; TC: transcervical); EA: early amniocentesis;
RR: relative risk; CI: confidence interval; NS: non-significant difference.
* Study group: women 20–34 years of age having amniocentesis for increased risk of aneuploidy or maternal infection; control group: women 20–34 years of age at low risk but having amniocentesis

Table 1. Summary of studies with mid-trimester amniocentesis population

3.5 Early amniocentesis

The desire for a first-trimester diagnosis stimulated interest in the feasibility of performing amniocentesis under 15 weeks gestation including first trimester. The major advantage of early amniocentesis (9 to 14 weeks' gestation) is that results are known much more earlier. This procedure which was introduced in the late 1980s, is technically the same as a 'late' procedure except that less amniotic fluid is removed. The 15ml amniotic fluid at this week of pregnancy is a significant amount, while the extremities are in a critical period for the development. Ultrasound needle guidance is considered to be an essential part of the procedure because of the relatively small target area. The presence of two separate membranes (amnion and chorion) until 15 weeks' gestation creates an additional technical difficulty. Only the amniotic (inner) sac should be aspirated, because the outer sac does not contain sufficient numbers of living fetal cells. It has been reported that there is a culture failure ranging from o,5-2,5%. The karyotyping success rate may be increased by using filter techniques in which amniotic cells are retained on a filter after aspiration while the rest of the amniotic fluid (cell free) is reinjected into the amniotic cavity (Alfirević et al.,2007).

Fetal complications related to early amniocentesis were expected to be higher than those related to mid-trimester amniocentesis because of the higher amount of removed amniotic fluid (Johnson et al., 1999). Since a controlled trial has not yet been done, the complications following early amniocentesis has been compared to that following chorionic villus sampling (CVS) or amniocentesis in week 16-18. To determine the safety and accuracy of early amniocentesis, a randomized, multicenter Canadian study (Meier et al.,2005) compared the procedure to second-trimester amniocentesis.Among the women in the early amniocentesis group, 1% gave birth to infants with a foot anomaly. By comparison, only 0.1% of those in the second-trimester group gave birth to infants with this deformity a proportion similar to that found within the general population.Both the U.K. and Danish studies (Tabor et al., 1986) found an increase in respiratory distress syndrome and pneumonia in neonates from the mothers who underwent early amniocentesis. It may be that altered amniotic fluid volume after amniocentesis or subsequent chronic amniotic fluid leakage interferes with normal lung development and lung structure at term, thus giving rise to pulmonary hypoplasia and consequently to RDS in the newborn. Whether these antenatal and neonatal changes have any longterm impact on lung development remains to be shown. The study, funded by the National Institute of Child Health and Human Development (Philip et al.,2004) compared the rate of fetal loss between early amniocentesis and CVS. The combined outcome of spontaneous loss before 20 weeks and procedure-related termination occurred slightly more often after amniocentesis than after CVS, with risk most increased when amniocentesis was performed during week 13. In addition, incidence of talipes equinovarus (clubfoot) was fourfold higher after amniocentesis than after CVS , again, most cases occurred when amniocentesis was performed during week 13.

Early amniocentesis appears to be as accurate as CVS and mid-trimester amniocentesis. Amniocentesis at 13 weeks gestation carries a significantly increase risk of talipes equinovarus and respiratory illness compared with CVS and mid-trimester amniocentesis and also suggests an increase in early, unintended pregnancy loss. The safety of amniocentesis before 14 weeks gestation is uncertain. Until its safety can be ensured, it is best to delay routine sampling until week 15 or 16 of pregnancy.

4. Cordocentesis

Cordocentesis is an invasive method of obtaining fetal blood from umbilical cord using transabdominal approach. This method first described in 1983 by Daffos and coworkers offers advantage in efficacy and safety over the fetoscopic methods previously used to obtain fetal blood and nowdays almost completely abandoned (Daffos et al.,1985). The main target for obtaining fetal blood is the umbilical vein. Other possible targets for fetal blood sampling are fetal heart ventricles and the intrahepatic tract of the umbilical vein (Antsaklis et al., 1992)

4.1 Timing and technique

Depending on the indication, cordocentesis can be performed from about 18 completed weeks of gestation until the end of the pregnancy. When imaging and placental conditions are optimal, it can be done as early as 15 completed weeks. It is usually performed on an ambulatory basis. It requires a high-resolution ultrasound scanner, an experienced team and a laboratory specializing in fetal blood analysis (Sirirchotiyakul et al.,2000). The most favorable puncture site is the placental insertion of the umbilical cord, as the cord is the least mobile at that location. A 20-22 gauge needle is used. A stable needle is important, especially with the posterior placenta, so that the needle will not bend on the relatively long path to the umbilical cord insertion (Ghezzi et al.,2001). Blood is drawn from the umbilical vein with a 1ml syringe. Blood samples must be immediately examined to identify to purity of the sample and the results of the analysis can be significantly altered in case it has been contamined by maternal blood or amniotic fluid. A free loop of umbilical cord or the fetal insertion of the cord can also be used for puncture. Intra-abdominal puncture of the umbilical vein is yet another option. It is most difficult to puncture a free loop of umbilical cord. Attempts to puncture free loops often result in the cord being pushed away by the needle (Liaou et al.,2006). Besides the large-caliber vein, it is also possible to sample blood from one of the two smaller-caliber umbilical arteries. This procedure, however, carries a risk of vasospasm with subsequent fetal bradycardia and/or profuse afterbleedind and therefore puncture of the umbilical vein is always preferred. Fetal heart is an alternative sampling site and this technique can be used when access to the fetal circulation must be obtained at gestational age less than 17-18 weeks gestation or if an emergency blood transfusion is required.

4.2 Indications

Indications for cordocentesis have changed regarded to past decade. In fact the list is shorter than a decade ago because the noninvasive methods have rendered cordocentesis less important. However, some specific metabolic, hematologic or gene disorders are still testable only by fetal blood sampling. Cordocentesis is most commonly used for rapid fetal karyotyping (Shah et al., 1990). This is done in cases with ambiguous chromosomal findings from amniotic cell culture or CVS. The results can be obtained in 48-72 hours by leukocyte culture of the fetal sampled blood. This advantage of rapid karyotyping can also be used when ultrasound reveals an abnormality that is associated with chromosome disorders or in cases of an abnormal triple test. On the other hand some essentials blood tests are replaced by amniocentesis due to PCR techniques for gene amplification and the emergence of many new genetic markers. Various fetal infections can be diagnosed in the fetal blood: rubella, cytomegalovirus, toxoplasmosis, varicella and parvovirus B19 (Valente et al., 1994). For detection a fetal infection cordocentesis is not performed before 22 weeks of gestation because IgM antibodies occur in fetal blood after 20 weeks of gestation. Various blood diseases can be diagnosed using cordocentesis: hemoglobinopathies, coagulopathies, immune deficiencies and trombocytopenias (Burrows and Kelton, 1993). Determination of the platelet count in congenital thrombocytopenias provides important information on the intrauterine risk to the fetus which is particularly applies to alloimune thrombocytopenia. If this disease is confirmed intrauterine therapy with platelets should be performed to avoid fetal cerebral hemorrhage. In disorders that can lead to severe fetal anemia as a result of hemolysis (Rh or Kell alloimmunisation, parvovirus B19 infection) cordocentesis can directly determine the degree of anemia and provide a specific basis for planning an intrauterine transfusion (Bowman, 1991). The use of Doppler peak velocity to assess the degree of fetal anemia reduce the need for fetal blood sampling. However, cordocentesis is always indicated when history, maternal titers or MCA Doppler show a risk of anemia.

Correlation between biophysical profile scoring (BPS) and fetal PH on cordocentesis, reduce percentage of fetal blood sampling in the determination of fetal blood gases and acid-base status, because BPS can be safely use to indicate fetal PH without invasive method. But because neither the BPS patterns nor Doppler findings provide clear-cut evidence of fetal compromise in all cases, cordocentesis can be a useful adjunct to the noninvasive tests, especially in cases of severe growth retardation. In cases with abnormal Doppler flow with a normal BPS score, cordocentesis can confirm or exclude chronic fetal asphyxia.

4.3 Complications

The overall complication rate of cordocentesis is slightly higher than that of amniocentesis. Besides the risk that are the same as for amniocentesis such as: abortion, membrane rupture and chorioamnionitis, there are additional risks that are specific for cordocentesis. Fetal loss rate related to cordocentesis reported to be as high as 6-7% in centers with low experience, but in experienced hands the rate is as low as 1-2%. Overall pregnancy loss rate depends largely on the fetal condition for which cordocentesis is done. The rate of pregnancy loss is worse in cases of fetal anomalies and abnormal karyotype (Tongsong et al.,2001).Unfortunately no controlled trials are yet available and it is not quite clear what is the fetal loss rate to quote to patients, because most clinical series contain many high risk cases such as stated before. The most common complication of cordocentesis is fetal bradycardia. The rate of fetal bradycardia reported in literature is 6,6%. In most cases it is transient, self-limited and with no long-term concequences. It is related to uterine contraction directly at the cord insertion or fetal movement against the umbilical cord by the contraction. Profound or prolonged bradycardia occurs in less than 3% of cases and it is associated with umbilical artery vasospasm after puncture of the umbilical cord or tetanic uterine contraction, which is rar. Early gestational age and hydrops fetalis correlated significantly with the development of bradycardia at cordocentesis. The other risk groups, including fetuses with intrauterine growth retardation, the puncture site, and the number of puncture attempts did not correlate with fetal bradycardia (Preis et al.,2004). Transient bleeding from the umbilical cord puncture, called the "jet phenomenon" is a relatively common, innocuous finding after cordocentesis and it lasts no more than 2 minutes.The bleeding from the artery is reported to be longer than that from the vein. Differences among centers with respect to bleeding may relate to the size of the needle used and the technique employed.Bleeding over 300 seconds or massive hemorrhage occurs less than once per 200 cordocentesis. When this occurs a viable fetus should be delivered by emergency cesarean section. Hematomas of the cord have been observed in pathologic specimens with the freehand technique, although most are not associated with adverse sequelae (Kay et al.,2011). The incidence of symptomatic cord hematoma causing significant fetal bradycardia is very low. The risk of amnionitis is approximately 1% when the freehand technique is used and less than 0.3% when the needle-guided technique is used. Rarely, chorioamnionitis can lead to the development of maternal sepsis and adult respiratory distress syndrome.

Maternal complications are also seen. Cordocentesis lasts longer than amniocentesis, so the mother will more likely be anxious and have more discomfort. On the other hand, cordocentesis is less uncomfortable than CVS, so the patients will less complain of pain and contractions.Acute rupture of membranes and preterm labor are very rare complications.

Fetal-maternal transfusion has been reported after both cordocentesis and amniocentesis, especially when the placenta was anterior. It is imperative that Rh-negative women be given Rh immunoglobulin after a procedure unless the fetus is known to be Rh-negative or the patient is already sensitized (Rujiwetpongstorn et al.,2005)

The safety of cordocentesis is believed to be both technique-dependent and experience-dependent. Fewer punctures are reported with the freehand technique, but a lower fetal/neonatal loss rate is reported with the needle-guided technique. The rate of bleeding is reported to be reduced with the needle-guided technique and with the use of smaller gauge needles. Several investigators have found a greater number of complications among their first 30 procedures.

5. Other invasive diagnostic procedures

On infrequent occasions, analysis of other fetal tissues may be required. Because they are only rarely required, their use is usually confined to only a few regional referral centers in hopes of limiting procedural risk. Fetal skin biopsy is indicated for diagnosis of some type of genodermatosis or congenital dermoepidermic disorders which is expected to be lethal in short or medium terms. Those disorders are: bullous epidermolysis, anhidrotic ectodermic dysplasias, keratinization disorders and pigmentary atopies (Elias et al.,1994). It can also be helpful in the workup of fetal mosaicism for some chromosomes, such as 22 chromososme, which are known not to be manifest in fetal blood. Fetal muscle biopsy is used to diagnose Duchenne's muscular dystrophy in a male fetus if DNA testing is not informative (Nevo et al.,1999). It can also be used to detect other hereditary myopathies as long as there is some clinical family history of these disorders. Fetal liver biopsy was the only means of diagnosing fetuses with inborn errors of the urea cycle such as ornithine transcarbamylase deficiency, carbamoylphosphate synthetase deficiency and other disorders expressed only in the liver such as von Gierke glycogen-storage disease type IA and primary hyperoxaluria type I (Haberle et al.,2004). However, most of these conditions are now diagnosable by DNA analysis (without the need for histology and enzymatic assays) of cells extracted from either chorionic villi or amniocytes. Direct genetic analysis of chorionic villi is feasible, fast and specific and can be regarded as the primary choice for prenatal diagnosis of these rare conditions. The procedure which is used more frequent than the previous described is aspiration and biochemical analysis of fetal urine for the evaluation of fetal renal function. This evaluation is essential in determination of fetuses whose kidneys are not irreversible damaged and who will have the benefit from intrauterine derived therapy.The biochemical markers that have close relation with the renal function are defined by Na,Cl, beta-2 microglobuline and osmotic urine (Troyano et al., 2002).Other punctures on fetal tumor formations such as teratomas or liquid collections such as pericardiocentesis do not have an acceptable justification from a diagnostic point of view, as the echographic evaluation and the present application of biophysical methods give an acceptable identification of their vascularisation and origin, including those of suspicious neoplasm.

6. Conclusion

More than 40-year history of invasive procedures has seen a rise and than a fall in the degree of invasiveness of the procedures. The decades of invasive diagnostic procedures have given us a unique opportunity to study the fetus. They have contributed to our understanding of human fetal physiology, metabolism, and disease. However, the introduction of non-invasive procedures has diminished the need for some invasive procedures, in the first place for cordocentesis. As molecular genetics shrinks the role of cordocentesis for prenatal diagnosis of hereditary disease and as cytogenetic techniques make inroads that supplant the need for fetal blood sampling to obtain a rapid karyotype, it is likely that there will be fewer indications for cordocentesis in the next decade. A diminished role for cordocentesis will demand further regionalization of care in order for some persons to maintain the skill and further the knowledge base of normal fetal physiology and fetal disease. On the other hand amniocentesis still remains the gold standard for karyotyping, especially now that rapid diagnostic methods are available. Will nowdays invasive proceduers suffer the same fate as fetoscopy—here one day, gone another—or will the indications for them gradually be refined, limiting its practice to situations not suitable for noninvasive fetal testing remains to be shown. Invasive procedures may become obsolete when reliable non-invasive prenatal diagnosis becomes available.

7. References

Allen, VM.; Wilson, RD.(2006). Pregnancy outcomes after assisted reproductive technology. Joint SOGC-CFAS Guideline . *J Obstet Gynaecol Can* ,vol.28,No.3,(March 2006),pp.220-233

Alfirevic Z, Sundberg K, Brigham S. Amniocentesis and chorionic villus sampling for prenatal diagnosis, Cochrane Database Syst Rev. 2003;(3):CD003252

Alfirević,Z.;Sunberg,K.;Brigham,S.(2007).Amniocentesis and CVS for prenatal diagnosis review. The Cohrane Collaboration. Issue 4.John Wiley&Sons,London

Antsaklis,A.;Papantoniou,N.;Vinzileos,A.(1992). An alternative method of fetal sampling for the prenatal diagnosis of hemoglobinopathies. *Obstetr Gynecol*,vol.73,No.4,(April 1992),pp.630

Antsaklis, A.; Papantoniou, N.; Xygakis, A.;Mesogitis, S.; Tzortzis ,E.;Michalas, S. (2000).Genetic amniocentesis in women 20–34 years old: associated risks. *Prenatal diagnosis*,vol.20,No.1,(January 2000),pp.247-250

Antsaklis,A.;Souka,AP.;Daskalakis,G.;(2002). Second trimester amniocentesis versus CVS in multiple gestations. Ultrasound Obstet Gynmecol, vol.20,No.5,(May2002),pp.476

Blessed ,WB.; Lacoste, H.;Welch RA.(2001). Obstetrician-gynecologists performing genetic amniocentesis may be misleading themselves and their patients. *Am J Obstet Gynecol* ,vol.184,No.3,(March 2001),pp.1340–1344.

Bianco, K.; Caughey, AB.; Shaffer, BL.; Davis, R.;Norton, ME.(2006). History of miscarriage and increased incidence of fetal aneuploidy in subsequent pregnancy. *Obstet Gynecol* ,vol.107,No.5-6,(June 2006),pp.1098-1102

Boulot, P.; Deschamps, F.; Lefort, G(1990). Pure fetal blood samples obtained by cordocentesis: Technical aspects of 322 cases. *Prenat Diagn* ,Vol.10,No.5, (May 1990),pp.93

Brambati, B.; Terzian, E.;Tognoni, G.(1991). Randomized clinical trial of transabdominal versus transcervical chorionic villus sampling methods. *Prenat Diagn* , vol.11,No.2,(February 1991),pp.285-293.

Brambati, B.; Simoni, G,.;Travi, M. (1992).Genetic diagnosis by chorionic villus sampling before 8 gestational weeks: efficiency, reliability, and risks on 317 completed pregnancies. *Prenat Diagn* ,vol.12,No.4,(April 1992),pp.789-799.

Brambati,B.;Tului,L.;Guercilena,S.(2001).Outcome of first trimester CVS for genetic investigation in multiple pregnancy. *Ultrasound Obstet Gynecol*,vol.17,No.4,(April 2001),pp.714

Brambati,B.;Tului,L.;Camurri,L.(2004). First trimester fetal reduction to a singleton infant or twins:outcome in relation to the final number and karytyping before reduction by CVS, *American Journal Obstet Gynecol*,vol.191,No.5,(May 2004),pp.2035

Brun,JL.;Mangione,R.;Gangbo,F.(2003). Feasibility,accuracy and safety of chorionic villus sampling:a report of 10741 cases.*Prenatal Diagnosis*,vol.23,No.4,(April 2003),pp.295-301

Bowman, JM. Rh immune disease: Diagnosis, management and prevention. (1991).In:Gynecology and Obstetrics, Sciarra JJ ,Vol 3, Chap 66. Philadelphia, JB Lippincott

Burrows,RF.;Kelton, JG.(1993). Pregnancy in patients with idiopathic thrombocytopenic purpura: Assessing the risks for the infant at delivery. *Obstet Gynecol Surv* ,vol.48,No.2,(February 1993),pp.781

Caughey, AB.; Hopkins, LM.; Norton, ME.(2006). Chorionic villus sampling compared with amniocentesis and the difference in the rate of pregnancyloss. *Obstet Gynecol*, vol.108,No.12,(December 2006),pp.612–616

Cederholm,M.;Haglund,B.;Axelsson,O.(2003).Maternal complications following amniocentesis and CVS for prenatal karyotyping. *BJOG*,vol.110,No.4,(April 2003),pp.392-399

Department of Obstetrics and Gynecology THoAIaSCA, China:Fetal sex prediction by sex chromatin of chorionic villi during early pregnancy. (1975). *Chin Med J*, Vol.1,pp.117-126

Daffos, F.;Capella-Pavlosky,M.;Forestier,F.(1983). A new procedure for pure fetal blood sampling in utero. Preliminary results at fifty-three cases. American Journal Obstetric Gynecology, vol.146,No.4,(April 1983),pp.985-987

Eddleman, KA.; Malone, FD.; Sullivan, L.; Dukes, K.; Berkowitz,RL.; Kharbutli Y.(2006). Pregnancy loss rates after midtrimester amniocentesis. *Obstet Gynecol* ,vol.108,No.7, (July 2006),pp.1067–1072

Elias,S.;Emerson,DS.;Simpson,JL.(1994).Ultrasound-guided fetal skin sampling for prenatal diagnosis of genodermatoses. *Obstet Gynecol*, vo.83,No.4, (April 1994),pp.337-341

Elias,S.;Simpson,JL.(1993).Amniocentesis.In:Essentials of prenatal diagnosis. Simpson, Jl.Churchill Livingstone:New York,pp.27-44

Fergal, D.;Malone, FD.; Jacob,A.; Canick, JA.; Ball, RH.; Nyberg, DA.(2005). First-trimester or second-trimester screening, or both, for Down'ssyndrome. *N Engl J Med* , Vol.353, No.6, (June 2005), pp.2001–2011

Finegan ,AK.; Sitarenios, G.; Bolan, PL.(1996).Children whose mothers had second trimester amniocentesis: follow-up at school age. *Br J Obstet Gynaecol* ,Vol.103,No.3, (March 1996),pp.214-218

Finegan, AK.; Quarrington, BJ.; Hughes, HE.(2000). Child outcome following mid-trimester amniocentesis: Development, behavior and physical status at age 4 years. *British Journal Obstetrics Gynaecology* , Vol97,No.3-4,(April 2000),pp425-435

Froster ,UG.; Jackson, L.(1996). Limb defects and chorionic villus sampling: results from an international registry, 1992–94. *Lancet* , vol.347,No.1,(January 1996),pp.489–94.

Ghezzi, .;, Maymon, E.; Redman, M.; Blackwell, S.; Berry, SM.; Romero, R.(2001). Fetal blood sampling.In:Sonography in obstetrics and gynecology: principle and practice, Fleischer AC. pp.775-804, McGraw-Hill; New York

Gratacós, E.; Devlieger, R.; Decaluwé, Wu J.; Nicolini ,U.; Deprest ,JA.(2000). Is the angle of needle insertion influencing the created defect in human fetal membranes? Evaluation of the agreement between specialists' opinions and ex vivo observations. *Am J Obstet Gynecol* ,vol.182,No.6, (June 2000),pp.646-649

Haberle,J.;Koch,Hg. (2004). Genetic approach to prenatal diagnosis in urea cycle defects. *Prenatal Diagnosis*,vol.24, No.5,(May 2004),pp.378-383

Hanson ,FW.;Happ, RL.; Tennant, FR.(1990) Ultrasonographically-guided early amniocentesis in singleton pregnancies. *Am J Obstet Gynecol* , Vol.162,No.9,(October 1990), pp.1376-83.

Horger, EO.;Finch ,H.; Vincent ,VA. (2001).A single physician's experience with four thousand six hundred genetic amniocentesis. *Am J Obstet Gynecol,* Vol.185, No.11,(November 2001), pp.279-288

Johnson, JM.; Wilson, RD.;Winsor, EJ.;Singer, J.; Dansereau ,J.; Kalousek DK. (1999).The early amniocentesis study: a randomized clinical trial of early amniocentesis versus midtrimester amniocentesis. *Fetal Diagn Ther*, vo.11,No.4, (April 1996),pp.85-93

Johnson, JM.; Wilson, RD.; Singer, J.;Winsor, E.; Harman, C.;Armson,BA. (1999).Technical factors in early amniocentesis predict adverse outcome. Results of the Canadian early (EA) versus mid-trimester (MA) amniocentesis trial. *Prenat Diagn* , vol.19,No.6, (June 1999),pp.732–738

Jackson, GL.; Zachary, JM.; Fowler SE.(1992). A randomized comparison of transcervical and transabdominal chorionic villus sampling. *N Engl J Med* , vol.327,No.5,(May 1992),pp.594–98

Jacobson, B.;Ladfors, L.; Milson, I.(2004). Advanced maternal age and adverse perinatal outcome. *Obstet Gynecol,* vol.104,No.7,(July 2004), pp.727-733

Kalousek,DK.;Vekemans,M.(2000).Confined placental mosaicism and genetic imprinting: *Baillieres Best Practice Results Clin Obstet Gynaecol*, vol.14,No.4,(April 2000),pp.723-730

Kay,H.;Nelson,M.;Wang Y.(2011).Cordocentesis and fetoscopy.In:The placenta:from development to disease.Kay,H,pp.147, Blackwell publication;ISBN:978-1-4433-3366-4;UK

Karp, LE.; Hayden, PW.(1977). Fetal puncture during midtrimester amniocentesis. *Obstetrics Gynecology* ,vol.115,No.12, (December 1977),pp.15-19

Kleinhaus, K.; Perrin, M.; Friedlander, Y.; Paltiel, O.; Malaspina, D.; Harlap, S.(2006). Paternal age and spontaneous abortion. *Obstet Gynecol* , vol.108,No.2,(February 2006),pp.369-377

Kong, CW.; Leung, TN.; Leung, TY.; Chan, LW.;Sahota, DS.; Fung, TY.(2006). Risk factors for procedure-related fetal losses after mid-trimester genetic amniocentesis. *Prenat Diagn* ,vol.26,No.6, (June2006), pp.925–930

Kotzot,D.(2001). Complex and segmental uniparental disomy; review and lessons from rare chromosomal complements. *J Med Genet*,vol.38,No.8,(August 2001),pp.497-507

Liao, C.; Wei, J.;Li, Q.; Li, L. Li ,J.; Li, D. (2006). Efficacy and safety of cordocentesis for prenatal diagnosis. *Int J Gynecol Obstet* , vol.93,no.4, (April 2006),pp.*13–17.*

Los,Fj.;van den BC.;Wildschut,HI.(2001). The diagnostic performance of cytogenetic investigation in amniotic fluid cells and chorionic villi. *Prenatal Diagnosis,* vol.21,No.12,(December 2001),1150-1158

Mariona, FG.; Bhatia, R.; Syner, FN.(1986). Chorionic villus sampling changes maternal serum alpha-fetoprotein. *Prenat Diagn* ,vol.6,No.5,(May 1986),pp.69-73

Meier,C.;Huang, T.; Owolabi, T.; Summers, A.;Wyatt PR. The identification of risk of spontaneous fetal loss through second-trimester maternal serum screening. *Am J Obstet Gynecol* , vol.193,No5-6,(June 2005),pp.395-403

Monni,G.;Ibba,RM.;Lai,R.(1993).Early transabdominal chorionic villus sampling in couples at high genetic risk. *Am J Obstet Gynecol,* vol.168,No.1,(January 1993),pp.170-171

Medical Research Council working party on amnio-centesis. (1978).An assessment of the hazards of amniocentesis. *Br J Obstet Gynaecol* ,vol.85,No.2,(February 1978),pp.1-41

Muller, F.;Thibaud, D.; Poloce, F.; Gelineau, MC.; Bernard, M.; Brochet, C.(2002). Risk of amniocentesis in women screened with positive for Down syndrome with second trimester maternal serum markers. *Prenatal Diagnosis,* vol.22,No.11,(November 2002),pp.1036–1039

Milner, AD.; Hoskyns, EW.; Hopkin, IE. (1992).The effects of midtrimester amniocentesis on lung function in the neonatal period. *Eur J Pediatr* ,vol.151,No.3, (March 1992), pp.458-460

Millaire, M.; Bujold, E.; Morency, AM.; Gauthier, RJ.(2006). Mid-trimester genetic amniocentesis in twin pregnancy and the risk of fetal loss. *J Obstet Gynaecol Can* ,vol.28,No.1,(January 2006),pp.512-518

Milunsky,A.(2010).Complications of amniocentesis,In:Genetic disorders and the fetus,Milunsky J,pp1184-1185,Wiley-Blackwell,ISBN 978-1-4051-9087-9;Oxford UK

MRC Working Party: An assessment of the hazard of amniocentesis. *British Journal Obstetric Gynecology* , vol.85,No.6, (June 1992),pp.1-41

Nadel, A.(2007).Letter to Editor: Pregnancy loss rates after midtrimester amniocentesis. *Obstet Gynecol* ,vol.109,No.7-8,(July 2007),pp.451

Nicolaides, K.; Brizot, ML.; Patel, F.(1994).Comparison of chorionic villus sampling and amniocentesis for fetal karyotyping at 10-13 weeks' gestation. *Lancet* ,vol.344,No.3, (March 1994),pp.435-439

Nevo,Y.;Shomrat,R.;Yaron,Y.;Harel,S,Legum,C. (1999). Fetal muscle biopsy as a diagnostic tool in Duchenne muscular dystrophy. *Prenatal Diagnosis,* vol.19,No.10,(October 1999),pp.921-926

Odibo,AO.;Dicke,JM,Gray,DL.(2008). Evaluate the rate and risk factors for fetal loss after CVS. *Obstet Gynecol*,vol.112,No.5,(May 2008),pp.813

Papantoniou, NE.; Daskalakis, GJ.; Tziotis, JG.; Kitmirides ,SJ.; Mesogitis, SA.;Antsaklis, AJ.(2001). Risk factors predisposing to fetal loss following a second trimester amniocentesis. *BJOG* ,vol.108,No.6 ,(June2001),pp.1053–1056

Paz,A.;Gomen,R.;Pokasman,I.(2001).Candida sepsis following transcervical CVS. *Infect Dis Obstet Gynecol*.vol.9,No.3,(March 2001),pp.147-148

Pijpers,L.; Jahoda, MGJ.; Vosters ,RPL.(1988). Genetic amniocentesis in twin pregnancies. *Br J Obstet Gynaecol*,vol.95,No.4,(April 1988),pp.323-326

Phipps,S.;Zinn,A.;Opitz,J.;Reynolds,J.(2005).Psychological response to amniocentesis:Effects of coping style.*American Journal of medical genetics*,vol.25,No.6,(June 2005),pp.143-148

Philip,J.;Silver,RK.;Wilson,RD.;Thom,EA.(2004).Late first trimester invasive prenatal diagnosis:results of an international randomized trial. *Obstet Gynecol*,vol.103, No.6,(June 2004),pp.1164-1173

Phupong,V.;Ultchaswadi,P.(2006).Spontaneus reseal of ruptured membranes after genetic amniocentesis.*Journal mediacal association Thai*,vol.89,No.7,(July 2006),pp.1033-1035

Pergament ,E.(2000).The application of fluorescence in- situ hybridization to prenatal diagnosis.*Current opinion obstet gynecology*, vol.72,No.12,(December 2000),pp.41-43

Preis,K.; Ciach,K.,Swiatkowska-Freun,M. (2004). The risk of complications of diagnostic and therapeutic cordocentesis. Ginekol.Pol.vol.75,No.10,(October 2004),pp.765-769

Rhoads,GG.;Jacson,LG.;Scheslleman,SE.(1989). The safety and efficacy of CVS for early prenatal diagnosis of cytogenetic abnormalities. *N Engl J Med,* Vol.320,No.5,(May 1989),pp.609-612

Reid ,KP.; Gurrin, LC.; Dickinson, JE.; Newnham, JP.; Phillips, JM.(1999). Pregnancy loss rates following second trimester genetic amniocentesis. *Aust NZ J Obstet Gynaecol* ,vol.39,No.2,(February 1999),pp.281-285

Rujiwetpongstorn, J.; Tongsong, T.; Wanapirak, C.(2005) Feto-maternal hemorrhage after cordocentesis at

Maharaj Nakorn Chiang Mai Hospital. *J Med Assoc Thai* ,vol.88,No.5,(May2005),pp.145-9.

Summers ,AM:, Langlois, S.; Wyatt, P.; Wilson,RD.(2007). Prenatal Screening for Fetal Aneuploidy. Joint SOGC–CCMG Clinical Practice Guideline.*J Obstet Gynaecol Can* ,Vol.29,No.6,(June 2007),pp.146-161

Sundberg,K.; Smidt-Jensen, S., Philip, J. (1997).Amniocentesis with increased cell yield, obtained by filtration and reinjection of the amniotic fluid. *Ultrasound Obstet Gynecol* ,vol.1,No.2,(February 1991),pp.91-94

Sawa, R.; Hayashi, Z.; Tanaka, T.(2001). Rapid detection of chromososme aneuploidies by prenatal interphase FISH and its clinical utility in Japan.*J apan obstetric gynecology*, vol.41,No.2,(February 2001),pp.13-15

Savva, GM.;Morris, JK.; Mutton, DE.; Alberman, E.(2006). Maternal age-specific fetal loss rates in Down syndrome pregnancies. *Prenat Diagn* ,vol.26,No.6,(June 2006),pp.499-504

Seeds, JW.(2004). Diagnostic mid trimester amniocentesis: how safe? *Am J Obstet Gynecol* ,vol.191,No.7,(July 2004),pp.608-616

Swift ,PG.; Driscoll, IB.; Vowles, KD.(1979). Neonatal small bowel obstruction associated with amniocentesis. *British Medical Journal* ,vol.720,No.2,(February 1979),pp.54-56

Sirirchotiyakul, S.; Piyamongkol, W.; Chanprapaph, P.(2000). Cordocentesis at 16-24 weeks of gestation: experience of 1,320 cases. *Prenat Diagn* vol.20,No.5,(May 2000),pp.224-228

Schreck, L. After early amniocentesis chances of fetal loss and foot deformity rise.(1998). *Family planning perspectives*,vol.30,No.6,(June 1998),pp.249-251

Smith, L.(2007). Letter to Editor: Pregnancy loss rates after midtrimester amniocentesis. *Obstet Gynecol* , vol.109,No.7,(July 2007),pp.452

Smidt-Jensen, S.; Permin, M.; Philip, J.(1992). Randomised comparison of amniocentesis and transabdominal and transcervical chorionic villus sampling. *Lancet,* vol.340,No.4,(April 1992),pp.1237-1244

Sunberg, K.; Bang, J.; Smidt-Jensens, S.; Brocks ,V.(1997). Randomised study of risk of fetal loss related to early amniocentesis versus CVS. *Lancet*,vol.350,No.11,(November 1997),pp.697-703

Shulman, LP.; Elias, S.; Phillips, OP. (1994). Amniocentesis performed at 14 weeks' gestation or earlier: comparison with first-trimester transabdominal chorionic villus sampling. *Obstet Gynecol* ,vol.83,No.9,(September 1994),pp.543-548.

Shah, DM.;Roussis, P.; Ulm, J. (1990). Cordocentesis for rapid karyotyping. *Am J Obstet Gynecol* , vol.162,No.6,(June 1990),pp. 1548

Sepulveda, W.; Donaldson, A.; Johnson ,RD.(1995). Are routine a-fetoprotein and acetylcholinesterase determinations still necessary at second-trimester amniocentesis? Impact of high-resolution ultrasonography. *Obstet Gynecol,* vol.85, No.1,(January 1995),pp.107-112

Tepperberg, J.;Pettenati ,MJ.; Rao, PN.(2001).Prenatal diagnosis using interphase fluorescence in situ hybridization (FISH):2-year multi-center retrospective study and review of the literature. *Prenatal diagnosis*,vol.21,No.6,(June 2001)pp.293

Tabor, A.; Philip, J.; Madsen, M.(1986). Randomise controlled trial of genetic amniocentesis in 4606 low-risk women. *Lancet* ,vol.1,No,5,(May 1986),pp.86-88

Tabor ,A.;Jerne, D.; Bock, JE.(1987). Incidence of rhesus immunization after genetic amniocentesis. *British Medical Journal*,vol.293,No.3,(March 1987),pp.533-536

Toth-Pal, E.; Papp, C.;Beke, A.; Ban, Z.; Papp, Z.(2004). Genetic amniocentesis in multiple pregnancy. *Fetal Diagnosis and Therapy* , vo.19,No.6,(June 2004),pp.138-144

Tongsong ,T.; Wanapirak, C.; Kunavikatikul, C.; Sirirchotiyakul, S.; Piyamongkol, W.; Chanprapaph ,P. (2001).Fetal loss rate associated with cordocentesis at midgestation. *Am J Obstet Gynecol* , vol. 184, no.1, (January 2001),pp.*719–723*

Thompson, PJ.; Greenough, A.; Nicolaides, KH.(1992). Lung volume measured by functional residual capacity in infants following first trimester amniocentesis or chorionic villus sampling. *British Journal of Obsterics and Gynecology* , vol.99,No.7-8,(August 1992),479-482

The NICHD National Registry for Amniocentesis Study Group.(1976). Midtrimester amniocentesis for prenatal diagnosis. Safety and accurancy. *JAMA* ,vol.5, (May1976),pp.1471-1476.

The Canadian Early and Mid-trimester Amniocentesis Trial (CEMAT) Group. (1998).Randomised trial to assess safety and fetal outcome of early and midtrimester amniocentesis. *Lancet,* vol.351,No.7,(July 1998),pp.242–247

Troyano,JM.;Clavijo,MT.;Clemente,I.;Marco,QY.;Rayward,J.;Mahtani,VG. (2002). Kidney and urinary tract diseases: Ultrasound and biochemical markers. *The ultrasound Review of Obstetrics and Gynecology*,Vol.2,No.2,(February 2002),pp.92-109

Vaughan,J.;Rodeck,C.Interventional procedures.In:Ultrasound in obstetrics and gynaecology,Dewbury,KC,Meire,HB.pp.557-606.London:Churchill Livingstone,2001

Valente, P.; Sever, JL.(1994). In utero diagnosis of congenital infections by direct fetal sampling. *Isr J Med Sci* ,vol.30, No.10,(October1994),pp.414

Von Dadelszen,P.;Sermer,M.; Hillier,J.(2005).A randomized controlled trial of biopsy forceps and cannula aspiration for transcervical chorionic villus sampling. *Br J Obstet Gynaecol,* vol.112,No.5,(May 2005),pp.559-566

Wapner, RL.; Johnson, A.; Davis, G.; Urban, A.; Morgan, P.; Jackson, L.(1993). Prenatal diagnosis in twin gestations: a comparison between second-trimester amniocentesis and first-trimester chorionic villus sampling. *Obstet Gynecol,* vol.82,No.1-2, (February 1993),pp.49

Wilson, RD.(2005) Amended Canadian Guideline for prenatal diagnosis (2005) change to 2005—techniques for prenatal diagnosis. SOGC Clinical Practice Guidelines.*Journal of Obstetrics and Gynecology Canada* , vol.27,No. 11, (November 2005). pp.1048–1054

Weiner, S. (1991).Indications, complications ,safety,reliability, and assessment of quality of fetal blood.*Ultrasound Obstet Gynecol,* vol.1,No.5,(May 1991),pp.17

Welch, RA.; Soha-Salem, EM.;Wiktor, BS.; Van Dyke, DL.; Blessed, WB.(2006). Operator experience and sample quality in genetic amniocentesis. *American Journal of obstetrics and gynecology* ,vol.194,No.12,(December 2006),pp.189-191

Wilson, RD. (2007).Letter to Editor: Pregnancy loss rates after midtrimester amniocentesis. *Obstet Gynecol* ,vol.109,No.1,(January 2007),pp.451-452

Wurster,KG.;Roemer,VM.;Decker,K.;Hirsch,HA.(1982).Amniotic infection syndrome after amniocentesis.*Geburtshilfe Frauenheilkd*.vol.42,No.9,(September 1982),pp.676-679

Yukobowich, E,.;Anteby ,EY,.;Cohen, SM.; Lavy, Y.;Granat, M.; Yagel, S.(2001). Risk of fetal loss in twin pregnancies undergoing second trimester amniocentesis. *Obstet Gynecol,* vol.98,No.11,(November 2001),pp.231–234

2

Prenatal Diagnosis of Severe Perinatal (Lethal) Hypophosphatasia

Atsushi Watanabe, Hideo Orimo,
Toshiyuki Takeshita and Takashi Shimada
Department of Biochemistry and Molecular Biology, Nippon Medical School
Division of Clinical Genetics, Nippon Medical School Hospital
Department of Obstetrics and Gynecology, Nippon Medical School
Japan

1. Introduction

Hypophosphatasia (HPP) is an inherited disorder characterized by defective mineralization of the bone and low activity of alkaline phosphatase (ALP; EC 3.1.3.1) (Mornet, 2008). Screening for mutations in the *ALPL* gene allows genetic counseling and prenatal diagnosis of the disease in families with severe forms of HPP.

2. Hypophosphatasia

HPP is a clinically heterogeneous disease and classified into at least six forms according to severity and age of onset: perinatal (lethal), perinatal (benign), infantile (MIM [Mendelian Inheritance in Man] # 241500), childhood (MIM# 241510), adult (MIM# 146300), and odontohypophosphatasia (Mornet, 2008) (Table 1). All forms of HPP display reduced activity of unfractionated serum ALP and the presence of either one or two pathologic mutations in the liver/bone/kidney alkaline phosphatase gene (*ALPL,* MIM# 171760), the gene encoding ALP, the tissue-nonspecific isozyme (TNSALP). There is no curative treatment for HPP to date.

2.1 *ALPL* gene

ALPL is the only gene known to be associated with HPP. *ALPL* consists of 12 exons: 11 coding exons and one untranslated exon. More than250 *ALPL* mutations have been described in persons from North America, Japan, and Europe (The Tissue Nonspecific Alkaline Phosphatase Gene Mutations Database). HPP is frequently caused by p.E191K and p.D378V in Caucasian, whereas p.F327L and c.1559delT are more common in Japanese(the first nucleotide (+1) corresponds to the A of the ATG initiation codon using the *ALPL* cDNA number of the standard nomenclature). This variety of mutations in *ALPL* results in highly variable clinical expression and in a great number of compound heterozygous genotypes.

2.2 Perinatal (lethal) form of hypophosphatasia

The perinatal (lethal) form of HPP (pl-HPP) is the most severe HPP with an autosomal recessive mode of inheritance (Gehring et al., 1999) In the lethal perinatal form, the patients show markedly impaired mineralization *in utero* (Fig.1). Pregnancies may end in stillbirth. Some infants survive a few days with pulmonary complication due to hypoplastic lungs and rachitic deformities of the chest. Hypercalcemia is common and may be associated with apnea or seizures.

Type	Inheritance	MIM	Symptoms
Perinatal (lethal)	AR		Hypomineralization, osteochondral spurs
Perinatal (benign)	AR or AD		Long-bone bowing, benign postnatal course
Infantile	AR	241500	Craniosynostosis, Hypomineralization, rachitic ribs, hypercalciuria, Premature loss, deciduous teeth
Childhood	AR or AD	241510	Short stature, skeletal deformity, bone pain/fractures, Premature loss, deciduous teeth
Adult	AR or AD	146300	Stress fractures: metatarsal, tibia; chondrocalcinosis
Odontohypophosphatasia	AR or AD		Exfoliation (incisors), dental caries , Alveolar bone loss

Table 1. Clinical Features of Hypophosphatasia by Type. AD; autosomal dominant, AR; autosomal recessive

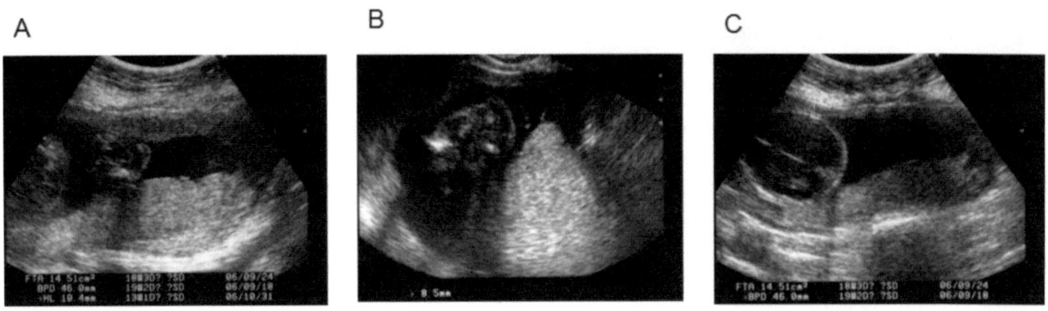

Fig. 1. Ultrasonography examination at 19 weeks' gestation of pl-HPP fetus
The upper limb(A) femur(B) at 19 weeks' gestation was shortened with no evidence of fractures. The cranium(C) at 19 weeks' gestation was thin with marked hypomineralization.

pl-HPP is more common in Japan than in other countries (Satoh et al. 2009). Parents of pl-HPP are heterozygous carriers of *ALPL* mutations. They show no clinical symptoms, but have reduced serum ALP activity and increased urinary phosphoethanolamine (PEA).

2.3 c.1559delT in *ALPL*, a common mutation resulting in the perinatal (lethal) form of hypophosphatasia in Japan

c.1559delT in *ALPL* is a common mutation resulting in pl-HPP in Japan and has only been found in Japanese to date (Orimo et al., 2002; Michigami et al., 2005). Symptoms caused by deletions and insertions of nucleotides that change the reading frame will be highly deleterious. Some patients with pl-HPP are homozygous for c.1559delT, with parents who are heterozygous carriers for the mutation but with no evidence of consanguinity (Fig. 2) (Sawai et al. 2003). Patients who are homozygous for the c.1559delT mutation differed in the severity of HPP, including both their symptoms and serum ALP activity. In the c.1559delT mutation, the symptom in HPP of homozygous mutation is responsible for a severe phenotype, but that of compound hetero varies from severe to mild that depends on mutation position in other allele.

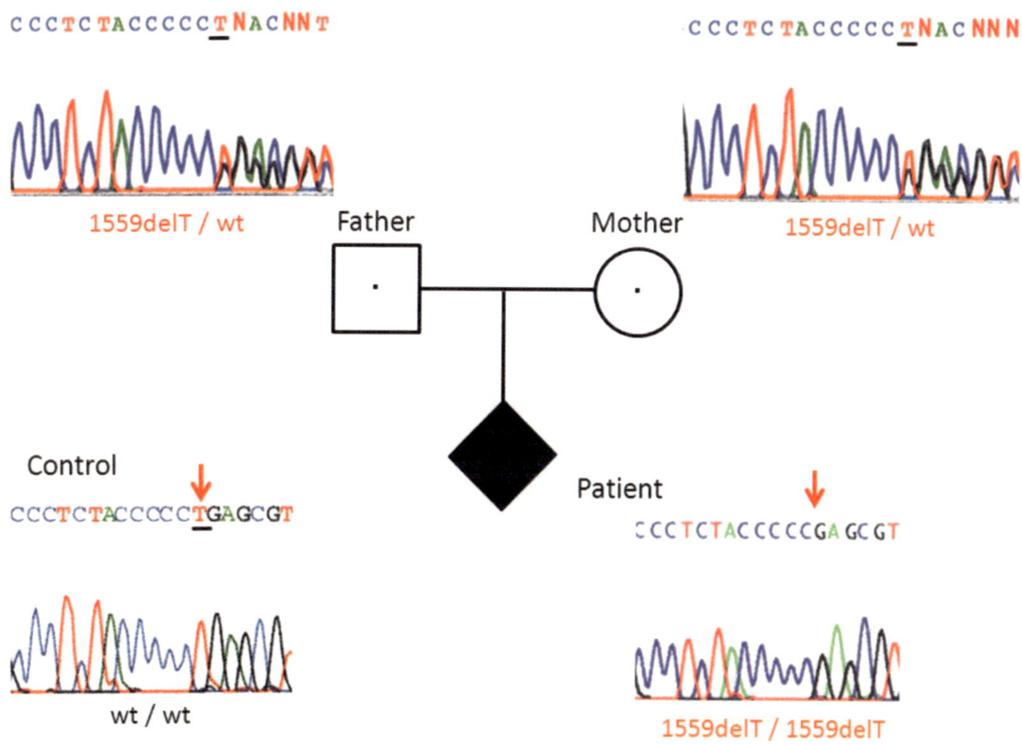

Fig. 2. Direct sequencing results around 1559delT in *ALPL* from a pl-HPP patient both parents, and healthy control. The sequence of the parents could not be determined in progress at cDNA number 1559 of the *ALPL* and these results indicate both parents were heterogenous carriers for 1559delT. The sequence of the pl-HPP patient could be determined in progress containing the deletion of T at nucleotide 1559, which was different from that of a healthy control and indicates that the fetus is homozygous for a 1559delT of the *ALPL.*

c.1559delT, a deletion of T at 1559, which caused a frameshift downstream from leucine (Leu) at codon 503, resulted in the elimination of the termination codon at 508 and the addition of 80 amino acid residues at the C-terminus. The mutant protein caused by 1559delT formed an aggregate, was polyubiquitinated, and was then degraded in the proteome (Komaru et al., 2005), thus allowing us to directly correlate the phenotype (perinatal type) and the genotype (1559delT).

The c.1559delT carrier frequency is 1/480 (95% confidence interval, 1/1,562-1/284) in Japanese (Watanabe et al. 2011). This indicates that approximately 1 in 900,000 individuals to have pl-HPP caused by a homozygous c.1559delT mutation. The majority of c.1559delT carriers had normal values of HPP biochemical markers, such as serum ALP and urine PEA. The only way to reliably detect the pl-HPP carriers is to perform the *ALPL* mutation analysis.

2.4 Prenatal diagnosis for perinatal (lethal) form of hypophosphatasia

pl-HPP has been diagnosed in *utero* by ultrasonography performed with careful attention to marked hypomineralization of the limbs and the skull (Fig.1) (Tongsong & Pongsatha, 2000). The differential diagnosis of HPP depends on the age at which the diagnosis is considered. Ultrasonography examination in prenatal stage may lead to a consideration of osteogenesis imperfecta type II, campomelic dysplasia, and chondrodysplasias with defects in bone mineralization, as well as pl-HPP. Experienced sonographers usually have little difficulty in distinguishing among these disorders. However, pl-HPP is occasionally not diagnosed with sonographic examination in the first trimester because incomplete ossification is a normal finding at this stage of development (Zankl, 2008).

Prenatal assessment for pregnancies at increased risk of severe HPP by mutation analysis is possible if two HPP causing *ALPL* mutations of an affected family member are identified (Watanabe et al., 2007). Most of pl-HPPs are related to c.1559delT in Japan (Watanabe et al., 2011), but to usually compound heterozygotes, carrying two distinct mutations in US and France (Simon-Bouy et al., 2008). In Japan,screeing of c.1559delT is important to diagnose pl-HPPs. In out of Japan, mutations occur throughout the entire gene without hot spots. To detect different mutations, all exon screening of *ALPL* is needed. In prenatal genetic diagnosis, fetal genomic DNA was extracted from chorionic villus at approximately ten to 12 weeks' gestation or cultured cells of amniotic fluid at approximately 15 to 18 weeks' gestation.

A prenatal genetic diagnosis for HPP gives a couple important information about the fetus. Prenatal genetic diagnosis for HPP in combination with ultrasonography is thus considered useful for confirming a diagnosis of HPP, which presents with a wide variety of phenotypes.

2.5 Genetic counseling for perinatal (lethal) form of hypophosphatasia

Genetic counseling for pl-HPP has two situations, family with an affected first child (index case) or fortuitous prenatal skeletal dysplasia in a family without history of HP (no index case) (Fig. 3) (Simon-Bouy et al., 2008). First, a couple with an index case with recessive form of pl-HPP will have in subsequent pregnancies affected children similar to the index case with a 25% chance of recurrence. However, the severity of symptoms in HPP may differ from one child to another even in the same mutation (Nakamura-Utsunomiya, 2010). Second, in pl-HPP, pregnancies with clinical symptoms could be detected by ultrasound with no familial history of pl-HPP (no index case). The screening for c.1559delT in *ALPL* may be useful for diagnosis of pl-HPP in Japanese. Detection of 1559delT mutation confirms the diagnosis of severe HPP, and an attempt to predict the severity of the disease. Postnatal molecular genetic analysis using the cord tissue can provide a diagnosis of pl-HPP allows time for parental counseling and delivery planning. In addition, Enzyme replacement therapy (Millán JL et al., 2008) and gene therapy (Yamamoto et al., 2011) will be certainly the most promising challenge. Confirmation of the diagnosis of HPP by *ALPL* genetic testing will be indispensable before starting the treatment, and perhaps the characterization of the mutations will orient and personalize the treatment in future.

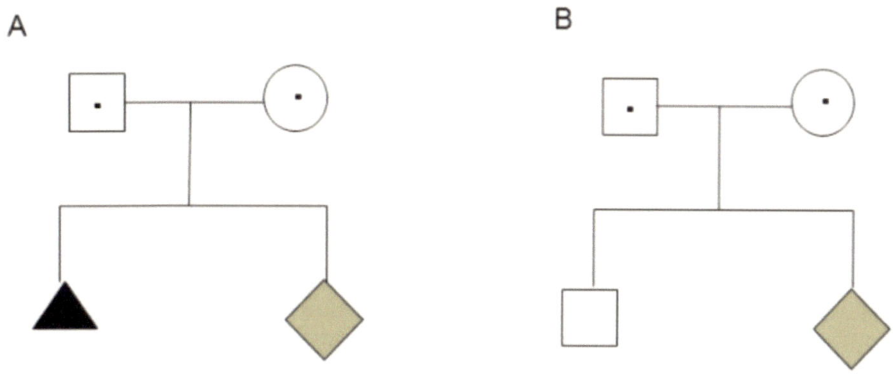

Fig. 3. Pedigree examples of two situations in genetic counseling for pl-HPP: A) family with an affected first child (index case) or B) fortuitous prenatal skeletal dysplasia in a family without history of HP (no index case)

A prenatal diagnosis should be provided in a supportive, noncoercive atmosphere that allows the couple to make informed choices regarding what is are best for them in view of their values and parenting goals. Genetic counseling is particularly important before prenatal diagnosis to enable parents to make an informed choice. Counseling before testing makes counseling after testing (for those with an affected fetus) less difficult because prospective parents are better prepared. Careful counseling regarding if and how to inform the parents about the child can help to overcome this potential problem. A prenatal genetic diagnosis may also help the professional team to prepare for a difficult delivery.

3. Conclusion

To diagnose pl-HPP in prenatal stage, collaborations between obstetricians and clinical geneticists are important and could provide support for parents of prenatal patients suspected of having skeletal dysplasia.

4. Acknowledgment

This work was supported in part by grants from the Ministry of Health and Welfare of Japan.

5. References

Gehring B., Mornet E., Plath H., Hansmann M., Bartmann P. & Brenner R. E. (1999). Perinatal hypophosphatasia: diagnosis and detection of heterozygote carriers within the family. *Clin. Genet.* 56, 313–317.

Komaru K., Ishida Y., Amaya Y., Goseki-Sone M., Orimo H. & Oda K. (2005). Novel aggregate formation of a frame-shift mutant protein of tissue-nonspecific alkaline phosphatase is ascribed to three cysteine residues in the C-terminal extension. Retarded secretion and proteasomal degradation. *FEBS J.* 272, 1704-1717.

Michigami T., Uchihashi T., Suzuki A., Tachikawa K., Nakajima S. & Ozono K. (2005). Common mutations F310L and T1559del in the tissue-nonspecific alkaline phosphatase gene are related to distinct phenotypes in Japanese patients with hypophosphatasia. *Eur. J. Pediatr.* 164, 277-282.

Mornet E. (2008). Hypophosphatasia. *Best Pract. Res. Clin. Rheumatol.* 22, 113-127.

Millán JL, Narisawa S, Lemire I, Loisel TP, Boileau G, Leonard P, Gramatikova S, Terkeltaub R, Camacho NP, McKee MD, Crine P, Whyte MP. (2008) Enzyme replacement therapy for murine hypophosphatasia. J Bone Miner Res. 23, 777-87.

Nakamura-Utsunomiya A, Okada S, Hara K, Miyagawa S, Takeda K, Fukuhara R, Nakata Y, Hayashidani M, Tachikawa K, Michigami T, Ozono K, Kobayashi M. (2010). Clinical characteristics of perinatal lethal hypophosphatasia: a report of 6 cases. *Clin. Pediatr. Endcrinol.* 19, 7-13.

Orimo, H., Goseki-Sone, M., Inoue, M., Tsubakio, Y., Sakiyama, T. & Shimada, T. (2002) Importance of deletion of T at nucleotide 1559 in the tissue-nonspecific alkaline phosphatase gene in Japanese patients with hypophosphatasia. *J. Bone Miner. Metab.* 20, 28-33.

Sawai H, Kanazawa N, Tsukahara Y, Koike K, Udagawa H, Koyama K, Mornet E. (2003). Severe perinatal hypophosphatasia due to homozygous deletion of T at nucleotide 1559 in the tissue nonspecific alkaline phosphatase gene. *Prenat. Diagn.* 23, 743-746.

Satoh N., Murotsuki A, & Sawai H. The birth prevalence rates for skeletal dysplasia in the registration system of the Japan Forum of Fetal Skeletal Dysplasia. *J. Jan. Perinat. Neonat. Med.* 45, 1005-1007 (2009). (Japanese)

Simon-Bou B, Taillandier A, Fauvert D, Brun-Heath I, Serre JL, Armengod CG, Bialer MG, Mathieu M, Cousin J, Chitayat D, Liebelt J, Feldman B, Gérard-Blanluet M, Körtge-Jung S, King C, Laivuori H, Le Merrer M, Mehta S, Jern C, Sharif S, Prieur F, Gillessen-Kaesbach G, Zankl A, Mornet E. (2008). Hypophosphatasia: molecular testing of 19 prenatal cases and discussion about genetic counseling.Prenat Diagn. 28 993-8.

The Tissue Nonspecific Alkaline Phosphatase Gene Mutations Database http://www.sesep.uvsq.fr/03_hypo_mutations.php#mutations

Tongsong T. & Pongsatha S. (2000). Early prenatal sonographic diagnosis of congenital hypophosphatasia. *Ultrasound Obstet. Gynecol.* 15, 252-255.

Zankl A., Morne, E. & Wong, S. (2008). Specific ultrasonographic features of perinatal lethal hypophosphatasia. *Am. J. Med. Genet.* 146A, 1200-1204.

Watanabe A., Yamamasu S., Shinagawa T., Suzuki Y., Takeshita T., Orimo H. Shimada T. (2007). Prenatal genetic diagnosis of severe perinatal (lethal) hypophosphatasia. *J. Nippon Med. Sch.* 74, 65–69

Watanabe A, Karasugi T, Sawai H, Naing BT, Ikegawa S, Orimo H, Shimada T. (2011). Prevalence of c.1559delT in ALPL, a common mutation resulting in the perinatal (lethal) form of hypophosphatasia in Japanese and effects of the mutation on heterozygous carriers. J Hum Genet.56, 166-8.

Yamamoto S, Orimo H, Matsumoto T, Iijima O, Narisawa S, Maeda T, Millán JL, Shimada T. (2011) Prolonged survival and phenotypic correction of Akp2(-/-) hypophosphatasia mice by lentiviral gene therapy. *J Bone Miner Res.* 26,135-142.

3

Skeletal Dysplasias of the Human Fetus: Postmortem Diagnosis

Anastasia Konstantinidou
University of Athens
Greece

1. Introduction

Congenital skeletal disorders comprise a heterogenous group of abnormalities of the bones related to their shape, growth and integrity. They are present at birth or become manifest during gestation causing abnormal development of the fetal skeleton that can be prenatally detected by ultrasonography. They make part of a large group of genetic skeletal disorders, formerly called constitutional disorders of bone. They all refer to abnormal skeletal development on the basis of a defective genetic background. Excluding chromosomal abnormalities affecting the skeleton, the large and heterogeneous family of genetic skeletal disorders comprise (1) disorders with significant skeletal involvement corresponding to the definition of skeletal dysplasias (alternatively called osteochondrodysplasias), (2) metabolic and molecular bone disorders, (3) dysostoses, (4) skeletal malformation and/or reduction syndromes and (5) multiple congenital malformation syndromes with a prominent skeletal involvement. . The genetic skeletal disorders, although individually rare, are not uncommon as a whole group. The latest 2010 Revision of the Nosology and Classification of Genetic Skeletal Disorders (Warman et al., 2011) includes 456 entities. Some 50 of them are perinatally lethal and can be diagnosed at birth (Nikkels, 2009), while some others, non lethal and compatible with short or long term survival, may present with abnormal phenotypic findings at birth or with abnormal ultrasonographic findings in utero and raise a prenatal diagnostic dilemma, as pertains to the possible lethality or morbidity of the affected fetus. With the advent of prenatal ultrasonographic examination, many of the affected fetuses are aborted at an early gestational age. A correct diagnosis and typing of the skeletal disorder is essential for the prognosis and genetic counselling of the family, as well as for the possibility of prenatal diagnosis in subsequent pregnancies. The molecular defects underlying the genetic skeletal disorders are increasingly being identified and have shed some light on the pathogeneses of these conditions. One important example is that of the fibroblast growth factor receptor (FGFR3) defects underlying skeletal dysplasias such as Thanatophoric dysplasia, Achondroplasia etc. Nevertheless, in only a restricted subgroup of fetal skeletal dysplasias is the molecular genetic analysis part of a routine prenatal control able to provide an accurate diagnosis. In most instances, the responsibility of the final diagnosis of a fetal skeletal dysplasia lies on the post-mortem examination and in many institutions it is largely or uniquely the task of the pathologist.

The objective of this chapter is to provide an overview on the role of the pathologist in the handling of the congenital skeletal disorders and enable the postmortem diagnostic approach. The chapter will summarize the principal postnatal diagnostic features of the more common subgroups of fetal genetic skeletal disorders to be used as diagnostic tools by the fetal pathologist at autopsy.

2. Current knowledge

General information on the definitions, frequency, classification, as well as the possibilities and restrictions of prenatal sonographic and genetic molecular diagnosis is given below.

2.1 Definitions

All the entities included in the latest classification of genetic skeletal disorders present a significant skeletal involvement corresponding to the definition of osteochondrodysplasias, dysostoses, metabolic bone disorders, and skeletal malformation and/or reduction syndromes.

The osteochondrodysplasias are disorders in the development and/or growth of cartilage and/or bone. The long bones are affected in a generalized manner with or without involvement of the membranous bone of the skull. The abnormalities are usually symmetric, and dwarfism is common and often disproportionate (Kornak & Mundlos, 2003).

A dysostosis is a disturbance in the pattern of the chondroid anlage as an organ. A dysostosis affects one or a few skeletal elements while the other bones remain normal. Dysostoses are caused by defects in signalling during organogenesis. These disorders can be asymmetric, there is usually no dwarfism and chondro-osseous histology is often normal.

2.2 Incidence – Frequency

The overall incidence of genetic skeletal disorders has been estimated to approximately 2 in 10,000 births (range according to the literature 2-5/10,000) (Rasmussen et al., 1996). Of those, the frequency of lethal skeletal dysplasias among stillborn and liveborn infants is 1 in 4,000 - 6,000 (Nikkels, 2009). A percentage of 23% of affected fetuses are stillborn, while a 32% die during the first week of life. The perinatal mortality rate due to skeletal dysplasias is estimated to 0.9% (Goncalves & Jeanty, 1994). The frequency among perinatal autopsies ranges from 1 in 50 to 1 in 100 (Konstantinidou, 2009; Nikkels, 2009). Overall, the skeletal dysplasias that are more frequently encountered are Thanatophoric dysplasia, Achondroplasia, Osteogenesis Imperfecta, Achondrogenesis, and the Short-Rib with or without Polydactyly syndromes (Jeanty et al., 2003, Konstantinidou et al., 2009). Thanatophoric dysplasia, Osteogenesis Imperfecta and Achondrogenesis constitute the majority of lethal skeletal dysplasias (Konstantinidou et al., 2009). Achondroplasia is the more frequent nonlethal skeletal dysplasia.

2.3 Classification

Since the mid-1960s the knowledge of skeletal dysplasias has significantly expanded and numerous new entities have been identified (Gilbert-Barness, 2007). Before then, a disproportionately short stature was called without any distinction by clinicians as "achondroplasia" (attributed to short limbs) or "Morquio disease" (attributed to a short trunk). The lack of knowledge and the scarcity of individual skeletal dysplasias, in association with the large heterogeneity, phenotypic variability and overlapping features of skeletal dysplasias led to a significant diagnostic controversy surrounding the skeletal dysplasias. The terminology has been basically descriptive, based on the clinical evolution (e.g. thanatophoric dysplasia - greek thanatos = death, phero = to bear: the dysplasia that bears death), the clinical description (e.g. campomelic dysplasia - greek campsis = curving, benting / meli = limbs: the dysplasia with curved or bent limbs), the assumed pathogenesis (e.g. osteogenesis imperfecta, achondrogenesis), or the name of investigators that first described the disease (e.g. Ellis-van Creveld syndrome).

With time, acquired knowledge in the field of molecular and clinical genetics has significantly contributed to the distinction and classification of skeletal disorders. A first significant classification was created in 1970 in Paris, and was subsequently revised in 1978 and 1983, while a substantial classification took place in 1998 and was revised in 2002, 2006 and 2010 (INCO, 1998; Hall, 2002; Superti-Furga & Unger, 2007; Warman et al., 2011). However, in the recent years, the number of recognized genetic disorders with a significant skeletal component is growing and the distinction between dysplasias, metabolic bone disorders, dysostoses and malformation syndromes is blurring. Molecular evidence leads to confirmation of individual entities and to the constitution of new groups but also allows for delineation of related but distinct entities and indicates a previously unexpected heterogeneity of molecular mechanisms. Thus, accumulating molecular evidence does not necessarily simplify the Nosology, and a further increase in the number of entities and growing complexity is expected. For classification purposes, in the latest revision, the 456 genetic skeletal disorders included are placed in 40 groups defined by molecular, biochemical and/or radiographic criteria. For classification purposes, pathogenetic and molecular criteria are integrating with morphological ones, but disorders are still identified by clinical and radiographic criteria (Warman et al., 2011).

According to our experience in diagnosing fetal skeletal dysplasias, the latest Revisions of the Nosology and Classification placing the genetic skeletal disorders in groups, have proved most useful in providing a list of conditions entering the differential diagnosis, once the main group has been recognized. In our cases of fetal autopsy, the diagnostic approach is still based on morphological features, radiographic appearance, pathological and histological findings.

2.4 Prenatal ultrasonography in skeletal dysplasias

Prenatal diagnosis is initially based on the sonographic detection, most commonly during the second gestational trimester. Several previously published series have emphasized on the diagnostic and prognostic implications of prenatal ultrasonography in fetal skeletal disorders (Doray et al., 2000; Parilla et al., 2003; Krakow et al., 2008; Witters et al., 2008). Two-dimensional ultrasonography may detect the majority of skeletal dysplasias, however, difficulties in the diagnosis as well as in the differential diagnosis are frequently arising. The use of further imaging modalities or invasive procedures is sometimes necessary in order to detect or exclude an underlying chromosomal or singe gene disorder. An accurate diagnosis is essential to allow adequate genetic counseling as well as further management of the case. For this approach, the three-dimensional ultrasonography and three-dimensional computed tomography may provide more detailed imaging results, whereas the role of fetal MRI may prove to be useful in the future. Despite the indisputable progress that has been achieved in the last years, in some cases the antenatal detection delays and is feasible only at the late second or even at the third gestational trimester. This may generate serious bioethical concern as well as difficulties in the management and the genetic counseling, particularly in cases of lethal skeletal dysplasias.

Prenatal ultrasound can detect cases of dwarfism and several other skeletal malformations, while there are sonographic measurements that serve as good predictors of lethality (Parilla et al., 2003). Lethality is usually due to thoracic underdevelopment and lung hypoplasia. Sonographic markers of lethality are mainly based on the assessment of lung biometry, measurements of chest circumference (CC) and its relation to the abdominal circumference (AC), femur length (FL), and finally assessment of the pulmonary arteries by Doppler ultrasonography. Thus, measurements of CC lower than the 5th centile, CC/AC $<5^{th}$ centile, chest/trunk length ratio <0.32, lung area $<5^{th}$ centile, right lung area/thoracic area ratio <0.11, and FL/AC <0.16, are considered as markers of lethality of high predictive value (Parilla et al., 2003). The presence of curved or bent femora should be taken into consideration when estimating the femur length in order to assess lethality, as in such conditions the bone may be longer than it appears. In the lethal skeletal dysplasias, the femur length is shorter with a deviation of 6.7 weeks from the 50th centile during the second trimester of gestation, whereas in those compatible with life the deviation is of 4.2 weeks (Parilla et al., 2003). The discordance between lethal and non lethal dysplasias is raised with advancing gestation. In achondrogenesis, the femur length is 30% of the normal mean, in osteogenesis imperfecta type 2 and thanatophoric dysplasia type 1 it measures 40-60% of the normal mean, while in the nonlethal achondroplasia and hypochondroplasia is as high as 80% (Goncalves et al., 1994).

Despite the accuracy in predicting lethality, however, in cases of skeletal malformations, as in all cases of fetal malformations, a specific diagnosis is necessary not only for the prognosis of the current pregnancy, but also to assess recurrence risk in subsequent pregnancies and enable genetic counseling and future prenatal diagnosis. Given that prenatal ultrasound accuracy in the final diagnosis of genetic skeletal disorders remains relatively low, ranging from 18% to 65% in published series (Doray et al., 2000; Parilla et al., 2003; Krakow et al., 2008; Witters et al., 2008; Konstantinidou et al., 2009; Hatzaki, et al., 2011), the impact of the specific diagnosis is still dependent on the molecular genetic or postmortem examination.

2.5 Prenatal molecular genetic control in skeletal dysplasias

Out of 456 entities included in the latest Revision of the Nosology (Warman et al., 2011), 215 are associated with one or more of 226 different genes. The nosologic status has been classified as final (mutations or locus identified), probable (pedigree evidence), or bona fide (multible observations and clear diagnostic criteria, but no pedigree or locus evidence yet). Among the skeletal dysplasias that can be encountered in the fetus at autopsy, several have a known underlying molecular defect. Examples include type 1 collagenopathies (e.g. osteogenesis imperfecta type 1, 2 and 3 with *COL1A* defects), type 2 collagenopathies (e.g. achondrogenesis type 2 and hypochondrogenesis with *COL2A* defects) and the group of fibroblast growth factor receptor defects (e.g. thanatophoric dysplasia, achondroplasia and hypochondroplasia with *FGFR3* mutations). This last group comprises practically the vast majority of the cases that are prenatally diagnosed by molecular genetic method (Hatzaki et al., 2011). The possibility of molecular analysis for mutations in selected exons of the *FGFR3* gene by PCR amplification of fetal DNA extracted from amniotic fluid cells has led to an increased demand for *FGFR3* testing. This has become part of a routine prenatal control when a preliminary diagnosis of "skeletal dysplasia" is set by ultrasonography, regardless of the phenotypic relevance to the *FGFR3* group of skeletal disorders. Thus, in many instances, the prenatal *FGFR3* molecular control proves to be irrelevant with the case, and should be substituted by molecular confirmation of other underlying defects, as indicated by the postmortem diagnosis.

3. Postmortem examination: The role of the pathologist

More than 50 skeletal dysplasias are identifiable at birth, the list being rapidly expanding (Krakow et al., 2008). Fetuses with skeletal disorders are frequently subjected to postmortem examination following prenatal ultrasonographic pathological findings and interruption of pregnancy or after intrauterine fetal demise.

Despite the scarcity of individual skeletal dysplasias, our experience is that the fetopathologist frequently deals with this group of disorders at fetal or perinatal autopsy and is responsible, in everyday practice, for the correct identification of such conditions. In the department of Pathology of Athens University, where consult cases of fetal autopsies are received from central and district hospitals in Greece, the frequency of fetal/perinatal skeletal dysplasias has raised to 1 in 40 over a 15-year period. Affected fetuses of the second trimester of gestation form the majority in the series of our patients. Liveborn infants affected with perinatally lethal skeletal dysplasias on the other hand are only a small minority, usually the offspring of families with a low socio-economic background that have not received prenatal follow-up. Increasing expertise in prenatal ultrasound has led to increased and more accurate early identification of fetal skeletal dysplasias. Prenatal identification of a presumably lethal skeletal dysplasia raises the option of termination of the pregnancy. Molecular characterization is often carried out prenatally, particularly for the family of FGFR3 gene mutations. In the case of positive results for a FGFR3 gene mutation, termination of pregnancy is often decided by the parents and the fetus is sent for autopsy. Postmortem examination in the context of a known molecular defect, apart from the confirmation of the diagnosis, may also be of scientific interest: the pathologist may observe and record phenotypic variability under the same molecularly defined entity with a single mutation, or contribute to a phenotype-genotype correlation in entities with mutational variability. When there is no molecular diagnosis preceding autopsy, the fetopathologist is responsible for the diagnostic approach, given that the prenatal ultrasonographic evaluation can usually predict lethality, but very often fails to identify the particular type of skeletal dysplasia, which is necessary for genetic counseling and future prenatal diagnosis. Significant phenotypic overlapping and relatively limited knowledge of the genetic background are the main sources of controversy in the diagnosis of these disorders. Thus, in everyday practice, the diagnosis and prognosis still depend on the postmortem radiographical, pathological and histopathological findings.

Although the assistance of an experienced paediatric radiologist or clinical geneticist in the interpretation of the postmortem radiography is desirable, this is not always feasible in many countries, because of lack of expertise. Under these circumstances, the fetopathologist should be able to deal with the radiographic interpretation of, at least, the more common among skeletal dysplasias and refer the remaining cases to specialized referral centers. Radiological diagnosis in very young fetuses may occasionally be very difficult, as some bones are not yet mineralized and only the chondroid anlage is present. Genetic metabolic diseases and malformation syndromes involving the skeleton are also difficult to diagnose at autopsy, demanding from the pathologist knowledge and skills of clinical dysmorphology and clinical genetics. The diagnostic difficulties are obvious, such as the restricted or incomplete phenotype at an early gestational age and the eventual lack of typical morphological or clinical hallmarks of the syndrome in utero (e.g. mental retardation, hearing deficit, hair loss etc). Despite these restrictions, however, there are many examples where an alert and experienced fetopathologist has first provided the affected family with a correct diagnosis of a genetic syndrome, based on the postmortem examination of an affected fetus.

4. Methods

In a combined retrospective and prospective study, we have gathered radiological, physical, gross pathological and histopathological data on 50 cases of genetic skeletal disorders diagnosed among 2250 fetal and perinatal autopsies carried out at the Department of Pathology of the University of Athens over a 12-year period.

The methodology for postmortem examination of the fetus with skeletal dysplasia included radiographic control, photographs, external inspection, gross inspection of all organs including the brain, organ dissection and sampling for microscopical examination, and, finally, sampling from the bones and cartilage for histological, histochemical and occasionally immunohistochemical staining.

4.1 Radiography

X-rays/babygram both anteroposterior and lateral, using a Faxitron Cabinet X-Ray System, were taken in the following instances: in all cases identified as possible "skeletal dysplasias" on prenatal ultrasonographic examination; in cases suspect of skeletal dysplasia on external inspection; in cases of external deformities. Measurements of the length of the long bones and spine on the X-ray were compared to normal values of fetal long bone growth and spine (van der Harten, 1990).

4.2 Autopsy - Histopathology

Detailed autopsy with histological sampling from various organs was performed in all cases. Bone samples included the head of the femur or humerus with the metaphysis and part of the diaphysis in all cases. A midsagittal section of lumbar vertebral bodies and the costochondral junction of the ribs were occasionally available. After fixation in 10% formalin and decalcification in 0,5M EDTA, paraffin sections were stained with Hematoxylin-Eosin, Periodic-acid-Schiff (PAS) and PAS after diastase predigestion, and occasionally additional Alcian blue and Masson trichrome stains were used. The bones were cut longitudinally to include the resting cartilage, growth plate, and primary spongiosa of the metaphysis .

4.3 Molecular genetic analysis

Molecular genetic control was available and confirmed the diagnosis in 12 cases. Of those, 6 referred to mutations of the FGFR3 gene, prenatally or postnatally tested by PCR amplification analysis. The mutations tested included R248C and S249C for Thanatophoric dysplasia, G380R for Achondroplasia and N540K for Hypochondroplasia, as previously published (Konstantinidou et al., 2009; Hatzaki et al., 2011). Molecular genetic control was also available in selective cases of Osteogenesis Imperfecta, Greenberg dysplasia and Cranioectodermal dysplasia (Konstantinidou et al., 2009).

5. Results

In our series of 2250 autopsied fetuses and infants, 50 cases could be identified as genetic skeletal disorders and were grouped under 13 of the 40 groups included in the 2010 Revision of the Nosology (Warman et al., 2011). The various types of skeletal dysplasias included in our series are shown in Table 1.

Among the overall group of fetal genetic skeletal disorders, the skeletal dysplasias (osteochondrodysplasias) were the more common (87.5%), followed by the limb hypoplasia/reduction group (12%) and the dysostoses (10%). The larger group of osteochondrodysplasias was the group of FGFR3 defects (20%). The more common types of osteochondrodysplasia were Thanatophoric dysplasia (16%), Osteogenesis Imperfecta (14%), and the group of Short-Rib dysplasia - with or without polydactyly (14%). Achondrogenesis/Hypochondrogenesis cases, although perinatally lethal, were not common in our series of autopsies (4%), in contrast with other published autopsy series (Nikkels et al., 2009). Fetal age at autopsy ranged from 12 to 37.4 weeks with a mean of 20.5 weeks. There was a predilection for male gender among skeletal disorders (male to female ratio 3:1). Lethal osteochondrodysplasias represented a majority of 58% among the diagnosed genetic skeletal disorders. The remaining 42% belonged to groups that are known to be non lethal or not always lethal, presenting, however, severe morbidity in most cases. Lethality could be accurately predicted by prenatal ultrasonography, based on the identification of thoracic underdevelopment and severe limb shortening.

The main ultrasonographic findings that led to a presumptive prenatal diagnosis of "skeletal dysplasia" were short limbs, curved femora, narrow thorax, fractures and acrania (lack of skull ossification). At postmortem examination, several cases of short femora were attributed to intrauterine growth restriction (IUGR), with no signs of a genetic skeletal disorder. Short and/or curved limbs were seen in a variety of skeletal dysplasias other than thanatophoric dysplasia. Fractures were seen in the context of osteogenesis imperfecta, achondrogenesis type 1A, hypophosphatasia and gracile bone dysplasia (osteocraniostenosis, osteocraniosplenic syndrome). Acrania was a feature of osteogenesis imperfecta type 2A, achondrogenesis type 2A and osteocraniostenosis.

Correct typing coinciding with the final postmortem diagnosis was achieved in only 25% of cases by ultrasonography. Lack of knowledge of the large variety of the less common skeletal dysplasias was the main reason of prenatal ultrasonographic diagnostic failure. Curved or angular bent femora were occasionally mistaken for fractured limbs, misleading the presumptive prenatal diagnosis towards the conditions that appear with fractures, such as osteogenesis imperfecta.

6. Description of the more common genetic skeletal disorders

The more common among the fetal skeletal disorders encountered in our series will be presented briefly below. The group number refers to the order of the 2010 Revision of the Nosology and Classification of Genetic Disorders of Bone (Warman et al., 2011).

1. *FGFR3 group*	21. *Chondrodysplasia punctata (CDP) group*
Thanatophoric dysplasia type 1 Achondroplasia heterozygous	Chondrodysplasia punctata (CDPX2) HEM (Greenberg) dysplasia
Hypochondroplasia	25. *Dysplasias with decreased bone density*
2. *Type 2 collagen group*	Osteogenesis Imperfecta type 2a
Achondrogenesis type 2 Spondyloepiphyseal dysplasia	Osteogenesis Imperfecta type 2b Osteogenesis Imperfecta type 2c
7. *Filamin group*	26. *Abnormal mineralization group*
Atelosteogenesis type 1	Hypophosphatasia
9. *Short-rib dysplasia (with or without polydactyly) group:SR(P)*	27. *Lysosomal storage diseases with skeletal involvement (dysostosis multiplex group)*
SR(P) 2 (Majewski)	Mucopolysaccharidosis
SR(P) 1/3 (Saldino-Noonan/Verma-Naumoff)	35. *Dysostoses with predominant vertebral involvement, with and without costal involvement*
Chondroectodermal dysplasia (Ellis-van Creveld)	Spondylocostal dysostosis /Jarcho-Levin syndrome
15. *Acromelic dysplasias*	38. *Limb hypoplasia-reduction defects group*
Cranioectodermal dysplasia (Sensenbrenner)	Roberts syndrome
18. *Bent-bone dysplasia group*	De Lange syndrome
Campomelic dysplasia	Ectrodactyly-radial defect
19. *Slender bone dysplasia group*	Split Hand-Foot malformation with tibial hypoplasia
Gracile bone dysplasia (Osteocraniostenosis) IMAGE syndrome	Femoral hypoplasia - Unusual facies

Table 1. The various types of genetic skeletal disorders in our series

6.1 Group 1: FGFR3 mutations group

Index cases: Thanatophoric dysplasia type 1, Achondroplasia

6.1.1 Thanatophoric dysplasia type 1 (TD1)

This type of congenital skeletal dysplasia was the most common in our series (8/50 cases, 16%). Prenatal ultrasonography detected all these cases as "skeletal dysplasias", but the correct labelling of *thanatophoric dysplasia* was suggested by the ultrasonographic findings in four of them, all belonging to the latest chronological period of our series. As the name suggests, the condition is invariably lethal in the perinatal period. It is attributed to mutations in the gene encoding the Fibroblast Growth Factor Receptor (FGFR3). Most cases occur sporadically as a result of a *de novo* autosomal dominant mutation. Three of our cases were molecularly confirmed to host the 742C>T mutation, resulting in aminoacid change R248C within exon 7 of the FGFR3 gene (Konstantinidou et al., 2009; Hatzaki et al., 2011). The mean age at autopsy was 21.3 weeks, ranging from 20 to 24 weeks of gestation.

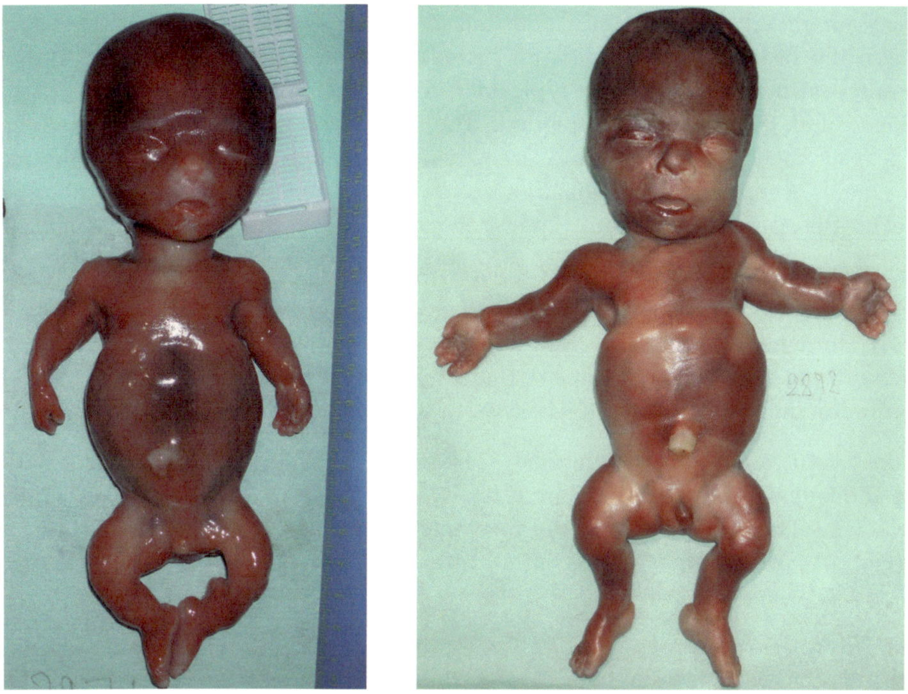

Fig. 1. Fetuses with Thanatophoric Dysplasia type 1 at 20 weeks (left) and 22.5 weeks (right)

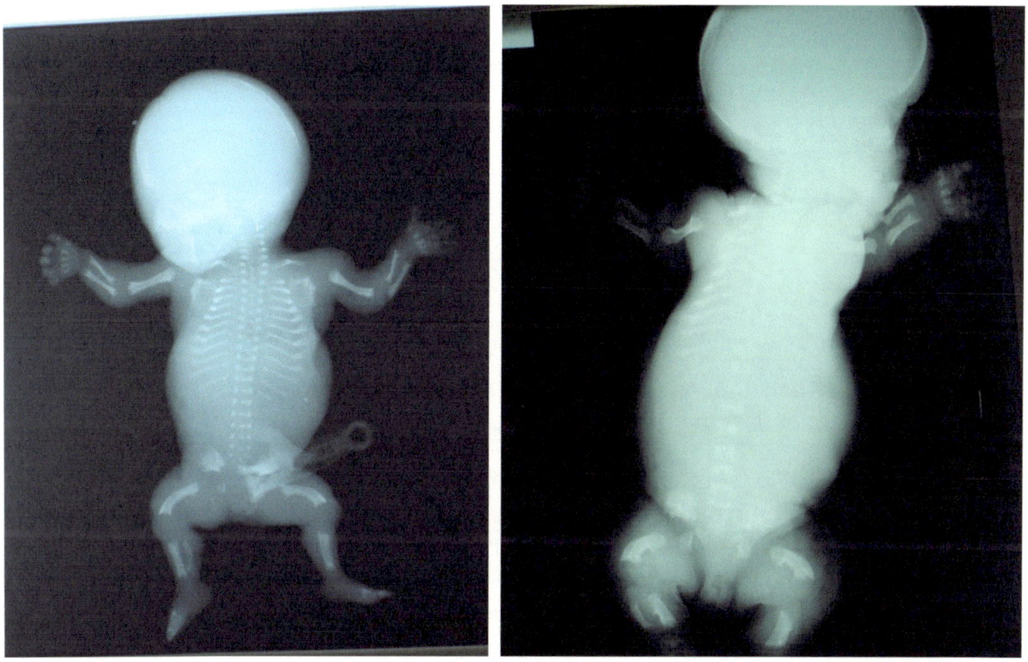

Fig. 2. Thanatophoric dysplasia type 1 at 20 and 32 weeks: Platyspondyly, short ribs, short tubular bones, curved femora with metaphyseal spikes, horizontally shortened ilia

All cases presented the following constant typical characteristics (Fig. 1): At external inspection the head was large with an increased fronto-occipital diameter. A flat nasal bridge and protruding tongue were typical facial characteristics. The thorax was narrow and bell-shaped and the abdomen distended. The upper and lower limbs were short in all respects (rhizomelic, mesomelic and acromelic shortening). All the linear somatometric measurements were affected in thanatophoric dysplasia, particularly the crown-heel and toe-heel lengths, as well as the cranial perimeter, chest and abdominal circumferences.

X-rays (Fig. 2) show severe platyspondyly with H-shaped or U-shaped vertebral bodies, relatively short ribs, small horizontally shortened iliac bones with sacrosciatic notches and markedly shortened upper and lower limb bones. Short and curved "telephone receiver-like" femora are a hallmark of type 1 thanatophoric dysplasia, but curving may be less pronounced in the younger fetuses. The femora show small metaphyseal spikes.

At autopsy, fetuses with thanatophoric dysplasia type 1 have a large head with small cranial sutures and megalencephaly. The brain is heavy, the temporal lobe is enlarged and there are multiple transverse grooves along the inferomedial surface of the temporal and occipital lobes (Fig. 3). Hippocampal dysplasia is also part of the temporal lobe dysplasia in this condition.

Temporal dysplasia was present in all the examined fetal brains in our sample of fetuses with thanatophoric dysplasia type 1. The finding could not be confirmed in severely macerated brains.

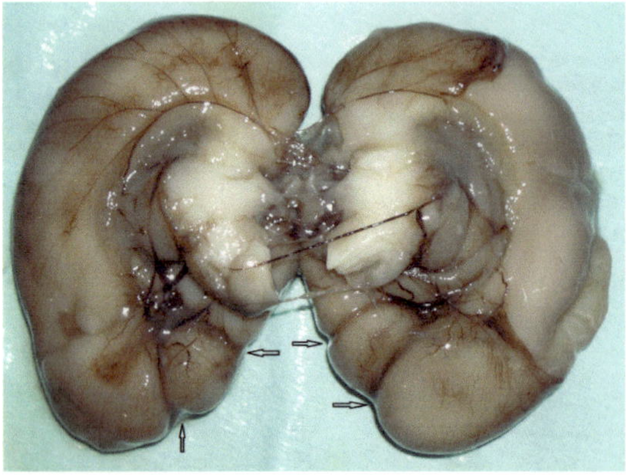

Fig. 3. The brain in Thanatophoric dysplasia at 22 weeks: transverse sulci along the inferomedial surface of the temporal and occipital lobes (arrows)

In one unique case of a fetus with otherwise typical TD1 findings, organ inspection and dissection revealed intestinal malrotation, renal tubular cysts and persisting ductal plate of the liver. These findings are frequent in other forms of skeletal dysplasias, particularly in the family of Short-Rib-Polydactyly dysplasias (referred to later in this chapter). The findings are unique in that they have never been reported in cases of TD1 to our knowledge. Molecular analysis in that case confirmed the presence of a typical R248C mutation in the *FGFR3* gene. A possible explanation for this unusual association of abnormal findings could be the presence of a second mutation or microdeletion in a different part of the genome.

Histopathologic examination of the epiphyseal growth plate in TD1 shows retardation and disorganization of the growth plate with irregular borders of the periphysis. There is fibrous extension of the ossification groove of Ranvier and periosteal expansion of bone formation at this site. These alterations correspond to the metaphyseal spikes seen on radiography (Fig. 4).

FGFR3 molecular genetic analysis showed the R248C mutation in four examined cases, while in the remaining cases the diagnosis of TD1 was based on the typical external, radiographic and histopathologic findings provided by the postmortem examination.

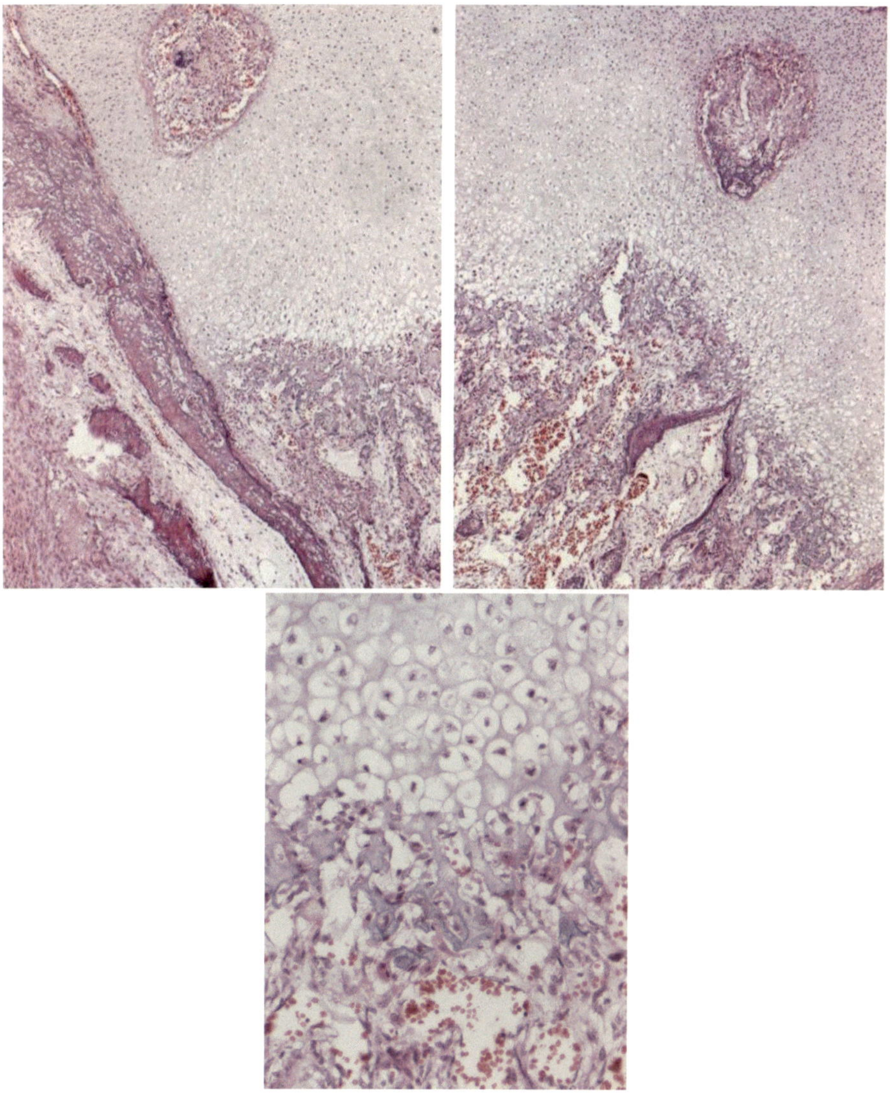

Fig. 4. Epiphyseal growth plate from the femoral head of a fetus with Thanatophoric dysplasia type 1. TOP: The borders between the cartilage and the primary spongiosa are irregular. Extension of the ossification groove of Ranvier (corresponding to the metaphyseal spikes seen on radiography) are seen on the left. BOTTOM: The growth plate is disorganized, without column formation.

6.1.2 Achondroplasia

This condition is the most common nonlethal osteochondroplasia. It is autosomal dominant due to mutations in the FGFR3 gene. In our case, there was a *de novo* heterozygous G380R mutation. The facial appearance is typical with a prominent forehead, small maxillary area and flat nasal bridge. The trunk is of almost normal length and there is rhizomelic shortening of limbs.

Radiographic features include platyspondyly, short ribs, squared iliac wings with horizontal acetabular roofs and spurs (trident appearance), splayed upper femoral metaphyses, metaphyseal flaring and short metacarpals (Fig. 5).

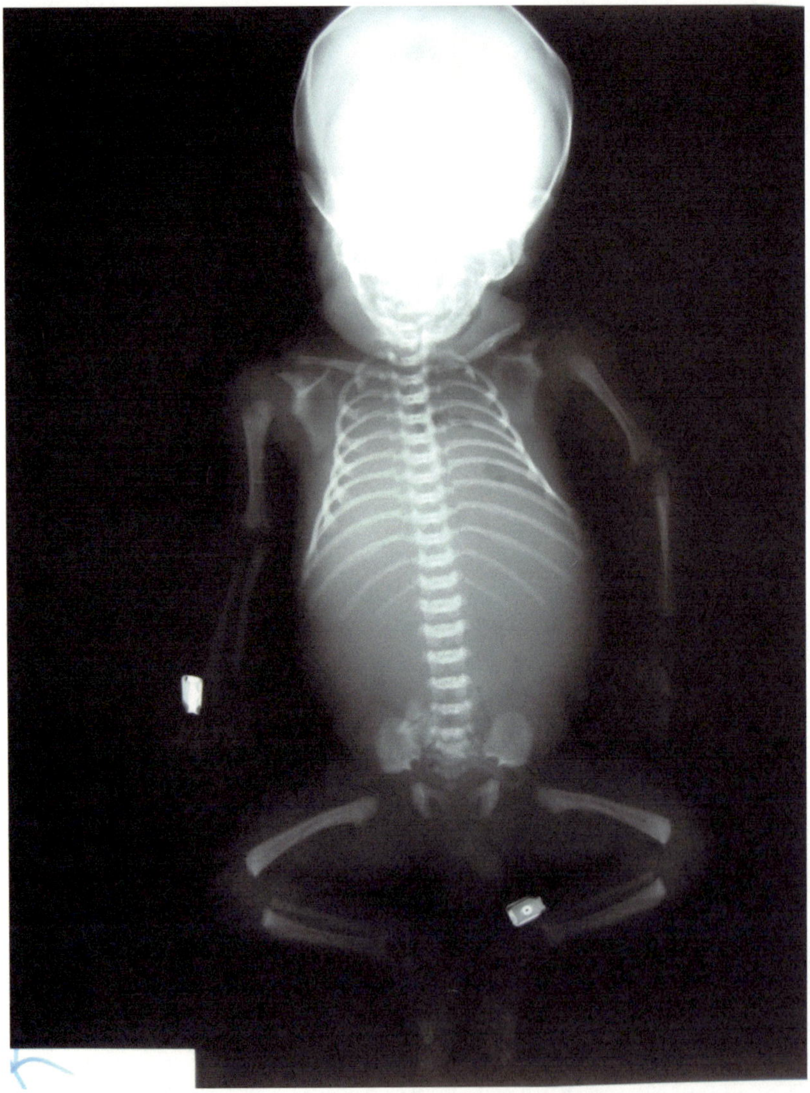

Fig. 5. Achondroplasia at 37 weeks: narrow thorax, rhizomelic limb shortening, splayed upper femoral metaphyses and trident appearance of iliac bones.

6.2 Group 2: Type II collagen group

Index case: Achondrogenesis type II

Achondrogenesis is the most severe lethal form of osteochondrodysplasia. This condition, commonly encountered in European published series of lethal skeletal dysplasias (Nikkels et al., 2009), was uncommon in our Greek series (1/50 cases). Achondrogenesis type II, as all type II collagenopathies, is an autosomal dominant disorder caused by mutations in the *COL2A1* gene.

Major radiographic features and clinical presentation are similar in achondrogenesis type I and type II (Fig. 6). Deficient skull ossification and rib fractures are present only in type Ia.

Histologically, the growth plate is severely disorganized. The resting cartilage is cellular with many prominent blood vessels and perivascular fibrosis. The chondrocytes may appear ballooned.

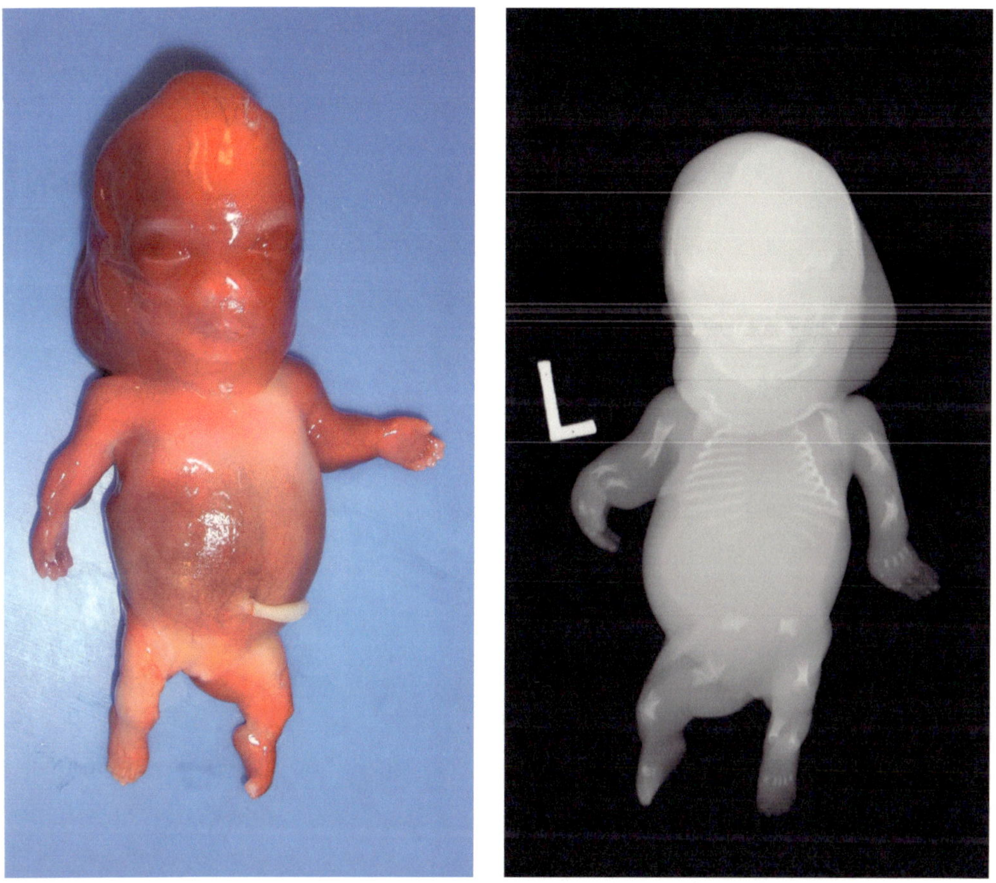

Fig. 6. Achondrogenesis: The trunk and extremities are extremely short. Hydrops is present. There is complete absence of ossification in the vertebrae, sacrum and pubis in the young fetus. The limb bones are extremely short and there are metaphyseal spike-like spurs. (Images kindly ceded by Dr. I. Scheimberg; Barts and The London NHS Trust)

6.3 Group 25: Osteogenesis Imperfecta and dysplasias with decreased bone density

Index cases: Osteogenesis Imperfecta type IIa and type IIb

6.3.1 Osteogenesis Imperfecta (O.I.) type II

The lethal type 2 is the most commonly met in the fetus. It is mostly a dominantly inherited condition due to mutations in the *COL1A1* and *COL1A2* genes. Some severe cases of O.I. are caused by compound heterozygote mutations in the *CRTAP* and *LERPE* genes and follow recessive inheritance. Based on morphological features radiology or histology, it is not yet possible to discriminate between the O.I. cases caused by mutations in the collagen I gene and the autosomal recessive cases (Nikkels et al., 2009).

Two index cases of Osteogenesis Imperfecta type IIa and IIb are shown below (Figure 7). Both cases had dominant mutations in the *COL1A1* gene. The fetus with O.I. type IIa has a large membranous skull (acrania) (Figure 7, left). There is deficient ossification of the skull but not complete acrania in type IIb (Figure 7, right). The femora are bent and shortened as a result of multiple recurrent fractures. The characteristic "blue sclera" recognised in infancy or later are not a feature of the fetus at autopsy. Brain heterotopias have been described in O.I. and were present in both of these index cases with O.I type IIa and IIb.

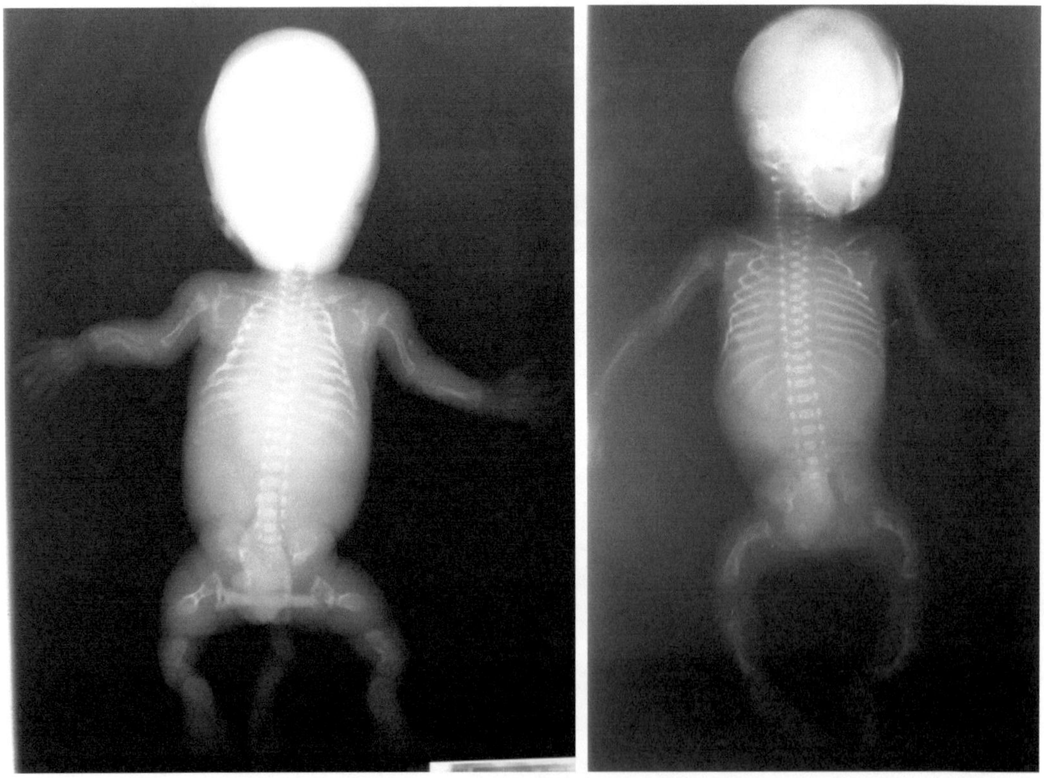

Fig. 7. Osteogenesis Imperfecta type IIa at 26 weeks (left) and type IIb at 20 weeks (right) Rib fractures are present in type IIa but there are hardly any in type IIb. The femora are deformed. The spine is normal.

Radiography (Fig. 7) of the 2nd trimester fetus shows multiple fractures with beaded ribs and crumbled femora in the more severe O.I. type IIa (Fig. 7, left) or bowed femora with fewer or no rib fractures in the less severe type IIb (Fig. 7, right). The humeri are usually straight without fractures, but they may appear bowed in severe forms of O.I. later in pregnancy. The spine is normal in the fetus.

Histopathology of the bone and cartilage is comparable in types IIa and IIb of Osteogenesis Imperfecta (Fig. 8, 9). The bony spicules in the metaphysis are narrow, hypercellular, and covered by basophilic meager primitive woven bone. They are markedly reduced in number and size in the diaphysis. The osteocytes are closely arranged around the bony trabeculae and in the subperiosteal area (Fig. 9). The growth plate is normal.

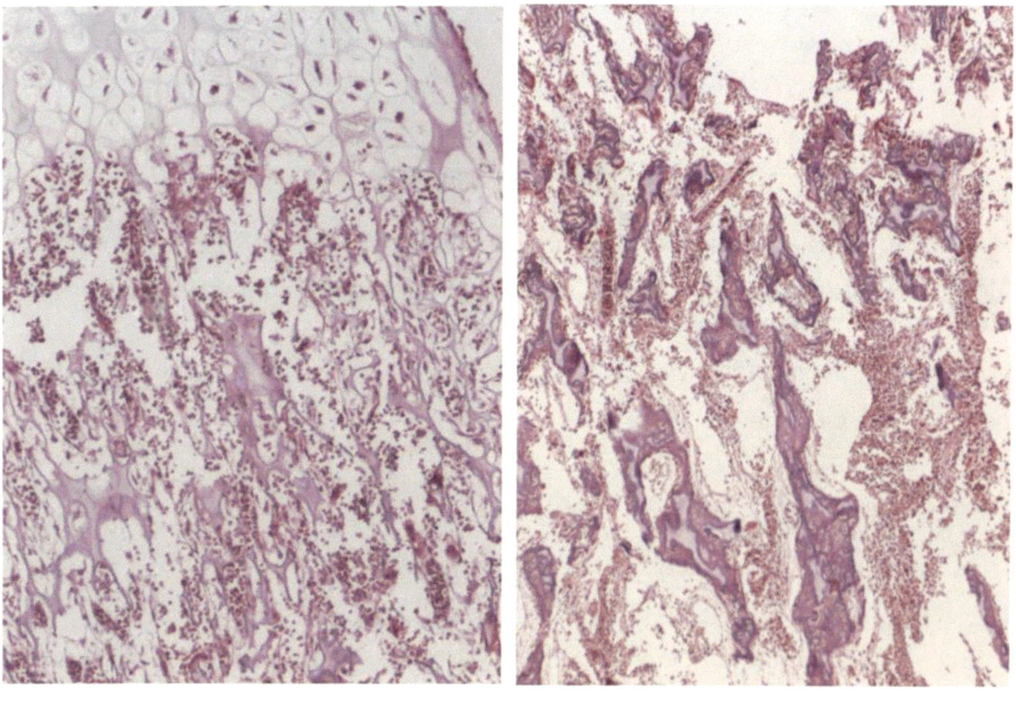

Fig. 8. Histology is comparable in Osteogenesis Imperfecta type 2a (left) and type 2b (right). The bony spicules of the primary spongiosa are narrow and covered by meager basophilic woven bone. Part of the normal growth plate is seen on top left. Towards the diaphysis, the bone marrow predominates over the bony trabeculae (right).

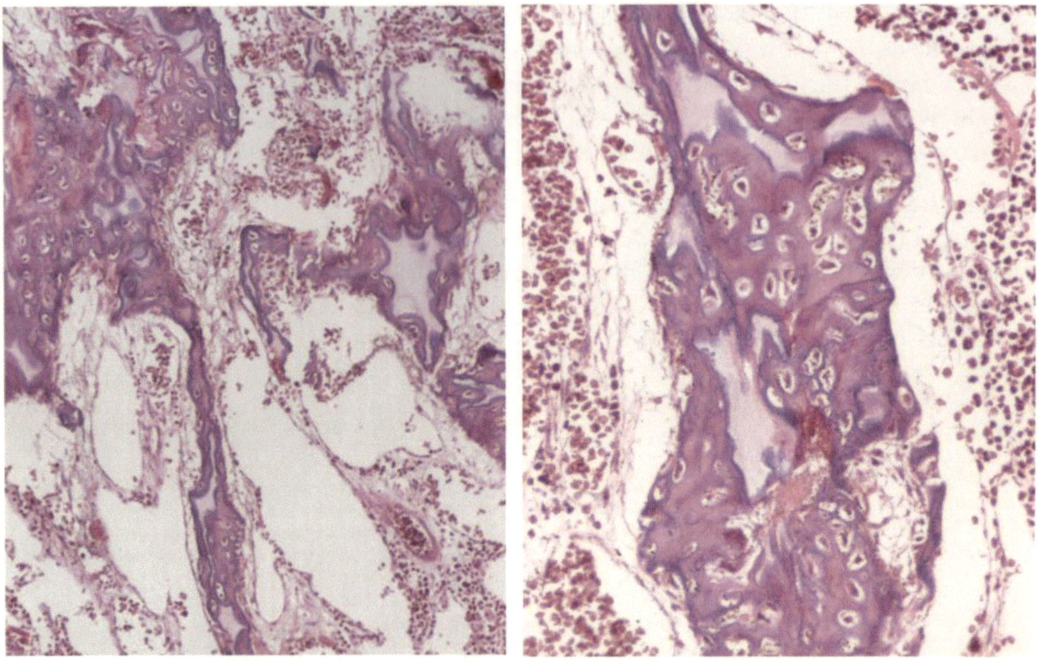

Fig. 9. Osteogenesis Imperfecta type 2b. There is increased number of osteocytes at the periphery of the bony spicules and at subperiosteal sites.

6.4 Group 9: Short-rib dysplasia (with or without polydactyly) - SR(P)

Index cases: SR(P) type II (Majewski), SR(P) type III (Verma-Naumoff), chondroectodermal dysplasia (Ellis-van Creveld)

6.4.1 Short-rib-polydactyly syndromes

There are at least 4 distinct types:

- Type I Saldino-Noonan
- Type II Majewski
- Type III Verma-Naumoff
- Type IV Beemer-Langer (polydactyly unlikely)

Types I and III may represent a phenotypic spectrum of the same entity as may types II and IV. Indeed, there are overlapping characteristics between all 4 types and several cases are described that cannot fit in a particular type (Gilbert-Barness, 2007).

All SRPs are autosomal recessive. Types I/III are caused by mutations in the *DYNC2H1* gene. The molecular background is not identified in the remaining ones. The association of SRP skeletal dysplasias with particular extraskeletal malformations, such as Dandy-Walker malformation, cardiovascular, gastrointestinal and genitourinary abnormalities, renal cysts and ductal plate malformation of the liver indicates that these syndromes probably belong to the expanding group of ciliopathies (Badano et al., 2006; Konstantinidou et al., 2009b).

In our series, 4 fetuses were diagnosed with SRP at autopsy, one with type II/Majewski (Fig. 10), two with type III/Verma-Naumoff, and one with SRP of undetermined type (aged 12 weeks of gestation).

External inspection in SRP dysplasias reveals a very narrow chest, very short limbs, and polydactyly (rare in type IV). The combination of these findings contributes to an early sonographic prenatal diagnosis, achieved as early as the 12th week of gestation in our series.

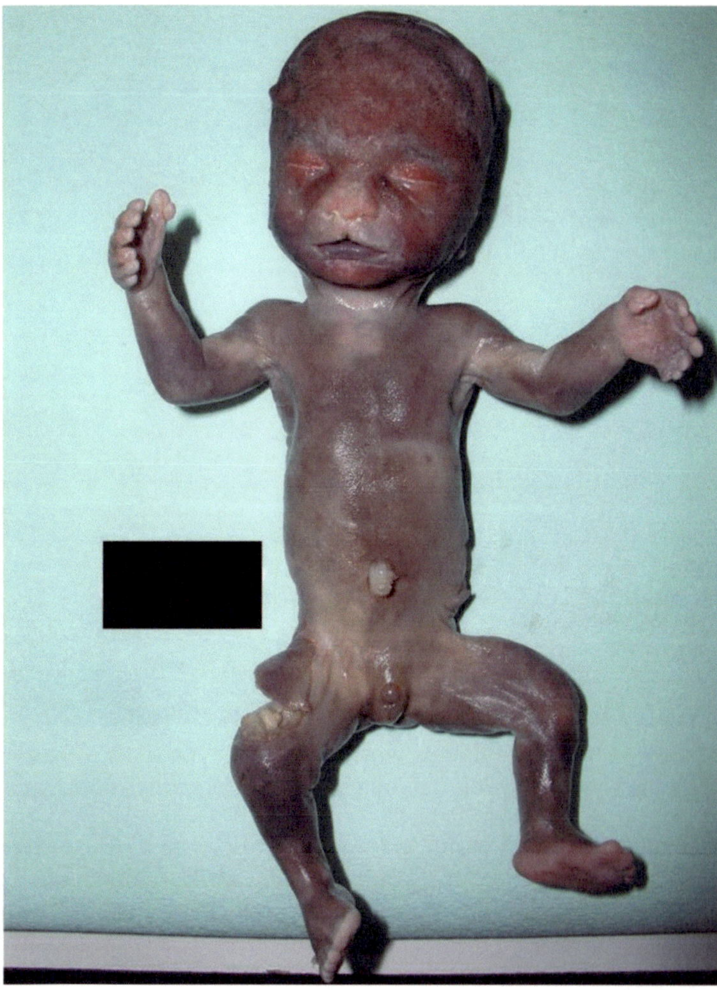

Fig. 10. Short-Rib-Polydactyly type II (Majewski) at 22 weeks. There is a median cleft lip, the chest is very narrow and the limbs are short. Micropenis and combined preaxial and postaxial polysyndactyly of hands and feet are also seen.

Radiographic features (Fig. 11): There is mild platyspondyly in types I/III, the ribs are very short and horizontal, and the long bones are short. Metaphyseal spurs are present in types I and III (Fig. 11 right), while in types II and IV the metaphyses are smooth. In our index case of type II (Majewski) the tibia is the shortest of all long bones (Fig. 11, left). Polydactyly is postaxial (in types I, II, III), preaxial (type II) or combined preaxial and postaxial (type II) and is common in all types, except type IV. Fusion of metacarpals is seen in type II-Majewski (Fig. 11 left), (as in chondroectodermal dysplasia Ellis-van Creveld).

Jeune syndrome and Ellis-van Creveld syndrome are also classified under the group of Short-Rib (with or without Polydactyly) dysplasias. These may be indistinguishable in the fetus.

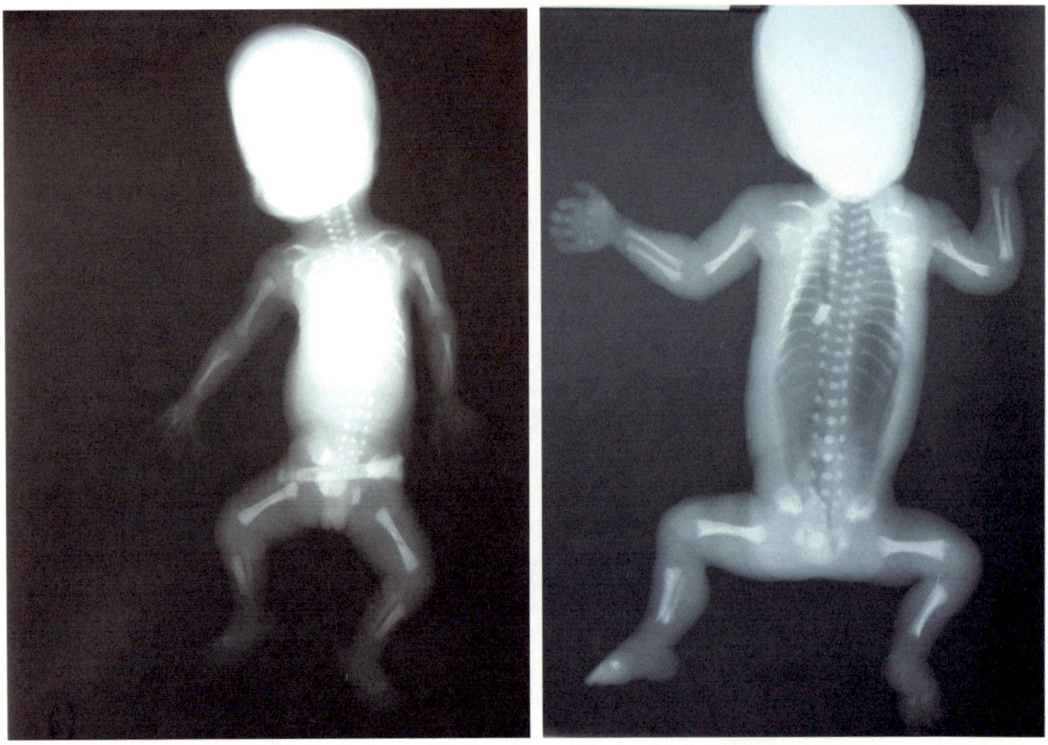

Fig. 11. Short-Rib-Polydactyly type II at 22 weeks (left) and type III at 23 weeks (right). The ribs are short. The tibia is the shorter long bone in type II. Metaphyses are spiked in type III.

Extraskeletal abnormalities noted in our index case of SRP type II (Majewski) consisted in a median cleft lip, micropenis and a Dandy-Walker malformation of the cerebellum. Microscopically, the kidneys showed renal tubular and glomerular cysts and in the liver persisting ductal plate was noted.

In our index case of SRP type III (Verma-Naumoff) there was mild hydrops, moderately hypoplastic lungs, a complex cardiovascular defect with atrioventricular canal defect type I and interruption of the aortic arch, intestinal malrotation, small kidneys with tubular cysts and portal fibrosis with persisting ductal plate of the liver, and there was no polydactyly.

6.4.2 Chondroectodermal dysplasia (Ellis-van Creveld)

Two fetuses in our series were diagnosed with Ellis-van Creveld (EvC) syndrome at post-mortem examination, both at 23 weeks of gestation (Fig. 12).

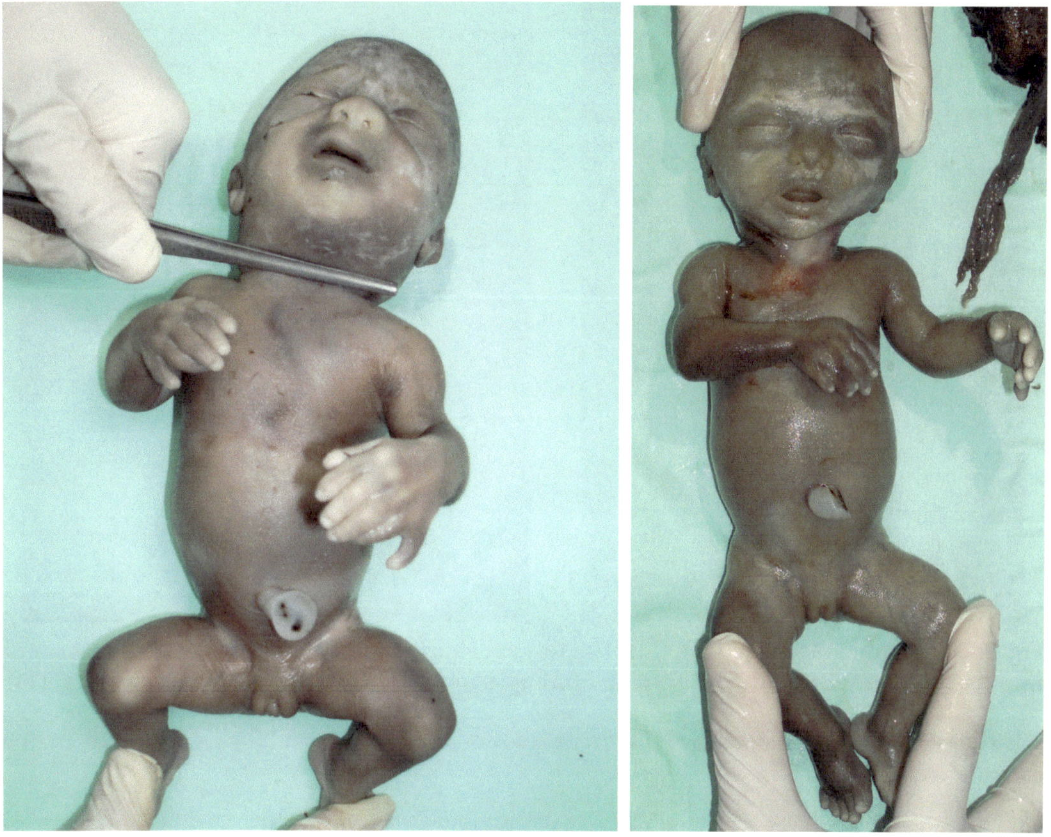

Fig. 12. Ellis-van Creveld syndrome (chondroectodermal dysplasia) at 23 weeks. There is postaxial polydactyly of both hands (left) and postaxial polysyndactyly (right). The chest is narrow and the limbs are moderately short.

At autopsy, organ dissection of the two female fetuses showed pulmonary hypoplasia, renal tubular cysts and persisting ductal plate in the liver. One fetus had postaxial hexadactyly and the other postaxial polysyndactyly of both hands (Fig. 12).

Molecular genetic analysis was not performed in either case. The presence of postaxial polydactyly favored the diagnosis of EvC versus Jeune Asphyxiating Thoracic Dysplasia (ATD), which in the fetus may be indistinguishable from EvC or SRP type II. In childhood, the typical disorders of ectodermal dysplasia, i.e. hypoplastic nails, thin hair and abnormal teeth combined with postaxial polydactyly would suggest the diagnosis of EvC versus Jeune ATD. Ellis-van Creveld and Jeune ATD are compatible with life; SRP type II is invariably lethal in the perinatal period.

Radiographic findings (Fig. 13) included short ribs, short long bones with rounded metaphyses, fibular hypoplasia in one case, vertically shortened ilia with notches and a V-shaped 3rd metacarpal in one case.

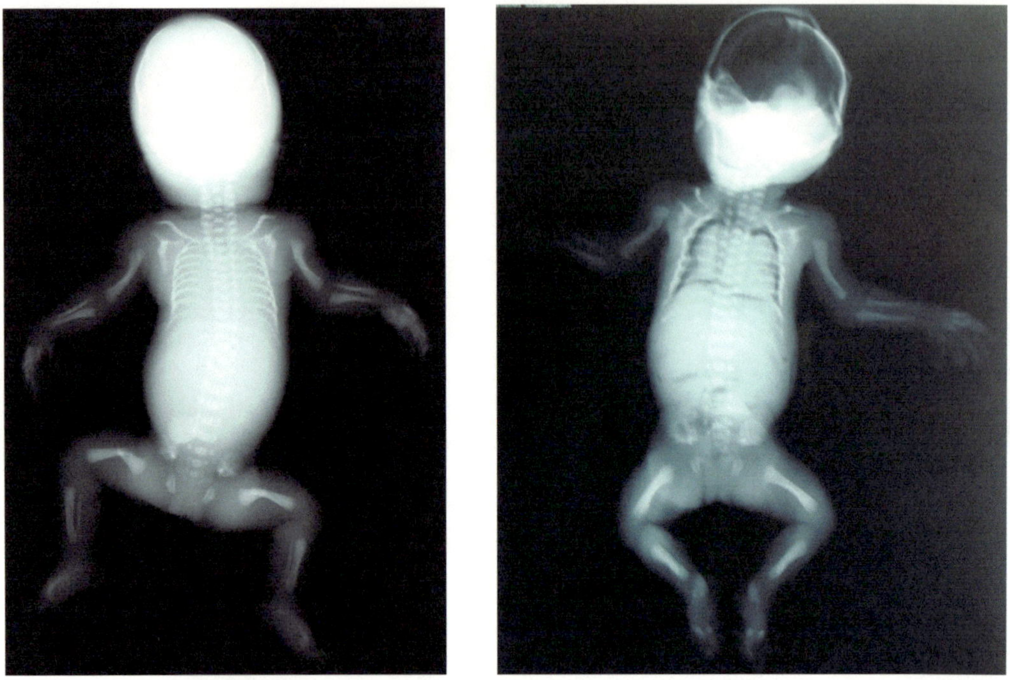

Fig. 13. EvC (same cases as in Fig. 12): The ribs are short. The long bones are short with rounded metaphyses. The radiographic findings may be indistinguishable from Jeune ATD.

Histology of the epiphyseal growth plate shows retardation and disorganization in the formation of columns (Fig. 14).

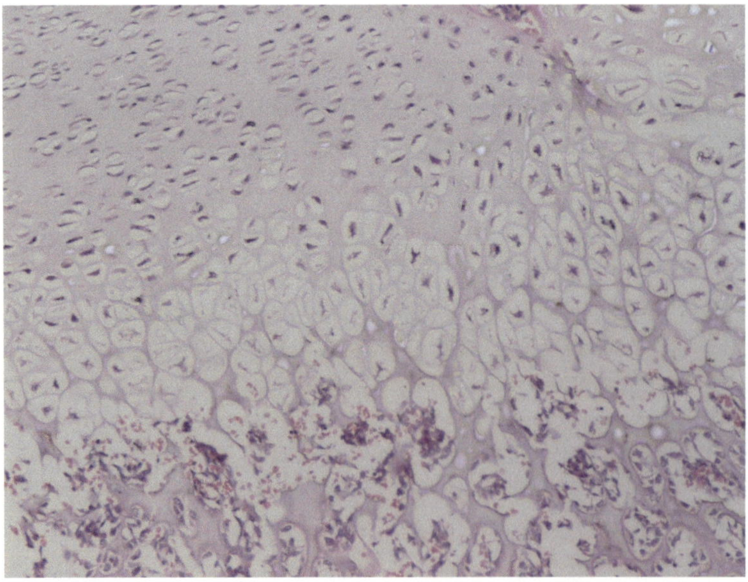

Fig. 14. Retardation and focal disorganization of the femoral epiphyseal growth plate in Ellis-van Creveld syndrome at 23 weeks.

6.5 Group 35: Dysostoses with predominant vertebral involvement with and without costal involvement

Index case: **Spondylocostal / Spondylothoracic dysostosis**

6.5.1 Spondylocostal / Spondylothoracic dysostosis

Various genetically distinct axial dysostoses with predominant vertebral and costal involvement were previously named as *Jarcho-Levin syndrome*, a label that has been eliminated by the 2010 revision of the Nosology. This heterogeneous group of disorders characterized by multiple spinal malsegmentation may be autosomal recessive, autosomal dominant or sporadic. It has been suggested that thoracic asymmetry characterizes Spondylothoracic dysostosis, whereas a short but overall symmetric thorax is a feature of Spondylocostal dysostosis (Solomon, 1978; O' Neill, 2011a).

There were 5 cases of spondylocostal /spondylothoracic dysostosis in our series (10%). Fetal age ranged from 13 to 37 weeks of gestation. One case referred to a liveborn neonate born to a mother who had not received prenatal sonographic control.

In all cases there were characteristic external, radiographic and pathological findings. The fetus with spondylocostal/spondylothoracic dysostosis has a short neck with low frontal and occipital hairline, short trunk in contrast to extremities of normal length, and scoliosis (Fig. 15).

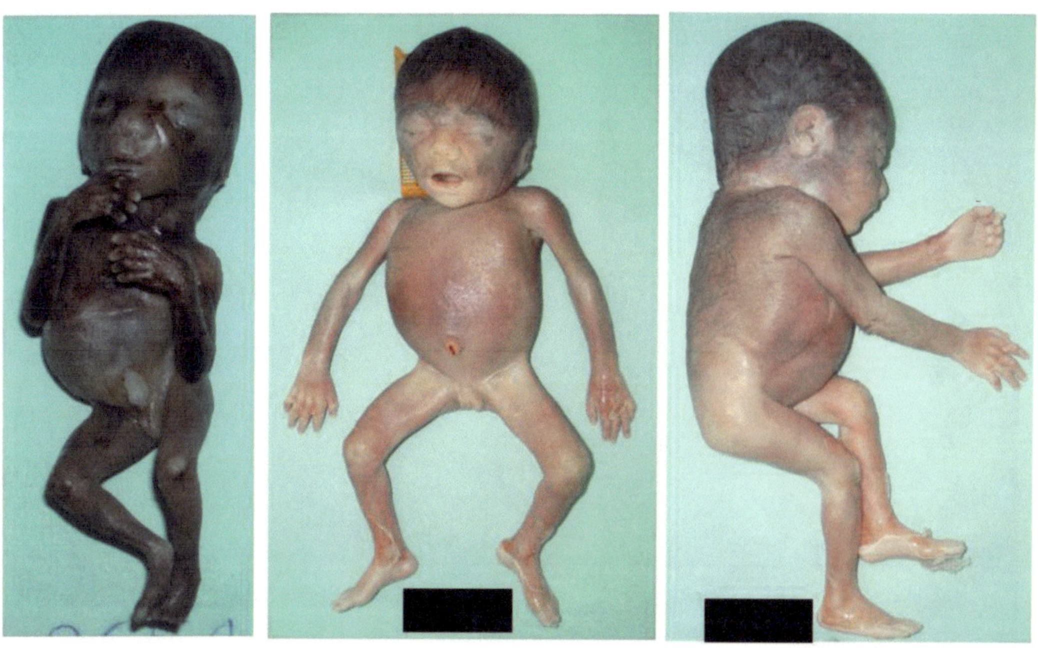

Fig. 15. Spondylothoracic / Spondylocostal dysostosis in two fetuses of 16.5 weeks (left - formalin-fixed) and 23.5 weeks (middle and right). Scoliosis, short neck, short deformed thorax and hirsutism in the older fetus are obvious.

Extraskeletal findings consisting in neural tube defects, hindbrain malformations, cardiovascular and genitourinary anomalies have been described in the former heterogeneous *Jarcho-Levin syndrome.* It is suggested that associated visceral anomalies are more common in sporadic cases of spinal malsegmentation than in the familial types of spondylocostal / spondylothoracic dysostosis (O' Neill, 2011a).

Our first index familial case is represented by a male fetus of 16.5 w, who was the second affected offspring of the family with features of spondylothoracic dysostosis (Fig. 15, left). At autopsy, we noted a Dandy-Walker variant of the cerebellum, asymmetry of thoracic and abdominal organs, hypospadias, and renal tubular microcysts.

The second index case, a female fetus of 23.5 w, offspring to consanguineous parents, had an atrial septal defect, a retroesophageal right subclavian artery and ectopic pancreatic tissue in the spleen.

Radiography shows the characteristic vertebral anomalies including vertebral segmentation with hemivertebrae and block vertebrae accompanied by deformity of the ribs. Fused ribs result in a typical 'crab-like' radiologic appearance of the thoracic skeleton (Fig. 16). The skeleton is otherwise normal.

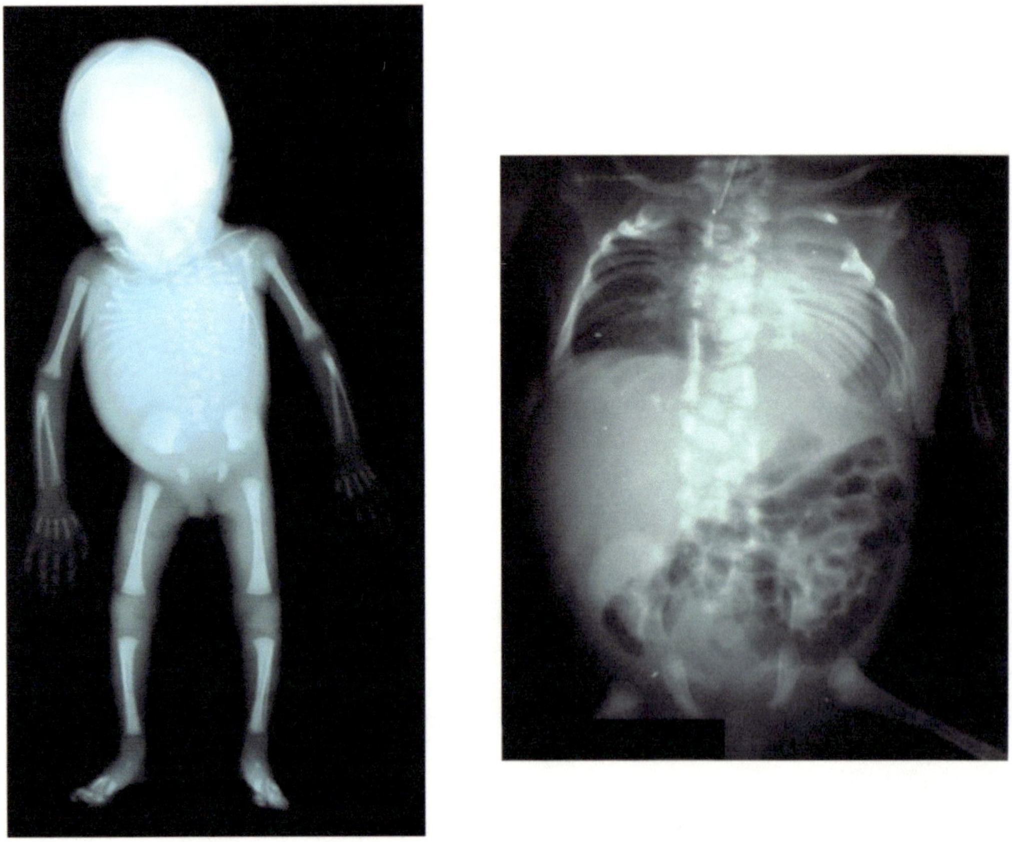

Fig. 16. Vertebral segmentation and deformity of the ribs with thoracic asymmetry in spondylothoracic dysostosis. Left: 23.5 w - Right: At term, crab-like appearance of the ribs

In the early lethal form of spondylocostal/spondylothoracic dysostosis patients die perinatally with respiratory complications; other forms of the syndrome allow survival to a later age.

6.6 Group 38: Limb hypoplasia-reduction defects group

Index cases: **Roberts syndrome, Split Hand-Foot malformation with tibial hypoplasia**

6.6.1 Roberts syndrome

Roberts syndrome is a rare autosomal recessive condition caused by mutation in the *ESCO2* gene, the protein product of which is required for the establishment of sister chromatid cohesion during S phase. In the fetus it is manifest with facial clefting and symmetrical limb defects, resulting in tetraphocomelia in most cases (Kniffin, 2010). Alternatively the syndrome is called "Long bone deficiencies associated with cleft lip-palate". Hypertelorism, facial hemangioma and clitoral or penile enlargement are also features of the syndrome. Another name of this condition often found in literature is "Roberts phocomelia" or "the (SC) pseudothalidomide syndrome", because of the resemblance to malformations seen in the thalidomide embryopathy. "Phocomelia" is an old term for nearly total deficiency of the long bones of a limb, (Greek *phoka* = seal, *melos* = limb; *phocomelia* = seal limb).

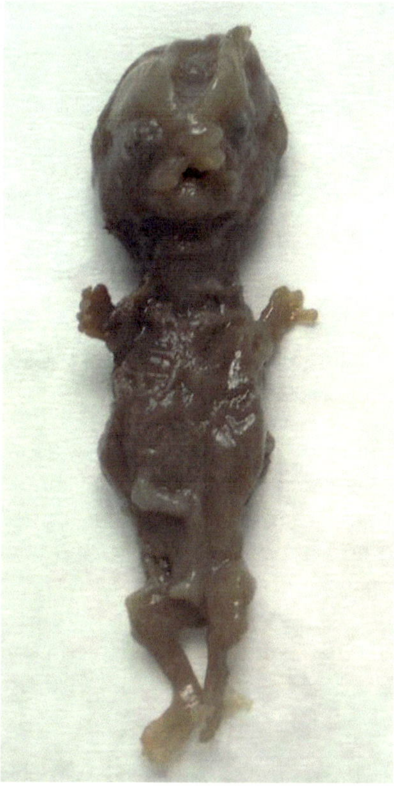

Fig. 17. Median cleft lip and palate, micrognathia, hypertelorism, upper limb phocomelia, ectrodactyly and syndactyly, hypoplastic femora, and penile enlargement in a 12.5-week male fetus with Roberts syndrome.

Karyotypic analysis shows in 50% of cases a characteristic centromeric abnormality of the chromosomes, namely, puffing and splitting of sister chromatides. The finding was present in one 25-week male fetus of our series, confirming the diagnosis of Roberts' syndrome (Pavlopoulos et al., 1998), and was absent from a second male fetus of 12.5 weeks (Fig. 17).

6.6.2 Split Hand-Foot malformation with tibial aplasia

The Split Hand-Foot malformations are a group of genetically heterogeneous disorders, presenting as isolated forms (five genetically different forms) or in combination with tibial hypoplasia or aplasia. The latter condition [OMIM #119100] is autosomal dominant, with a recently determined molecular defect mapping on chromosome 1q42.2-q43 (O' Neill, 2009b).

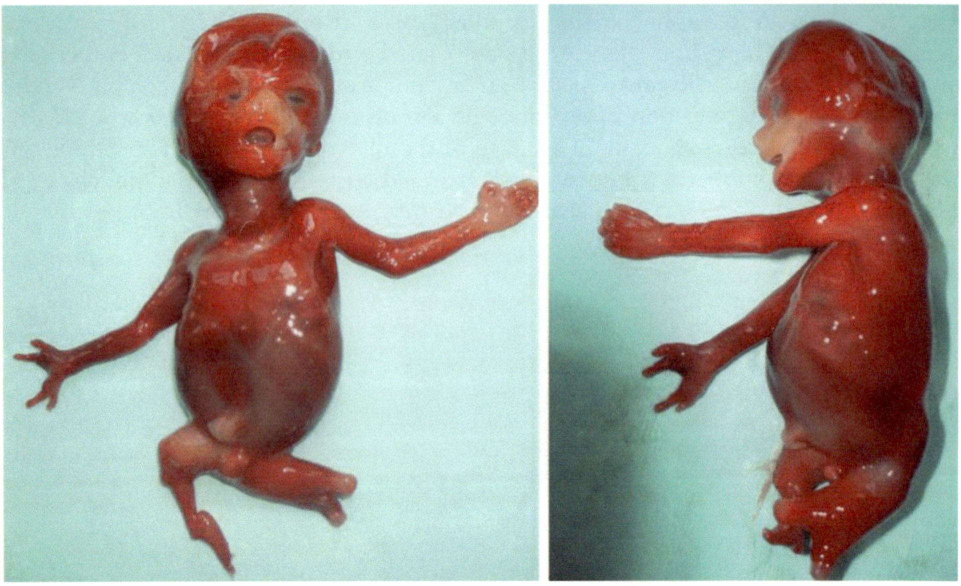

Fig. 18. Cleft hand, tibial aplasia, and bifid femur in a 16.5-week male fetus

Our index case refers to a male fetus of 16.5 weeks sent for autopsy after termination of pregnancy because of sonographically diagnosed limb reduction defects (Fig. 18). A possible secondary aetiology should be ruled out, given that limb defects are often sporadic, attributed to vascular disruptions or amniotic band syndrome. At autopsy, we noted a cleft hand, absent tibia, bifid femur and hypoplasia of other long bones. This led to the diagnosis of the genetic disorder *Split hand/foot malformation with tibial aplasia,* alternatively named *Split-hand/foot malformation with long bone deficiency* [OMIM #119100]. The postmortem diagnosis conducted the genetic investigation and enabled genetic counseling of the family.

7. Conclusion

The pathologist will perform the post-mortem examination of a fetus or infant affected by a genetic skeletal disorder in cases of intrauterine death caused by lethal skeletal dysplasias, or, more often nowadays, when the detection of skeletal abnormalities on prenatal ultrasound leads to the termination of pregnancy. The presence of skeletal abnormalities mandates an extended study of the fetus. Pediatric radiologists who have experience in radiologic assessment of skeletal disorders of infants and children can provide expertise in this area. However, in many institutions it is the task of the pathologist to deal with the skeletal disorders at autopsy. It is important that pathologists carrying out fetal and perinatal autopsies should be familiar with the phenotypic manifestations of the more common skeletal disorders, including the interpretation of radiologic findings. The association with extraskeletal abnormalities in particular settings also contributes to the diagnostic approach. The histology of the cartilage and bone and of the epiphyseal growth plate proves very useful in a restricted number of skeletal dysplasias. As specific diagnosis and classification of genetic skeletal disorders is difficult, a collaborative approach among pathological, radiological and genetic services is optimal to provide the parents with all available information regarding the diagnosis and prognosis of fetal and perinatal genetic skeletal disorders.

8. Acknowledgment

The study on fetal genetic skeletal disorders is financed by the *Kapodistrias* 70/4/6585 programme of the University of Athens and by "REA" Maternity Clinic, Athens, Greece, research programme 70/3/11191.

9. References

Badano, JL, Mitsuma, N, Beales, PL, & Katsanis, N. (2006). The ciliopathies: an emerging class of human genetic disorders. *Annual Review of Genomics & Human Genetics*, Vol. 7, pp. 125-148

Doray, B, Favre, R, Viville, B, Langer, B, Dreyfus, M, & Stoll, C. (2000). Prenatal sonographic diagnosis of skeletal dysplasias. A report of 47 cases. *Annals of Genetics,* Vol. 43, pp.163–169

Gilbert-Barness, E. (2007) Osteochondrodysplasias - constitutional diseases of bone. In: *Potter's Pathology of the fetus, Infant and Child*, second edition, Editor Gilbert-Barness, E, pp. 1836-1897, Mosby-Elsevier, 9780323034036, Philadelphia

Goncalves, L, Jeanty, P. (1994) Fetal biometry of skeletal dysplasias: a multicentric study. *Journal of Ultrasound Medicine,* Vol.13, pp. 767–775

Hall, CM. 2002. International nosology and classification of constitutional disorders of bone (2001). *American Journal of Medical Genetics,* Vol. 113, pp.65-77

van der Harten, HJ, Brons, JT, Schipper, NW, Dijkstra, PF, Meijer, CJ, & van Geijn, HP. (1990). The prenatal development of the human skeleton: a combined ultrasonographic and post-mortem radiographic study. *Pediatric Radiology,* Vol.21, pp. 52-56

Hatzaki, A, Sifakis, S, Apostolopoulou, D, Bouzarelou, D, Konstantinidou, A, Kappou, D, Sideris, A, Tzortzis, E, Athanassiadis, A, Florentin, L, Theodoropoulos, P, Makatsoris, C, Karadimas, C, & Velissariou, V. (2011). FGFR-3 related skeletal dysplasias diagnosed prenatally by ultrasonography and molecular analysis: Presentation of 17 Cases. *American Journal of Medical Genetics part A,* Sep 9. doi: 10.1002/ajmg.a.34189

Jeanty, P. (2003). Skeletal Dysplasias. In: *Diagnostic Imaging of Fetal Anomalies.* Editors Nyberg, DA, McGahan, J, Pretorius, D, Pilu G. Lippincott Williams & Wilkins, Philadelphia, p.661

INCO (1988). International nomenclature and classification of the osteochondrodysplasias (1977) *American Journal of Medical Genetics part A,* Vol. 79, pp. 376-382

Kniffin, C. (June 2010). #268300 Roberts Syndrome; RBS In: *Online Mendelian Inheritance in Man* [*OMIM*], 20.07.2011, Available from http://omim.org/entry/268300

Konstantinidou, AE, Agrogiannis, G, Sifakis, S, et al. (2009). Genetic skeletal disorders of the fetus and infant: Pathological and molecular findings in a series of 41 cases. *Birth Defects Research (Part A),* Vol. 85, pp. 811–821

Konstantinidou, AE, Fryssira, H, Sifakis, S, Karadimas, C, Kaminopetros, P, Agrogiannis, G, Velonis, S, Nikkels, PGH, & Patsouris, E. (2009). Cranioectodermal Dysplasia: a Probable Ciliopathy. *American Journal of Medical Genetics part A,* Vol. 149A, p.p. 2206-2211

Kornak, U, Mundlos, S. (2003). Genetic disorders of the skeleton: a developmental approach. *American Journal of Human Genetics,* Vol. 73, p.p. 447-474

Krakow, D, Alanay, Y, Rimoin, LP, Lin V, Wilcox, WR, Lachman, RS, & Rimoin, DL. (2008). Evaluation of Prenatal-Onset Osteochondrodysplasias by Ultrasonography: A Retrospective and Prospective Analysis. *American Journal of Medical Genetics part A,* Vol. 146A, p.p. 1917–1924

O' Neill, M. (January 2011). #277300 Spondylocostal Dysostosis 1, autosomal recessive SCDO1, In: *Online Mendelian Inheritance in Man [OMIM],* 23.07.2011, Available from http://omim.org/entry/277300#reference20

O' Neill, M. (November 2011). #119100 Split-hand/foot malformation with long bone deficiency 1; SHFLD1, In: *Online Mendelian Inheritance in Man [OMIM],* 23.07.2011, Available from http://omim.org/entry/119100

Nikkels, P.G.J. (2009). Diagnostic approach to congenital osteochondrodysplasias at autopsy. *Diagnostic Histopathology,* Vol.15, No.9 (September 2009), p.p. 413-424

Offiah, AC, Hall, CM. (2003). Radiological diagnosis of the constitutional disorders of bone. As easy as A, B, C? *Pediatric Radiology,* Vol. 33, p.p.153-161

Parilla, BV, Leeth, EA, Kambich, MP, Chilis, P, & MacGregor, SN. (2003). Antenatal detection of skeletal dysplasias. *Journal of Ultrasound Medicine,* Vol. 2, p.p. 255-258

Rasmussen, SA, Bieber, FR, Benacerraf, BR, Lachman, RS, Rimoin, DL, & Holmes, LB. (1996). Epidemiology of osteochondrodysplasias: changing trends due to advances in prenatal diagnosis. *American Journal of Medical Genetics,* Vol. 61, p.p. 49-58

Solomon, L., Jimenez, R. B., Reiner, L. (1978). Spondylothoracic dysostosis: report of 2 cases and review of the literature. *Archives of Pathology and Laboratory Medicine,* Vol.102, No.4, (April 1978), p.p. 201-205

Superti-Furga, A, Unger, S, and the Nosology Group of the International Skeletal Dysplasia Society. (2007). Nosology and Classification of Genetic Skeletal disorders: 2006 Revision. *American Journal of Medical Genetics part A,* Vol. 143A, p.p. 1–18

Pavlopoulos, PM, Konstantinidou, AE, Agapitos, E, & Davaris, P. (1998). Cell proliferation rate and nuclear morphology in Roberts syndrome. *Clinical Genetics,* Vol. 54, p.p. 512-516

Warman, ML, Cormier-Daire, V, Hall, C, Krakow, D, Lachman, R, LeMerrer, M, Mortier, G, Mundlos, S, Nishimura, G, Rimoin, DL, Robertson, S, Savarirayan, R, Sillence, D, Spranger, J, Unger, S, Zabel, B, & Superti-Furga, A. (2011). Nosology and classification of genetic skeletal disorders: 2010 revision. *American Journal of Medical Genetics part A,* Vol. 155A, p.p. 943–68

Witters, I, Moerman, P, Fryns, JP. (2008). Skeletal dysplasias: 38 prenatal cases. *Genetic Counseling,* Vol. 19, p.p. 267-275

4

Prenatal Sonographic Diagnosis and Evaluation of Isolated Macrodactyly

Hande Yağmur[1], Atıl Yüksel[2] and Hülya Kayserili[3]

[1]*Fulya Acıbadem Hastanesi, İstanbul*

[2]*İstanbul Faculty of Medicine, Department of Obstetrics and Gynecology, Division of Perinatology, İstanbul Üniversitesi*

[3]*İstanbul Faculty of Medicine, Department of Medical Genetics, İstanbul Üniversitesi*

Turkey

1. Introduction

Macrodactyly, defined as enlargement of one or several digits of the hands or feet, is a rare malformation. It may be due tumorous enlargement of a single tissue element, as in hemangioma, lymphangioma or enchondroma or it may be caused by overgrowth of all structures of the digit, including phalanges, subcutaneous tissue, nerves, vessels and skin as in 'true macrodactyly'(Barsky, 1967). Furthermore, it may either be isolated or associated with other anomalies such as hemihypertrophy, vascular malformations, lipomas, cutaneous lesions or visceral anomalies as a feature of a syndrome.

There is only one case report of prenatally diagnosed isolated macrodactyly till then by Yüksel et al. Macrodactyly of the second toe of the left foot was noted on a routine fetal anomaly scan at 24 weeks (Figure 1). The other toes were of normal size and there were no other associated anomalies on serial scans. The fetal karyotype was also normal. The baby was born at term and evaluations carried out at birth, 6 months and 2 years of age revealed no other additional abnormalities; neither hemihypertrophy, macrocephaly, lipomas nor vascular abnormalities were detected. Diagnosis of congenital isolated true macrodactyly was confirmed. Distal phalangectomy was performed at 6 months of age and due to progressive enlargement after the first operation, the digit had to be amputated at 9 months of age. Histopathological evaluation of the specimen was consistent with true macrodactyly, with enlargement of all mesenchymal tissues, mainly of fibroadipose tissue origin (Yüksel et al., 2009).

Macrodactyly is an isolated finding without evidence of other systemic involvement in the majority of cases. However, there is a well-established association of macrodactyly with overgrowth syndromes such as Proteus syndrome, Bannayan-Riley-Ruvalcaba syndrome, CLOVES (Congenital Lipomatous Overgrowth, Vascular malformations, Epidermal nevi, and Skeletal/Spinal abnormalities) syndrome, Maffucci syndrome, Ollier's disease, Klippel-Trenaunay-Weber syndrome, neurofibromatosis, tuberous sclerosis and Milroy disease (Alomari, 2009; Norman-Taylor & Mayou, 1994; Yüksel et al., 2009). Therefore, prenatal diagnosis of macrodactyly necessitates thorough evaluation of all systems to differentiate between isolated and syndromic macrodactyly, which have different prognostic implications.

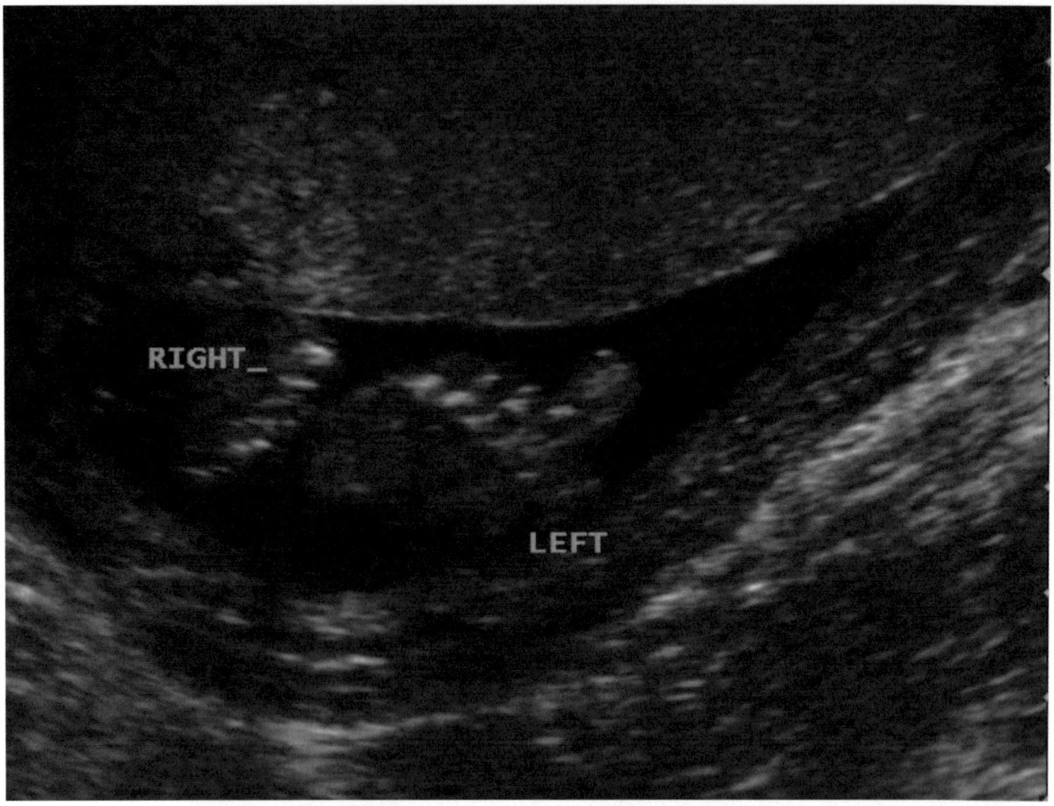

Fig. 1. Ultrasonographic scan of the fetus at 24 gestational weeks demonstrating the difference in size between two second toes. Macrodactyly of the left second toe is confirmed by comparable measurements. This is another image of the same case presented in 'Prenatal diagnosis of isolated macrodactyly' in Ultrasound in Obstetrics and Gynecology 2009; 33: 360-362.

2. Macrodactyly

2.1 True macrodactyly

Congenital true macrodactyly is a rare, nonhereditary malformation and appears to be more common in the hands than in the feet (Barsky, 1967). Overall, it constitutes around 1% of all congenital anomalies of the upper limb (Flatt, 1977, as cited in Kotwal & Farooque, 1998).

The disease is almost always unilateral and a single digit or several, usually adjacent digits may be involved (D'Costa et al., 1996, as cited in Singla et al., 2008; Syed et al., 2005). The second or third digit of the hand or foot are frequently involved in the majority of cases, corresponding to the median nerve and medial plantar nerve distribution (Krengel et al., 2000; Sone et al., 2000). The enlargement is most pronounced at the distal end of the digits on the volar side and therefore causes dorsal angulation (Singla et al., 2008). It may also be associated with syndactyly, polydactyly, or clinodactyly (Goldman & Kaye, 1977).

Two subtypes of true macrodactyly, namely, static and progressive types, have been described (Barsky, 1967). In the static type, the growth rate of the involved digit is the same as the normal digits whereas in the progressive type, growth is accelerated compared to the rest. The progressive type is less common and involvement of the metacarpal and metatarsal bones is more likely in the progressive type (Turkington & Grey, 2005). Abnormal accelerated growth usually ceases at puberty (Singla et al., 2008; Turkington & Grey, 2005).

Marked increase in adipose tissue within a mesh of fibrous tissue that involves the bone marrow, periosteum, muscles, nerve sheaths and subcutaneous tissues is the characteristic pathological finding in true macrodactyly (Kelikian, 1974 and Thorne et al., 1968 as cited in Goldman & Kaye, 1977). The most striking difference between macrodactyly of the hand and foot is neural involvement. Hypertrophy and tortuosity of the digital nerve is a notable finding in macrodactyly of the hand whereas it is rarely seen in the foot (Syed et al., 2005; Dennyson et al., 1977 as cited in Syed et al., 2005). The etiology is unclear and proposed mechanisms include lipomatous degeneration, neurofibromatosis, disturbed fetal circulation and local deficiency of growth inhibiting or overexpression of growth promoting factors (Syed et al., 2005; Gupta et al., 1992, as cited in Singla et al. 2008).

Macrodactyly causes cosmetic disfigurement and may also impair function due to secondary degenerative joint disease and nerve entrapment (Turkington & Grey, 2005). Treatment is usually not entirely satisfactory and may require several bulk reducing operations, carpal tunnel release, phalangectomy, and amputation (Kotwal & Farooque, 1998).

2.2 Macrodactyly due to tumorous enlargement

In contrast to true macrodactyly whereby all the structures of the digit are overgrown as a whole, there is tumourous enlargement of a single tissue element. Most of the tumors (95%) are benign and they may be classified according to the tissue of origin. Abnormal growth of vascular (hemangiomas, glomus tumors), osseous (enchondromas -multiple enchondromas as in Ollier disease-, osteoid osteomas, osteoblastomas, giant cell tumors, aneurysmal and unicameral bone cysts), neural (schwannomas, fibrolipomatous hamartomas, neurofibromas), cutaneous (mucous cysts, nodular fasciitis, pyogenic granulomas) and soft tissue (ganglions, lipomas, nodular tenosynovitis) elements cause localized masses of the hand and digits (Lin SJ et al., 2011).

Fibrolipomatous hamartoma is a rare, intraneural tumor characterized by fibrofatty infiltration around the nerve fascicles (Razzaghi & Anastakis, 2005). It is associated with macrodactyly due to overgrowth of bone and subcutaneous fat in more than one-third of the patients and it presents early in childhood with macrodactyly or later with a volar forearm mass and compressive neuropathy (Silverman & Enzinger, 1985, as cited in Razzaghi & Anastakis, 2005; Razzaghi & Anastakis, 2005).

Malignant tumors are rare. Primary malignant tumors may be of skin (most common site for malignant tumors), bone or soft tissue origin whereas metastatic tumors are mainly due to lung, kidney or head and neck cancers (Marrero IC et al., 2011).

3. Syndromes associated with macrodactyly

3.1 Proteus syndrome

Proteus syndrome (MIM 176920) is a sporadic disorder that may be caused by a somatic alteration in a gene, that probably controls local production or regulation of tissue growth factor receptors (Cohen MM Jr., 1993 and Samlaska et al., 1989, as cited in Jamis-Dow et al., 2004). The infants affected by the disorder usually appear normal or show only mildly asymmetric development at birth, but progressively develop the characteristic features of the syndrome during childhood. As the manifestations are highly variable, standard diagnostic criteria have been developed to minimise misdiagnosis (Biesecker et al., 1999, as cited in Jamis-Dow et al., 2004). Skeletal abnormalities such as macrodactyly, scoliosis, asymmetric overgrowth and limb length discrepancy, soft tissue abnormalities such as lipomas or regional absence of fat, asymmetric muscle development, connective tissue nevi and vascular malformations are common manifestations of the disease wheareas visceral anomalies such as splenomegaly, asymmetric megalencephaly, white matter abnormalities, nephromegaly, and masses other than fatty, muscular or vascular masses are uncommon (Jamis-Dow et al., 2004). Macrodactyly was encountered in 16 of 21 (76%) patients with Proteus syndrome in whom the diagnosis was based on standardized criteria (Jamis-Dow et al., 2004). Isolated macrodactyly has also been proposed as an extremely localized form of Proteus syndrome (van Bever & Hennekam, 1994).

Sigaudy et al. reported a prenatally diagnosed case of Proteus syndrome presenting with a large cystic mass on the right side of the abdomen and thorax and possible syndactyly of the fourth and fifth fingers at 26 weeks. The pregnancy was terminated at 28 weeks due to massive enlargement of the mass and autopsy revealed cystic lymphangioma on the right side, enlargement of the left arm, lateral deviation of the third to fifth fingers of the left hand with a large fixed gap between the second and the third finger, bilateral enlargement of the third toes, a small thymic cyst and left hemimegalencephaly confirming the diagnosis of Proteus syndrome (Sigaudy et al., 1998). Brasseur et al. reported a very similar case with antenatally diagnosed large, cervico-thoraco-brachial cystic lymphangioma at 22 weeks. After birth, macrodactyly of the first and second toes were noted and Proteus syndrome was diagnosed (Brasseur et al., 2009). Another prenatally diagnosed case with Proteus syndrome had a cystic enlargement of one limb and abnormal positioning of the toes (Richards et al., 1991, as cited in Sigaudy et al., 1998). These case reports show that severe cases of Proteus syndrome with early manifestations can be detected in utero. Most of the cases show at least one manifestation at birth and this finding can be either strongly suggestive of Proteus syndrome or more subtle (Sigaudy et al., 1998). Furthermore, as the phenotype develops over time, cases with apparently isolated findings such as macrodactyly may ultimately be diagnosed with Proteus syndrome (Lacombe & Battin, 1996, as cited in Sigaudy et al., 1998).

3.2 Bannayan-Riley-Ruvalcaba syndrome

Bannayan-Riley-Ruvalcaba (MIM 153480) syndrome is an autosomal dominant disorder, associated with mutations of the PTEN gene. Macrocephaly, lipomas, vascular malformations, intestinal polyps, and pigmented macules of the penis are the characteristic features of this syndrome. Macrodactyly of the right index finger along with a hamartoma of the small bowel mesentery with angiomatous, lipomatous and lymphangiomatous components has been reported by Zonana et al (Zonana et al., 1976).

There have been no reports regarding the prenatal diagnosis of Bannayan-Riley-Ruvalcaba syndrome; however, as it is characterized by hamartomatous changes leading to localized overgrowth, it may be included in the differential diagnosis of overgrowth syndromes like Proteus syndrome and macrodactyly (Jamis-Dow et al., 2004).

3.3 CLOVES syndrome

CLOVES syndrome (MIM 612918) is a disorder with complex truncal lipomatous mass, vascular malformations, epidermal nevi, acral deformities including large, wide feet and hands, macrodactyly and wide sandal gap and scoliosis and other musculoskeletal, neurologic, renal and cutaneous malformations (Alomari, 2009). Sapp et al. described 7 patients with progressive, primarily truncal vascular malformations, dysregulated adipose tissue, scoliosis and enlarged, but not severely distorted, bony structures without progressive overgrowth and designated the condition as a distinct entity, namely, CLOVE (Congenital Lipomatous Overgrowth, Vascular malformations, Epidermal nevi) syndrome (Sapp et al., 2007). They stated that bony distortion in these patients was limited to areas of the body that had undergone major surgery in contrast to patients with Proteus syndrome. Later in 2009, the acronym CLOVES syndrome was proposed to emphasize the association of Skeletal/Scoliosis and Spinal abnormalities with this syndrome (Alomari, 2009). Spinal-paraspinal fast-flow lesions within or adjacent to the truncal overgrowth or a cutaneous birthmark in 6 patients with CLOVES syndrome were also reported (Alomari et al., 2011).

There is one case report regarding antenatal findings of a multicystic abdominal wall mass, asymmetry of the cerebral hemispheres and face in a fetus, where postnatal clinical and imaging findings led to the diagnosis of CLOVES syndrome (Fernandez-Pineda et al., 2010).

3.4 Klippel-Trenaunay-Weber syndrome

Klippel-Trenaunay-Weber (KTW) (MIM 149000) syndrome is a rare disorder associated with large cutaneous capillary and venous malformations with hypertrophy of the related bones and soft tissues. The cutaneous lesions include one or several port-wine stains over the affected limb and large venous ectatic vessels and vesicular lymphatic lesions. The lower extremity is more commonly involved. The enlargement of the limb is due to muscle hypertrophy, thickened skin, excessive subcutaneous fat, abnormal vascular tissue and occasionally lymphedema (Requena & Sangueza, 1997, as cited in Gonçalves et al., 2000). Hypoplasia or aplasia of the venous system is also a feature of the syndrome although it is less commonly encountered (Jacob et al., 1998, as cited in Coombs at al., 2009).

The mosaic pattern and occasional familial cases of KTW syndrome have been explained by paradominant inheritance, whereby heterozygous individuals for the single gene defect are phenotypically normal and the trait is expressed when a somatic mutation occurs in the normal allele at an early stage of embryogenesis (Happle, 1993, as cited in Gonçalves et al., 2000).

Peng et al. have reviewed the prenatal findings of 21 cases with Klippel-Trenaunay-Weber syndrome involving the thigh until 2006. Asymmetric limb hypertrophy was the prominent prenatal finding and extensive involvement of other parts of the body such as the pelvis, abdomen, retroperitoneum or thorax was noted in around 70% of cases (Peng et al., 2006). Signs of high cardiac output probably due to the rapid development of numerous arteriovenous fistulas, such as cardiomegaly, polyhydramnios, non-immune hydrops fetalis and thick placenta have also been reported (Paladini et al., 1998; Peng et al., 2006).

There are two case reports demonstrating the association of Klippel-Trenaunay syndrome with macrodactyly. The first one presented antenatally with multiple distorted cystic areas involving the right leg and abdomen and cardiomegaly with early fetal heart failure who was found to have bilateral macrodactyly of the second toe as well after birth (Zoppi et al., 2001). The second one is a fetus with marked lower limb edema, cystic areas in the abdomen/pelvis/lower limbs and abnormal development of the feet demonstrating bilateral hypoplasia of the femoral and popliteal veins in whom postnatal clinical evaluation also revealed right foot hemihypertrophy/syndactyly and left hallux hypertrophy (Coombs at al., 2009).

3.5 Neurofibromatosis type 1

Neurofibromatosis type 1 (NF1) (MIM 162200) is a relatively common, autosomal dominant multisystem disorder that affects around one in 3500 individuals. Nearly half of the cases occur as a result of a new mutation (Freidman, 1998, as cited in McEwing et al., 2006) and expressivity is highly variable even among family members who carry the same mutation (Korf & Rubenstein, 2005, and Riccardi & Lewis, 1998, as cited in Boyd et al., 2009). It is characterized by cafe-au-lait macules, neurofibromas (plexiform neurofibroma being pathognomonic), axillary or inguinal freckling, optic glioma, iris hamartomas (Lisch nodules), and osseus lesions such as sphenoid dysplasia or thinning of long bone cortex. Macrodactyly in patients with neurofibromatosis is due to plexiform neurofibroma; it may be bilateral and involvement of the distal phalanx may not be as prominent as in true macrodactyly (Goldman & Kaye, 1977).

The prenatal diagnosis is very unlikely as the neonatal clinical features are usually solitary and cutaneous such as cafe-au-lait macules (McEwing et al., 2006) and spesific clinical findings increase in frequency with age (Freidman, 1998, as cited in McEwing et al., 2006). Nevertheless, there are a few cases with early and severe prenatal manifestations proven to be associated with neurofibromatosis postnatally. McEwing et al. reported a case presenting with a large oropharyngeal tumor, macrocephaly, ventriculomegaly, cardiomegaly, pleural and pericardial effusion, ascites and polyhydramnios. There was a positive paternal history of NF1 and after termination of pregnancy at 32 weeks, postmortem histologic evaluation was consistent with plexiform neurofibroma, confirming the diagnosis (McEwing et al., 2006). Another similar fetus with an oral tumor was also found to have NF1 postnatally (Hoyme et al., 1987, as cited in McEwing et al., 2006). Lastly, Drouin et al. reported a fetus with ambiguous genitalia, macrocephaly, shortened long bones and polyhydramnios in whom postnatal evaluation demonstrated a large abdominopelvic tumor and skeletal abnormalities consistent with NF1 (Drouin et al, 1997, as cited in McEwing et al., 2006).

3.6 Tuberous sclerosis

Tuberous sclerosis (MIM 191100/191092) is an autosomal dominant, hamartomatous disorder with variable expressivity. It affects about 1/6000 to 1/10000 live births and two thirds of the cases are considered to result from *de novo* mutations. It is associated with skin abnormalities such as hypomelanotic macules, facial angiofibromas, shagreen patches, fibrous facial plaques, and ungual fibromas, brain abnormalities like cortical tubers, subependymal nodules, astrocytomas causing seizures, intellectual disability, and mental retardation, renal anomalies such as angiomyolipomas and cysts, and cardiac rhabdomyomas (Northrup & Au, 1999). Bone changes also occur and macrodactyly has been reported in 11 patients with tuberous sclerosis complex (Aldrich et al., 2010; Ghalli, 2001; Norman-Taylor & Mayou, 1994; Sahoo et al., 2000; Sharma et al., 2011; Shin & Garay,1997; Tung & Shih, 2009; Kousseff, 1989, and Ortonne et al., 1982 and Wallis & Beighton, 1989, and Zaremba, 1968, as cited in Norman-Taylor & Mayou, 1994). Mesodermal dysplasia as a component of tuberous sclerosis complex is postulated to be responsible for the macrodactyly (Sahoo et al., 2000) and overgrowth of the tissues and bones of the forearm and wrist has also been reported (Webb et al., 1996, as cited in Sahoo et al., 2000).

The cases of tuberous sclerosis complex with macrodactyly were mainly in the infancy and childhood age group and in most of them the diagnosis of tuberous sclerosis was clinically obvious (Norman-Taylor & Mayou, 1994). The case reported by Sharma et al. developed macrodactyly of the index and middle finger of the right hand at 9 nine months of age along with a fibrous hamartoma at his right wrist whereas in Ghalli's case macrodactyly of the second left toe was present at birth.

Cardiac rhabdomyomas, arrhythmias, cerebral lesions such as cortical tubers and subependymal nodules, hydrops, and stillbirth are the most prevalent findings in the fetus (Isaacs, 2009). Although there are no reports of prenatal diagnosis of macrodactyly associated with tuberous sclerosis, regarding the highly variable phenotypic expression of the disease, it may be considered in the differential diagnosis.

3.7 Ollier disease and Maffucci syndrome

Ollier disease and Maffucci syndrome (MIM 166000) are rare, sporadic disorders characterized by multiple enchondromas of primarily small bones of the hands and feet, the long tubular bones, and also the flat bones like the pelvis. Maffucci syndrome is also associated with hemangiomas of the skin, mucosa and internal organs (Casal et al., 2010).

These two entities usually become manifest during childhood and adolescence and prenatal diagnosis has not been reported.

3.8 Milroy disease

Milroy disease (MIM 153100) is a rare, autosomal dominant disorder characterized by lymphedema of the lower extremities, either of the whole leg or limited to the feet or toes (Lev-Sagie et al., 2003). Although the associated localized overgrowth may mimic the clinical picture of macrodactyly, it is differentiated easily from true macrodactyly since the bony structures are of normal size in Milroy disease .

Prenatal diagnosis of Milroy disease has previously been reported; with edema of the dorsum of both feet in two cases, bilateral leg edema and hydrothorax in one case and bilateral edema of the lower extremities most marked in the calves and feet in another case (Lev-Sagie et al., 2003; Makhoul et al., 2002; Franceschini et al., 2001). Lymphedema has been

Syndrome	Mode of Inheritance	Common manifestations
Proteus syndrome	Sporadic	Macrodactyly, asymmetric overgrowth and limb length discrepancy, vertebral abnormalities, soft tissue abnormalities, connective tissue nevi, vascular malformations, visceral anomalies such as splenomegaly, asymmetric megalencephaly, white matter abnormalities and nephromegaly
Bannayan-Riley-Ruvalcaba syndrome	Autosomal dominant/*de novo* mutation	Macrocephaly, lipomas, vascular malformations, intestinal polyps, pigmented macules of the penis
CLOVES syndrome	Sporadic	Complex truncal lipomatous mass, vascular malformations, epidermal nevi, acral deformities including large, wide feet and hands, macrodactyly, and wide sandal gap, scoliosis and other musculoskeletal, neurologic, renal and cutaneous malformations
Klippel-Trenaunay-Weber syndrome	Paradominant inheritance	Cutaneous capillary and venous malformations with hypertrophy of the related bones and soft tissues, hypoplasia or aplasia of the venous system
Neurofibromatosis type 1	Autosomal dominant/*de novo* mutation	Cafe-au-lait macules, neurofibromas, axillary or inguinal freckling, optic glioma, iris hamartomas (Lisch nodules), osseus lesions such as sphenoid dysplasia or thinning of long bone cortex
Tuberous sclerosis	Autosomal dominant/*de novo* mutation	Hypomelanotic macules, facial angiofibromas, shagreen patches, fibrous facial plaques, ungual fibromas, brain abnormalities like cortical tubers, subependymal nodules, and astrocytomas, renal anomalies such as angiomyolipomas and cysts, cardiac rhabdomyomas
Ollier disease	Sporadic	Enchondromas, cerebral tumors
Maffucci syndrome	Sporadic	Enchondromas, vascular malformations
Milroy disease	Autosomal dominant/*de novo* mutation	Lymphedema of the lower extremities

Table 1. Characteristics of syndromes associated with macrodactyly.

associated with several other syndromes in early childhood such as lymphedema-distichiasis, Cholestasis-Lymphedema Syndrome (Aagenaes Syndromes) and Hennekam syndrome.

The main features of above named syndromes associated with macrodactyly are summarized in Table 1.

In addition to these syndromes which are well-known and more frequent, macrodactyly as a feature of several other rare conditions has also been observed. In this context, macrodactyly has been reported in association with minor tibial duplication (Adamsbaum et al., 1991), benign lipoblastomatosis with the relationship of this condition to Proteus syndrome being unclear (Colot et al., 1984), terminal osseous dysplasia with pigmentary defects (Brunetti-Pieri et al., 2010), macrocephaly-capillary malformation syndrome (reported as enlarged hands in one case) (Barnicoat et al., 1996), segmentary fibrous dysplasia (Keymolen et al., 1999) and a lethal skeletal dysplasia associated with ectopic digits (Morton et al., 1998). These conditions have overlapping features such as overgrowth and vascular malformations with well defined syndromes like Proteus syndrome and therefore, they should be kept in mind for the differential diagnosis of syndromic macrodactyly.

4. Conclusion

Although the majority of cases with macrodactyly are isolated, prenatal recognition of an enlarged digit mandates thorough evaluation of all systems in search for associated anomalies which may indicate syndromic involvement. Moreover, serial scans are recommended as some of the features such as hemihypertrophy may develop over time and indirect signs such as cardiac overload or hydrops fetalis may lead to recognition of an additional finding. In addition, fetal magnetic resonance imaging may be considered in cases with associated anomalies, although its contribution is controversial. As macrodactyly can be a clinical finding in several autosomal dominantly inherited disorders such as neurofibromatosis, tuberous sclerosis, Bannayan-Riley-Ruvalcaba syndrome and Milroy disease, family history and examination of further family members, prospect mother and father being the first ones to be evaluated, are mandatory to reveal the familial occurrence of a further case (Yüksel et al., 2009). Amniotic band syndrome, which causes swelling and edema distal to the point of constriction, should also be included in the differential diagnosis of prenatally diagnosed macrodactyly (Yüksel et al., 2009).

A practical algorythym for the prenatal evaluation of macrodactyly is depicted in Fig. 2. Further case reports/series and information on the outcome of isolated and syndromic macrodactyly cases will help to improve the evaluation and management of this entity.

It could be speculated that the most critical aspect in the management of isolated macrodactyly is its possible association with a syndrome which could become evident later in childhood, and emphasizing this possibility is mandatory when counselling the parents. Knowing that there is a significant clinical overlap between the overgrowth syndromes and that the phenotype may well develop in time, postnatal follow-up of the newborn during the first decade on a yearly basis by a multidisciplinary team consisting of a geneticist, dermatologist and orthopedic surgeon should be considered and the parents should be counselled accordingly.

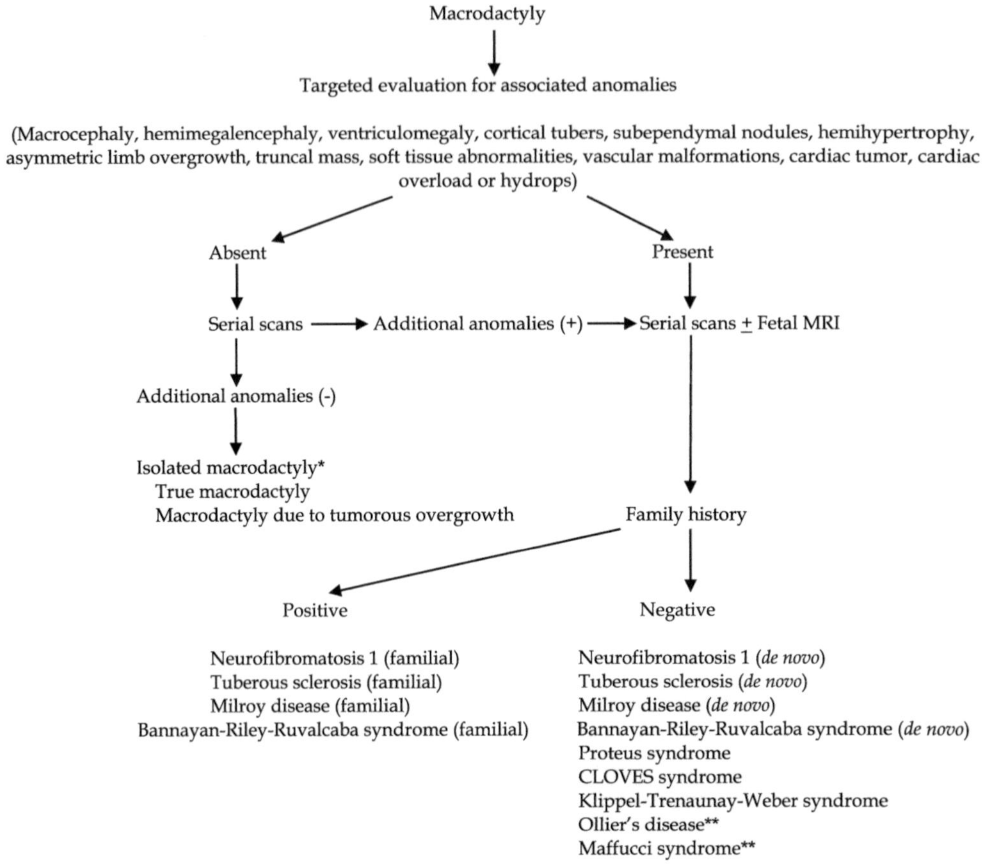

* Associated anomalies may become overt postnatally and may ultimately lead to the diagnosis of a specific syndrome associated with macrodactyly
** Prenatal diagnosis has not been reported previously.

Fig. 2. Algorythym for the management and work-up for differential diagnosis of prenatal finding of macrodactyly.

5. References

Adamsbaum C, Kalifa G, Seringe R & Bonnet JC. Minor tibial duplication: a new cause of congenital bowing of the tibia. *Pediatr Radiol.* 1991;21(3):185-8.

Aldrich CS, Hong CH, Groves L, Olsen C, Moss J & Darling TN. Acral lesions in tuberous sclerosis complex: insights into pathogenesis. *J Am Acad Dermatol.* 2010 Aug;63(2):244-51.

Alomari AI. Characterization of a distinct syndrome that associates complex truncal overgrowth, vascular, and acral anomalies: a descriptive study of 18 cases of CLOVES syndrome. *Clin Dysmorphol.* 2009 Jan;18(1):1-7.

Alomari AI, Chaudry G, Rodesch G, Burrows PE, Mulliken JB, Smith ER, Fishman SJ & Orbach DB. Complex Spinal-Paraspinal Fast-Flow Lesions in CLOVES Syndrome: Analysis of Clinical and Imaging Findings in 6 Patients. *AJNR Am J Neuroradiol.* 2011 Feb 10.

Barnicoat A, Salman M, Chitty L &Baraitser M. A distinctive overgrowth syndrome with polysyndactyly. Clin Dysmorphol. 1996 Oct;5(4):339-46.

Barsky AJ. Macrodactyly. *J Bone Joint Surg Am.* 1967 Oct;49(7):1255-66.
Boyd KP, Korf BR & Theos A. Neurofibromatosis type 1. *J Am Acad Dermatol.* 2009 Jul;61(1):1-14.
Brasseur A, Seryer D, Plancq MC, Krim G, Lanta S & Le Blanche A. [Thoraco-brachial cystic lymphangioma and Proteus syndrome: prenatal diagnosis and MR follow-up]. *J Radiol.* 2009 May;90(5 Pt 1):608-11.
Brunetti-Pierri N, Lachman R, Lee K, Leal SM, Piccolo P, Van Den Veyver IB &Bacino CA. Terminal osseous dysplasia with pigmentary defects (TODPD): Follow-up of the first reported family, characterization of the radiological phenotype, and refinement of the linkage region. *Am J Med Genet A.* 2010 Jul;152A(7):1825-31.
Casal D, Mavioso C, Mendes MM & Mouzinho MM. Hand involvement in Ollier Disease and Maffucci Syndrome: a case series. *Acta Reumatol Port.* 2010 Jul-Sep;35(3):375-8.
Colot G, Castermans-Elias S &Philippet G. Macrodactyly associated with benign lipoblastomatosis. *Ann Chir Main.* 1984;3(3):262-5.
Coombs PR, James PA & Edwards AG. Sonographic identification of lower limb venous hypoplasia in the prenatal diagnosis of Klippel-Trénaunay syndrome. *Ultrasound Obstet Gynecol.* 2009 Dec;34(6):727-9.
Fernandez-Pineda I, Fajardo M, Chaudry G & Alomari AI. Perinatal clinical and imaging features of CLOVES syndrome. *Pediatr Radiol.* 2010 Aug;40(8):1436-9.
Franceschini P, Licata D, Rapello G, Guala A, Di Cara G & Franceschini D. Prenatal diagnosis of Nonne-Milroy lymphedema. *Ultrasound Obstet Gynecol.* 2001 Aug;18(2):182-3.
Ghalli FE. Macrodactyly in tuberous sclerosis. *Pediatr Dermatol.* 2001 Jul-Aug;18(4):364-5.
Goldman AB & Kaye JJ. Macrodystrophia lipomatosa: radiographic diagnosis. *AJR Am J Roentgenol.* 1977 Jan;128(1):101-5.
Gonçalves LF, Rojas MV, Vitorello D, Pereira ET, Pereima M & Saab Neto JA. Klippel-Trenaunay-Weber syndrome presenting as massive lymphangiohemangioma of the thigh: prenatal diagnosis. *Ultrasound Obstet Gynecol.* 2000 Jun;15(6):537-41. Review.
Isaacs H. Perinatal (fetal and neonatal) tuberous sclerosis: a review. *Am J Perinatol.* 2009 Nov;26(10):755-60.
Jamis-Dow CA, Turner J, Biesecker LG & Choyke PL. Radiologic manifestations of Proteus syndrome. *Radiographics.* 2004 Jul-Aug;24(4):1051-68. Review.
Keymolen K, De Smet L, Kenis H &Fryns JP. Segmentary fibrous dysplasia manifesting as macrodactyly. *Genet Couns.* 1999;10(4):373-6.
Kotwal PP & Farooque M. Macrodactyly. *J Bone Joint Surg Br.* 1998 Jul;80(4):651-3.
Krengel S, Fustes-Morales A, Carrasco D, Vázquez M, Durán-McKinster C & Ruiz-Maldonado R. Macrodactyly: report of eight cases and review of the literature. *Pediatr Dermatol.* 2000 Jul-Aug;17(4):270-6.
Lev-Sagie A, Hamani Y, Raas-Rothschild A, Yagel S & Anteby EY. Prenatal ultrasonographic diagnosis of atypical Nonne-Milroy lymphedema. *Ultrasound Obstet Gynecol.* 2003 Jan;21(1):72-4.
Lin SJ et al., (updated May 18, 2011). Benign Hand Tumors, In: *Medscape,* January 10, 2012,Available from: http://emedicine.medscape.com/article/1286448-overview
Makhoul IR, Sujov P, Ghanem N & Bronshtein M. Prenatal diagnosis of Milroy's primary congenital lymphedema. *Prenat Diagn.* 2002 Sep;22(9):823-6.
Marrero IC et al., (updated Nov 17, 2011). Malignant Hand Tumors, In: *Medscape,* January 10, 2012, Available from: http://emedicine.medscape.com/article/1286560-overview
McEwing RL, Joelle R, Mohlo M, Bernard JP, Hillion Y & Ville Y. Prenatal diagnosis of neurofibromatosis type 1: sonographic and MRI findings. *Prenat Diagn.* 2006 Dec;26(12):1110-4.

Morton JE, Kilby MD & Rushton I. A new lethal autosomal recessive skeletal dysplasia with associated dysmorphic features. *Clin Dysmorphol.* 1998Apr;7(2):109-14.

Norman-Taylor F & Mayou BJ. Macrodactyly in tuberous sclerosis. *J R Soc Med.* 1994 Jul;87(7):419-20.

Northrup H & Au KS. Tuberous Sclerosis Complex. 1999 Jul 13 [updated 2009 May 7]. In: Pagon RA, Bird TD, Dolan CR, Stephens K, editors. *GeneReviews* [Internet]. Seattle (WA): University of Washington, Seattle; 1993-.

Online Mendelian Inheritance in Man, Web-based databases, Available from: www.ncbi.nlm.nih.gov/omim

Paladini D, Lamberti A, Teodoro A, Liguori M, D'Armiento M, Capuano P & Martinelli P. Prenatal diagnosis and hemodynamic evaluation of Klippel-Trenaunay-Weber syndrome. *Ultrasound Obstet Gynecol.* 1998 Sep;12(3):215-7.

Peng HH, Wang TH, Chao AS, Chang YL, Shieh SC & Chang SD. Klippel-Trenaunay-Weber syndrome involving fetal thigh: prenatal presentations and outcomes. *Prenat Diagn.* 2006 Sep;26(9):825-30.

Razzaghi A & Anastakis DJ. Lipofibromatous hamartoma: review of early diagnosis and treatment. *Can J Surg.* 2005 Oct;48(5):394-9.

Sahoo B, Handa S & Kumar B. Tuberous sclerosis with macrodactyly. *Pediatr Dermatol.* 2000 Nov-Dec;17(6):463-5.

Sapp JC, Turner JT, van de Kamp JM, van Dijk FS, Lowry RB & Biesecker LG. Newly delineated syndrome of congenital lipomatous overgrowth, vascular malformations, and epidermal nevi (CLOVE syndrome) in seven patients. *Am J Med Genet A.* 2007 Dec 15;143A(24):2944-58.

Sharma S, Sankhyan N, Gulati S, Kumar A, Srinivas M, Shukla B & Mathur SR. Macrodactyly and fibrous hamartoma in a child with tuberous sclerosis complex. *J Child Neurol.* 2011 Jan;26(1):95-8.

Shin AY & Garay AA. Unilateral insensate macrodactyly secondary to tuberous sclerosis in a child. *Am J Orthop (Belle Mead NJ).* 1997 Jan;26(1):30-2.

Sigaudy S, Fredouille C, Gambarelli D, Potier A, Cassin D, Piquet C & Philip N. Prenatal ultrasonographic findings in Proteus syndrome. *Prenat Diagn.* 1998 Oct;18(10):1091-4.

Singla V, Virmani V, Tuli P, Singh P & Khandelwal N. Case Report: Macrodystrophia lipomatosa - Illustration of two cases. *Indian J Radiol Imaging.* 2008 Nov;18(4):298-301.

Sone M, Ehara S, Tamakawa Y, Nishida J & Honjoh S. Macrodystrophia lipomatosa: CT and MR findings. *Radiat Med.* 2000 Mar-Apr;18(2):129-32.

Syed A, Sherwani R, Azam Q, Haque F & Akhter K. Congenital macrodactyly: a clinical study. *Acta Orthop Belg.* 2005 Aug;71(4):399-404.

Tung HE & Shih SL. Tuberous sclerosis with rare presentation of macrodactyly. *Pediatr Radiol.* 2009 Aug;39(8):878.

Turkington JR & Grey AC. MR imaging of macrodystrophia lipomatosa. *Ulster Med J.* 2005 May;74(1):47-50.

van Bever Y & Hennekam RC. Isolated macrodactyly or extremely localized Proteus syndrome? *Clin Dysmorphol.* 1994 Oct;3(4):351-2.

Yüksel A, Yagmur H & Kural BS. Prenatal diagnosis of isolated macrodactyly.*Ultrasound Obstet Gynecol.* 2009 Mar;33(3):360-2.

Zonana, J., Rimoin, D. L. & Davis, D. C. Macrocephaly with multiple lipomas and hemangiomas. *J. Pediat.* 89: 600-603, 1976.

Zoppi MA, Ibba RM, Floris M, Putzolu M, Crisponi G & Monni G. Prenatal sonographic diagnosis of Klippel-Trénaunay-Weber syndrome with cardiac failure. *J Clin Ultrasound.* 2001 Sep;29(7):422-6.

5

Prenatal Evaluation of Fetuses Presenting with Short Femurs

Funda Gungor Ugurlucan[1], Hülya Kayserili[2] and Atil Yuksel[1]
[1]*Department of Obstetrics and Gynecology, Istanbul Medical Faculty Istanbul University*
[2]*Department of Medical Genetics, Istanbul Medical Faculty Istanbul University*
Turkey

1. Introduction

Femur length (FL) is the measurement between the distal and proximal ossification centers of the femoral diaphysis. FL is one of the fetal biometry measurements which is measured ordinarily during the routine second trimester scanning and onwards in determining the gestational age and growth between ultrasound examinations.

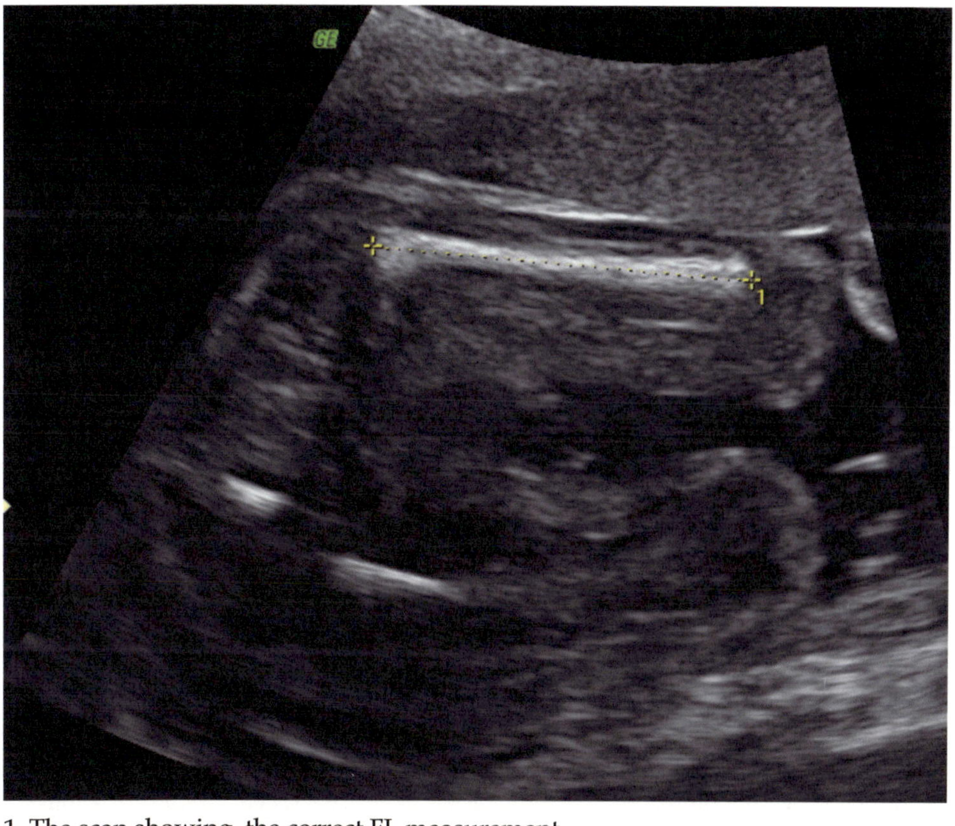

Fig. 1. The scan showing the correct FL measurement

Short FL is defined as below the 5th percentile or – 2 standard deviations (SD) appropriate for gestational age at the ultrasound examination. FL measurement is one of the easiest fetal biometry measurements. However; careful ultrasonographic measurement of only the ossified portions of the diaphysis is needed to obtain accurate measurements. The ossified portion of the femur is measured from the major trochanter to the distal end of the femoral shaft; the distal and proximal epiphyses are not included in the measurement. Oblique planes must be avoided and the femur closer to the transducer must be measured while the transducer is aligned parallel to the long axis of the bone. (*Figure 1*)

In most cases, short FL may be measured inaccurately or may be a variant of normal, especially if present as an isolated finding. However; short FL might be a diagnostic challenge for the examiner with various differential diagnoses. Short FL may be a part of a malformation such as a skeletal dysplasia or aneuploidies such as Trisomy 21 (Down Syndrome) or Monosomy X, and metabolic syndromes. (Kurtz et al.1990; Vergani et al. 2000; Bromley et al. 2002) Some studies have also suggested that a short FL is a feature of intrauterine growth restriction (IUGR) and small-for-gestational age (SGA) babies. (Todros et al. 1996; Zalel et al. 2002) Short FL may be associated with uteroplacental insufficiency and altered biochemical markers. (Weisz et al. 2008)

In this chapter, the abnormalities that might present with a short FL will be described in detail and then the management of short FL will be discussed.

2. Femur length and aneuplodies

The antepartum detection of fetal aneuploidy is one of the major goals of prenatal screening programs and aneuploidies are the most common genetic abnormalities detected by prenatal diagnosis. (Nyberg et al. 2008) The major screening method for aneuploidies in the antenatal period is detection of abnormalities during ultrasonography in addition to biochemical markers, maternal age, and genetic risk. However, for definitive diagnosis, karyotype analysis by amniocentesis or chorionic villus biopsy is needed.

Trisomy 21 (Down's syndrome) is an aneuploidy characterized by presence of an extra chromosome 21. It is named after John Langdon Down who first described the syndrome in 1866. (Down JLH; 1866) The condition was identified as an extra chromosome 21 in 1959 by Jerome Lejeune. (Lejeune et al. 1959) Characteristic dysmorphic features of trisomy 21 predominantly affect the head and neck and the extremities. Changes in the extremities include short broad hands, hypoplastic mid phalanx of fifth finger, incurved fifth finger, transverse palmar crease, space between the first and second toes (sandal gap deformity), hyperflexibility of joints. In addition, fetuses with trisomy 21 have slightly shorter long-bones than their normal counterparts. Actually, the mean length at birth is approximately 0.5 standard deviations (SD) less than normal babies in addition to decrease in birthweight and head circumference are less in babies with trisomy 21 when compared with normal counterparts. (Cronk CE; 1978)

In 1987, Lockwood et al and Benacerraf et al were the first ones to show that short FL was associated with increased risk of trisomy 21. (Lockwood et al. 1987; Benacerraf et al. 1987) The other biometric parameters were also evaluated, but the most significant changes were observed in the length of the extremities. (Barr Jr M.; 1994) Various criteria have been described for the determination of short FL. Lockwood and Brumsfield used the biparietal diameter (BPD) to FL ratio in order to evaluate the risk of Down syndrome. (Lockwood et al. 1987; Brumsfield et al. 1989) Lockwood chose an upper limit of 1.5 standard deviations above the mean. This led to a sensitivity of 50% and false- positive rate of 7% for identifying fetuses with Down syndrome. Brumsfield suggested a sensitivity of 40% and false positive rate of 2.2% using a BPD: FL ratio of ≥ 1.8 in the second trimester. (Brumsfield et al. 1989) But, it must be kept in mind that the BPD: FL ratio might differ depending on the gestational age of the fetus; second trimester seems to be the best time for evaluation. On the other hand, Grist used the measured-to-expected FL ratio and identified fetuses with Down syndrome with a sensitivity of 50% and false positive rate of 6.5%. (Grist et al. 1990)

It seems that most of the studies suggest that fetuses with trisomy 21 have slightly short FL. However the change in FL is only slight and therefore it is regarded as a soft marker for trisomy 21. Soft markers of trisomy 21 are ultrasonographic findings with the possibility of association with chromosomal abnormalities such as choroid plexus cysts, echogenic bowel, short FL, short humerus length (HL), pyelectasis. They are insufficient to be used as an isolated marker, but rather they are more likely to be useful when combined with each other. (Bethune, 2007) It must be remembered that isolated soft markers are identified in 11-17% of normal fetuses; however the prevalence is much higher in trisomy 21 and the risk of trisomy 21 increases more especially of there is more than one marker. (Breathnach et al., 2007) So a detailed fetal anatomy scanning should be performed to search for other markers when a short FL is encountered and if there is more than one marker a karyotype analysis should be obtained. Increased nuchal fold thickness, hypoplastic nasal bone and aberrant right subclavian artery are more powerful markers for Down Syndrome, and fetal chromosomal analysis might be offered in most cases with these findings even if they were isolated.

Short HL is also associated with trisomy 21 and it is suggested that the risk of trisomy 21 is higher with a short HL than a short FL. (Bethune, 2007) Therefore measurement of HL should be part of the routine whenever a short FL is measured.

Turner Syndrome (Monosomy X) is the only monosomy that is compatible with life. Turner syndrome was first described by Henry Turner in 1938 and was recognized to be secondary to karyotypic variation of 45,X in 1959. (Turner, 1938; Ford et al., 1959; Wiedemann & Glatzl, 1991) Although most conceptions with Turner syndrome die, 1% survive until term. (Cockwell et al., 1991) Its incidence is 1 in 2500 to 3000 live-born girls. Approximately half have monosomy X (45,X), and 5 to 10% have a duplication (isochromosome) of the long arm of one X (46,X,i(Xq)). (Sybert & McCauley, 2004) It is characterized by large cystic hygromata and fetal hydrops at the early stages of gestation in addition to short FL and short HL. (Chen & Chien, 2007) Live born fetuses may have minor problems such as short stature, widely spaced nipples, congenital lymphedema, webbed neck, and minor bone and cartilage abnormalities. Prenatal sonographic diagnosis is usually established in the late first and early second trimesters, secondary to cystic hygroma formation. (Weisz et al., 2008) One study evaluated the clustered ultrasonography findings in fetuses with Turner syndrome. (FitzSimmons et al., 1994) Thirteen fetuses with Turner syndrome were observed among 9348 early pregnancies (1/3086). Huge septated cystic hygroma, subcutaneous edema, and hydrops were observed in all cases. Short FL was detected in 12 of the 13 (92%) fetuses. Papp et al reported seven fetuses (10.1%) with short FL in 69 fetuses with Turner syndrome. The authors concluded that the addition of the soft marker of short FL to the second-trimester sonographic survey may increase the detection rate of Turner syndrome. (Papp et al.,2006)

Todros et al evaluated the outcome of pregnancy in 86 fetuses diagnosed with short FL in the second trimester ultrasonography scanning. (Todros et al., 2004) Twenty-eight of the fetuses (32.5%) were normal, 40 (46.5%) were structurally abnormal and 18 (21%) were small for gestational age. Of the 40 malformed fetuses, 16 (40%) were aneuploid. The structural malformations associated with aneuploidy included 10 cases of congenital heart disease with trisomy 21, three cases of multiple malformations with trisomy 18, one case of multiple malformations with trisomy 13 and two cases of Turner syndrome with aortic coarctation. None of the fetuses with isolated short FL was aneuploid. Therefore the authors suggested that short FL is not considered as an indication for karyotype analysis unless associated with other sonographic markers.

3. Femur length, skeletal dysplasias and other malformations

The skeletal dysplasias account for about 5% of the genetic disorders seen in the newborn period. (Orioli et al.,1986) They represent a significant burden to many families because of potential lethality, and short- and long-term medical complications, and recurrence risk. The fetal skeleton is easily visualized by ultrasound, however most series note a diagnostic accuracy for the skeletal dysplasias at less than 50%. (Doray et al., 2000; Parilla et al., 2003; Krakow et al., 2008)

Shortening of the FL is referred to as rhizomelia. When a short FL is identified before 24 weeks gestation, skeletal dysplasias must be considered and all long bones (each femur, humerus, radius, ulna, tibia, and fibula) must be measured to determine the relative length against normal values. In addition to measurement of the length, the long bones should be evaluated regarding changes in shape, mineralization, bowing, angulation, and metaphyseal flare. Although there is severe shortening of all limbs in the majority of skeletal dysplasias, the foot length is relatively normal. The normal FL: foot length ratio is 1.0 throughout the pregnancy, thus a ratio of less than 1 is useful in distinguishing skeletal dysplasia from other causes of short FL, such as IUGR or aneuploidy. (Campbell et al., 32)

Many skeletal dysplasias and specific syndromes are associated with short FL. These are listed in *Table 1;* however in most of these, it is possible to detect several additional ultrasonographic markers in a detailed ultrasonography scan.

Achondroplasia (OMIM Entry # 100800) is the most frequent form of short-limb dwarfism and most common form of skeletal dysplasia. (Horton et al., 2007) It occurs in one in 15,000 to one in 40,000 live births.

It is caused by mutation in the fibroblast growth factor receptor-3 gene (*FGFR3*), which is located at chromosome 4p16.3 and is inherited as an autosomal dominant fashion with essentially complete penetrance. (Superti-Furga & Unger, 2007) More than 99% of individuals with achondroplasia have one of two mutations in *FGFR3*. Over 80% of individuals with achondroplasia have parents with normal stature and have achondroplasia as the result of a *de novo* gene mutation. Affected individuals exhibit short stature caused by rhizomelic shortening of the limbs, characteristic face with frontal bossing and midface hypoplasia, exaggerated lumbar lordosis, limitation of elbow extension, bowed legs, and trident hand. (Nyberg, 2003) Head and abdominal circumference may be normal, but are often enlarged. But these signs are not specific. Prenatal sonographic diagnosis is often not possible as the length of long bones is well preserved until around 22 weeks' gestation, the time of the routine fetal anomaly scan. (Goncalves & Jeanty, 1994; Chitty et al., 2011) The FL is at the fifth percentile at this time and then below the first percentile at about 30 weeks. (Nyberg, 2003) Presentation and diagnosis of *de novo* cases often occurs at this period when the short limbs, frontal bossing and trident hand may be evident. Even then, misdiagnosis is common. (Modaff et al., 1996)

Alkyldihydroxacetonephosphate synthase deficiency
Atelosteogenesis type III
Barrow (1984)- short-limbed dwarfism; congenital heart defect
Baxova (1993)- micromelic bone dysplasia-humerus, femur, tibia type
Brachydactyl-type A1
Chondrodysplasia punctata-tibia metacarpal type
De la Chapelle-neonatal osseous dysplasia
Dysspondylochondromatosis
Gracile bone dysplasia
Hypochondroplasia
Hypochondroplasia (autosomal recessive)
Kyphomelic dysplasia
Metaphyseal acroscyphodysplasia
Metaphyseal chondrodysplasia- cone-shaped epiphyses
Omodysplasia
Omodysplasia type II
Patterson (1975)-rhizomelic dysplasia
Proximal femoral focal deficiency
Pseudoacondroplasia-like syndrome
Slaney (1999)- spondyloepimetaphyseal dysplasia-hypogammaglobulinaemia
Spondyloepimetaphyseal dysplasia-type Genevieve
Spondylometaphyseal dysplasia-type Borochowitz
Spondylometaphyseal dysplasia-type Sutcliffe
Silver-Russell syndrome

Table 1. The list of skeletal dysplasias and syndromes that might present prenatally with isolated short FL

Bowing of the femora have been reported in some cases. One study suggested that all the fetuses with achondroplasia had rounded metaphyseal–epiphyseal interface, with an angle connexion to diaphysis wider than expected at the ultrasonography scan. (Boulet et al., 2009)

Routine prenatal ultrasound examination may identify short FL and raise the possibility of achondroplasia in a fetus not known to be at increased risk. Krakow et al described the use of 3D ultrasonography in pregnancies from 16 to 28 weeks' gestation to enhance appreciation of the facial features and relative proportions of the appendicular skeleton and limbs for the diagnosis of achondroplasia. (Krakow et al., 2009) Ruano et al used a combination of 3D ultrasonography and intrauterine 3D helical computer tomography to enhance the diagnostic accuracy for intrauterine skeletal dysplasias. (Ruano et al., 2004)

Molecular testing can confirm the diagnosis in achondroplasia. DNA extracted from fetal cells obtained by amniocentesis or fetal cord blood sampling can be analyzed for *FGFR3* mutations if achondroplasia is suspected. (Francomano et al., 1993a)

Hypochondroplasia (OMIM Entry #146000) is also inherited in an autosomal dominant pattern and caused by mutation in the gene for *FGFR3* located on 4p, which is 98-99% mutated in achondroplasia. (Francomano et al., 1993b) The majority of the cases result from spontaneous mutations and that the unaffected parents of a child with hypochondroplasia have an extremely low risk (<0.01%) of having another affected child. Its prevalence is 1 in 50.000 births. (Hicks, 2003) The molecular testing strategies can detect only % 70 of the cases.

Not all patients with presumed hypochondroplasia have demonstrable mutations in the *FGFR3* gene, suggesting genetic heterogeneity. It is characterized by short stature, short arms and legs, and macrocephaly. The skeletal features are very similar to achondroplasia but usually tend to be milder. (Spranger, 1988) Shortening of long bones with mild metaphyseal flare is observed. The hands are relatively short but do not exhibit the "trident" appearance that is typical in achondroplasia. Facial features are usually normal and the classic facial features of achondroplasia (e.g., midface hypoplasia, frontal bossing) are not generally seen. Head size may be large without significant disproportion.

Hypochondroplasia shows some resemblance to achondroplasia, but is much milder and can be distinguished on clinical and radiographic grounds. Unlike achondroplasia, motor milestones are usually not significantly delayed and symptoms resulting from spinal cord compression (e.g., apnea, neuropathy) are less common. (Wyne-Davies et al., 1981)

The antenatal diagnosis is difficult as skeletal disproportion tends to be mild and the ultrasonography findings nonspecific. Prenatal molecular genetic testing is available if the mutations in the parents with hypochondroplasia have been identified. If the mutation causing hypochondroplasia cannot be identified, ultrasound examination is the only method of prenatal testing. It is often possible to detect an affected fetus early in the pregnancy if the fetus is at risk of being a heterozygote with another dominantly inherited skeletal dysplasia. (Francomano et al., 1993b) However, it is currently difficult to detect heterozygous hypochondroplasia or other milder phenotypes using ultrasonography. Signs of disproportionate growth may suggest the diagnosis of hypochondroplasia, but a "normal" third trimester ultrasound examination is not sufficient to rule out a diagnosis of hypochondroplasia. DNA banking may be offered to the family for future analysis. DNA-based diagnosis (*FGFR3* N540K and G380R mutation analysis) via chorion villus sampling, amniocentesis or fetal cord blood sampling may be helpful in ruling out lethal forms of skeletal dysplasia and establishing a more favorable prognosis for the fetus. (Francomano et al., 1993b)

Leroy I-cell disease is an autosomal recessive disorder first described in 1967 by Leroy and Demars and called I-cell disease due to the presence of phase dense intracytoplasmic inclusions in fibroblasts which were termed I cells. (Leroy et al., 1969) There is a biochemical defect in uridine diphospho-N-acetylglucosamine-1-phosphotransferase, which is the enzyme that catalyses addition of a mannose phosphate residue for lysosomal trafficking. (Wenger et al., 2002) Death from pneumonia or congestive heart failure usually occurs within the first decade of life. The most severely affected system is the skeletal system. Bone changes are similar to those observed in mucopolysaccharidoses. The classic finding is dysostosis multiplex, with a cloaking appearance of the long tubular bones due to periosteal new bone formation, anterior beaking and wedging of the vertebral bodies, widening of the ribs, proximal pointing of the metacarpals, and bullet shaped phalanges. Other findings are coarse facial features, developmental delay, growth failure, umbilical and inguinal hernias, hepatomegaly, and hypotonia. (Benacerraf, 1998) Lees et al have described polyhydramnios and short femurs in a case of Leroy I-cell disease that was diagnosed in the postnatal period. (Lees et al., 2001) The family had a history of Leroy I-cell disease. Yuksel et al reported two cases that both had short femurs and in one femoral bowing was additionally detected in the late second trimester and both were diagnosed as Leroy I-cell disease by enzyme analysis in the postnatal period. (Yuksel et al., 2007) None of the two families had a history of Leroy I-cell disease. Invasive prenatal diagnosis is possible by analysis of enzyme activity in chorionic villi or cultured amniocytes, but it is offered to families only known to be at risk for the metabolic disease.

For most of the other skeletal dysplasias presenting with short FL, other associated ultrasound findings such as bell-shaped thorax, protuberant abdomen, and polydactyl are present. (Nyberg, 2003)

Femoral-facial syndrome (FFS), also known as *femoral hypoplasia-unusual facies syndrome (FHUFS)* (MIM 134780), first described by Daentl et al, is a rare and sporadic multiple congenital anomaly syndrome comprising bilateral femoral hypoplasia and characteristic facial features, such as long philtrum, thin upper lip, micrognathia with or without cleft palate, and a short nose with broad tip. (Daentl et al., 1975; Nowaczyk et al., 2003) Nowaczyk et al reported an infant born with the disorder whose ultrasonography scan at 19 weeks was reported as normal. Review of the prenatal radiographs showed no diagnostic features in this child. These authors underlined the difficulties in identifying femoral abnormalities on 2D imaging and suggested that 3D imaging would be more effective for prenatal diagnosis. (Nowaczyk et al., 2003)

Acampomelic campomelic dysplasia (MIM 114290) is referred to cases without campomelia which is the bowing of the legs, especially the tibias. (Macpherson et al., 1989) However the other features of the syndrome such as ovarian dysgenesis, craniofacial changes, and defective tracheal bronchial cartilage are observed. (Rodriguez, 1993) Mutations in SOX-9 gene have been observed, 46, XY sex reversal is common. (Kwok et al., 1995)

Shprintzen syndrome (MIM 182212) is also associated with short FL. It is characterized by short stature, mild mental retardation, ear and hearing abnormalities, microcephaly, micrognathia, and cardiac and limb defects. The syndrome is autosomal dominantly inherited and is caused by mutations in the *fibrillin 1* gene, which cannot be tested easily in the antenatal period due to its size. (Biery et al., 1999)

The most important point in the antenatal diagnosis of skeletal dysplasias is the prediction of lethal disorders. It is crucial to measure the thoracic circumference and warn the parents when the thoracic circumference is well below the fifth centile. Multidisciplinary approach is necessary in the diagnosis and counselling of these cases. After delivery or termination of the pregnancy, the diagnosis should be confirmed by clinical, radiographic, and histopathological analysis and also by molecular testing strategies when available. Cell cultures and DNA should be banked to be used for future diagnostic molecular testing.

4. Femur length and intrauterine growth restriction

Several case series have shown an association between short FL and IUGR. Bromley et al, reported four fetuses with short femurs measuring more than 2 SD below the mean compared with the biparietal diameter. (Bromley et al., 1993) These fetuses were subsequently found to have severe IUGR with no evidence of skeletal dysplasia. Two other studies have described a short FL in cases with IUGR. (O'Brien et al., 1982)

In one study, 18 of the 86 fetuses (21%) referred for FL below the 10th percentile had SGA. (Todros et al., 2004) The diagnosis of SGA in fetuses was confirmed about 9 weeks after the initial finding of short FL. In another study short FL was associated with low birth weight and SGA, but not with gestational hypertension. These cases of isolated short FL were associated with significantly lower levels of pregnancy associated plasma protein- A (PAPP-A), but similar β-hCG, inhibin-A, and alpha-fetoprotein (AFP) when compared to fetuses with normal FL. (Qin et al., 2006)

Fetuses with short FL at the second trimester scanning might be considered as having an increased risk of IUGR. Maternal evaluation regarding blood pressure monitorization and follow-up for development of preeclampsia, ultrasonographic evaluation of the placenta, and Doppler analysis should be offered in this situation. In one study 50% of the women developed preeclampsia while undergoing follow-up for short FL and IUGR. (Todros et al., 2004)

The association between short FL and IUGR is unclear. It might be explained by the brain sparing effect with decreased flow to the lower body. It is likely that IUGR and short FL are linked to preeclampsia by the common mechanism of placental insufficiency. (Weisz et al., 2008)

Silver-Russell syndrome (SRS, MIM 180860) is a syndrome characterized by severe asymmetric IUGR, poor postnatal growth, craniofacial features such as a triangular shaped face and a broad forehead, body asymmetry, and a variety of minor malformations. It was reported independently by Silver et al. and Russell. (Silver et al., 1953; Russell, 1954) The long bones are short whereas the head measurements are within the normal range. The hallmark for the diagnosis of Silver-Russell syndrome is the demonstration of limb length asymmetry, which is unusual in other conditions. Yet there is no specific testing to confirm the diagnosis in the prenatal period. (Nyberg, 2003) In very near future testing strategies like chip-based next generation sequencing and methylation testing assays will be available for definitive diagnosis of SRS cases and many other sydromes having short femurs as the only clinical sign will be thoroughly evaluated during the antenatal period.

5. Femur length and normal variants

It must be considered that most of the fetuses presenting with isolated short FL are clinically normal. A short FL is defined as below the 5th percentile or below two standard deviations from the mean for the gestational age. That results in a pickup rate that exceeds the expected frequency of skeletal dysplasias. Various criteria have been published for the determination of short FL and HL. (Lockwood et al., 1987; Benacerraf et al., 1992) These criteria overlap the range observed in unaffected fetuses and vary widely among different populations; therefore, it would be prudent to develop standards for each population. Some authors have advocated the use of ethnic-specific FL growth charts. FL is observed to be shorter in Asian and oriental populations. (Nyberg, 2003; Down, 1866; Bromley et al., 1993; Shipp et al., 2001; Kovac et al., 2002a; Drooger et al., 2005) A significant difference in the mean expected FL among fetuses in the second trimester with regard to ethnicity was observed. It was stated that using ethnic-specific formulas for expected FL can have a considerable impact on the use of sonographic risk factors for trisomy 21 screening. (Kovac et al., 2002b) In another study, it was reported that short stature increased a woman's risk of having an abnormal BPD:FL ratio at the second trimester. They indicated that risk assessment for fetal trisomy 21 for such patients might be inaccurate. (Drooger et al., 2005) At 18 and 19 weeks' gestation, women shorter than one SD below the mean were twice as likely to have an abnormal BPD:

FL ratio compared with women taller than one SD above the mean (relative risk 2.38; 95% confidence interval 1.21, 4.69). (Drooger et al., 2005)

6. Management of short femur length

The differential diagnoses of short FL include normal variation, a false-positive measurement, IUGR, aneuploidy, and skeletal dysplasias. Very short FL is suggestive for skeletal dysplasias and other syndromes. (*Table 2*)

Diagnosis	**Down Syndrome**	**Achondroplasia**	**Skeletal Dysplasias/Syndromes**	**Intrauterine Growth Restriction**	**Constitutional**
Detailed anomaly scan	Markers of aneuploidy (echogenic intracardiac focus, pyelectasis, choroid plexus cysts, duodenal atresia, nuchal translucency , etc)	Frontal bossing, short fingers, trident hand short arms, narrow chest, macrocephaly	Abnormalities of other tubular bones, bowing, metaphyseal changes, abnormal posture/movements, thoracic circumference important	Small biometric measureme nts, possible abnormal Doppler findings	No obvious changes
Femur growth pattern	Often about 5th centile from early pregnancy on	Normal until 25 weeks, then falls in centiles	Severely short at second trimester or before	Variable onset, might begin with short FL weeks before small abdominal circumfe- rence	Often near 5th percentile, growth velocity is normal
Diagnosis	Down syndrome screening tests, karyotype analysis if > 1 soft marker	Molecular testing (Family history may be positive, *de novo* mutations common)	Depends on diagnosis and inheritance pattern. Postnatal diagnosis is possible. . Cell culture and DNA banking must be offered.	Karyotype analysis if > 1 soft marker, growth restriction develops during follow-up	Mother and/or father has short stature. History of short stature

Table 2. Differential Diagnosis of short femur length

Detailed ultrasonography scanning should be performed in patients presenting with short FL to exclude fetal malformations. Other tubular bones should be evaluated in addition to FL.

It must be remembered that the majority of isolated short FL are normal or constitutionally short and 13-61% of the fetuses diagnosed with isolated short FL at the second trimester scanning are classified as normal eventually on the follow-up. (Todros et al., 2004; Papageorghiou et al., 2008) In contrast, severely shortened (<5th percentile) or abnormal appearing long bones may be a sign of a skeletal dysplasia or early onset fetal growth restriction. (Weisz et al., 2008)

Counselling should be given to cases with isolated short FL; however a more conservative approach is more appropriate. Serial ultrasonography examinations should be performed in order to exclude skeletal dysplasias, IUGR, and uteroplacental insufficieny. Karyotype analysis should be offered if there are other sonographic markers suggesting aneuploidies. In cases where the karyotype analysis is normal, it is wise to store the DNA for future analysis in cases of sporadic skeletal dysplasias and syndromes. Isolated short FL cases should be followed up. Short FL due to IUGR should be suspected if during follow-up a small abdominal circumference, or abnormal Doppler parameters develop. If the FL falls further from the mean in the three-four weeks of follow-up skeletal dysplasia or severe IUGR should be suspected. (Kurtz et al., 1990)

Mild shortening of FL may suggest chromosomal abnormality or a syndrome. (Benacerraf et al., 1987; LaFollette et al., 1989; Perella et al., 1988; Nyberg et al., 1990) If mildly short FL (defined as length < 90% of the predicted FL) is present, there is a 1% risk of trisomy 21 in a high risk population (1/250 trisomy 21) and 3% risk of trisomy 21 in a low risk population (1/700 trisomy 21). (Nyberg et al., 1990) Short HL is even more specific than short FL in predicting trisomy 21. If short HL (defined as length < 90% of the predicted HL) is identified, there is a 3% risk of trisomy 21 in a high-risk population and a 1-2% risk of trisomy 21 in a low-risk population. (Benacerraf et al., 2001)

In the third trimester, one should remember that the FL is subject to the same 'biologic variability' as other biometric markers. It is not unusual for the FL measurement to be slightly less than other biometric markers in the absence of morphologic abnormality. This is particularly true if the remainder of the sonographic evaluation of the fetus is normal.

Evaluation of fetal posture and fetal movements are very important in prenatal ultrasound. Abnormal posture or movement may be the first clues to either focal or generalized musculoskeletal abnormality. Some skeletal dysplasias may develop additional features during the follow-up. The family must be clarified about the fact that some of the sydromes cannot be ruled out despite detailed sonographic evaluation.

7. Key points

1. Most of the fetuses with isolated short FL are normal or constitutionally short.
2. Detailed sonographic evaluation regarding additional markers for aneuploidy, measurement of other tubular bones, Doppler analysis should be performed.
3. If there are additional markers, karyotype analysis should be performed. The DNA may be banked for future analysis.
4. If the fetal karyotype analysis is normal, serial follow-up scans should be scheduled.
5. If, during follow-up the FL falls more from the mean, skeletal dysplasias or severe IUGR should be suspected. Molecular analysis must be performed for the diagnosis of

skeletal dysplasias with known molecular teiology, such as achondroplasia and hypochondroplasia . Preeclampsia must be ruled out.

6. Findings more suggestive for skeletal dysplasias include FL 2 SD below the mean for gestational age; FL/ foot length <1; and FL/ abdominal circumference < 0.16 .
7. Despite detailed sonographic evaluation, some of the syndromes cannot be ruled out and postnatal clinical genetic evaluation of fetuses or newborns should be considered.

8. References

Barr Jr M. Growth profiles of human autosomal trisomies at midgestation. Teratology 1994; 50:395.

Benacerraf B, Gelman R, Frigoletto F. Sonographic identification of second trimester fetuses with Down's syndrome. N Engl J Med 1987; 317: 1371.

Benacerraf BR, Neuberg D, Frigoletto FD Jr. Humeral shortening in second trimester fetuses with Down syndrome. Obstet Gynecol 1991; 77: 223.

Benacerraf BR, Neuberg D, Bromley B, Frigoletto FD Jr. Sonographic scoring index for prenatal detection of chromosomal abnormalities. J Ultrasound Med 1992;11(9):449.

Benacerraf BR: Ultrasound of Fetal Syndromes. New York, Churchill Livingstone, 1998.

Bethune M. Literature review and suggested protocol for managing ultrasound soft markers for Down syndrome: thickened nuchal fold, echogenic bowel, shortened femur, shortened humerus, pyelectasis and absent or hypoplastic nasal bone. Australas Radiol. 2007; 51(3):218.

Biery NJ, Eldadah ZA, Moore CS, Stetten G, Spencer F, Dietz HC: Revised genomic organization of FBN1 and significance for regulated gene expression. Genomics 1999; 56: 70–77.

Boulet S, Althuser M, Nugues F, Schaal J-P, Jouk PS. Prenatal diagnosis of achondroplasia: new specific signs. Prenat Diagn 2009; 29: 697-702.

Breathnach FM, Fleming A, Malone AD. The second trimester genetic sonogram. Am J Med Genet C Semin Med Genet 2007; 145C (1): 62.

Bromley B, Brown DL, Benacerraf BR. Short femur length associated with severe intrauterine growth retardation. Prenat Diagn 1993; 13: 449–452.

Bromley B, Lieberman E, Shipp TD, Benacerraf BR. The genetic sonogram: a method of risk assessment for Down syndrome in the second trimester. J Ultrasound Med 2002;21:1087- 1096.

Bronshtein M, Zimmer EZ, Blazer S. A characteristic cluster of fetal sonographic markers that are predictive of fetal Turner syndrome in early pregnancy. Am J Obstet Gynecol 2003; 188(4): 1016- 1020.

Brumsfield CG, Hauth JC, Cloud GA et al. Sonographic measurement and ratios in fetuses with Down syndrome. Obstet Gynecol 1989; 73: 644

Campbell J, Henderson A, Campbell S. The fetal femur/ foot length ratio: a new parameter to assess dysplastic limb reduction. Obstet Gynecol 1988; 72 (2): 181

Chen CP, Chien SC. Prenatal sonographic features of Turner syndrome. J Med Ultrasound 2007;15(4):251–257

Chitty LS, Griffin DR, Meaney C, Barrett A, Khalil A, Pajkrt E, Cole TJ. New aids for the non-invasive prenatal diagnosis of achondroplasia: dysmorphic features, charts of fetal size and molecular confirmation using cell-free fetal DNA in maternal plasma. Utrasound Obstet Gynecol 2011; 37(3): 283-289.

Cockwell A, MacKenzie M, Youings S, et al. A cytogenetic and molecular study of a series of 45,X fetuses and their parents. J Med Genet 1991;28:151–5.

Cronk CE. Growth of children with Down's syndrome: birth to age 3 years. Pediatrics 1978; 61(4): 564.

Daentl, D. L., Smith, D. W., Scott, C. I., Hall, B. D., Gooding, C. A. Femoral hypoplasia--unusual facies syndrome. J. Pediat 1975; 86: 107-111.

Doray B, Favre R, Viville B, Langer B, Dreyfus M, Stoll C. Prenatal sonographic diagnosis of skeletal dysplasias.A report of 47 cases. Ann Genet 2000;43:163–169.

Down JLH. Observations on an ethnic classification of idiots. London Hosp Clin Lect Rep 1866; 3: 259.

Drooger JC, Troe JW, Borsboom GJ, Hofman A, Mackenbach JP, Moll HA, Snijders RJ, Verhulst FC, Witteman JC, Steegers EA, Joung IM. Ethnic differences in prenatal growth and the association with maternal and fetal characteristics. *Ultrasound Obstet Gynecol* 2005; 26: 115–122.

FitzSimmons J, Fantel A, Shepard TH. Growth parameters in mid-trimester fetal Turner syndrome. Early Hum Dev 1994; 38(2): 121-129.

Ford CE, Jones KW, Polani PE, et al. A sex-chromosome anomaly in a case of gonadal dysgenesis (Turner's syndrome). Lancet 1959;1:711–3.

Francomano CA. Achondroplasia. In: Pagon RA, Bird TD, Dolan CR, Stephens K, editors. GeneReviews [Internet]. Seattle (WA): University of Washington, Seattle; 1993-. 1998 Oct 12 [updated 2006 Jan 09].

Francomano CA. Hypochondroplasia. Pagon RA, Bird TD, Dolan CR, et al., editors. GeneReviews [Internet]. Seattle (WA): University of Washington, Seattle; 1993-1998.

Goncalves L, Jeanty P. Fetal biometry of skeletal dysplasias: a multicentric study. *J Ultrasound Med* 1994; 13: 977–985.

Grist TM, Fuller RW, Albiez KL et al. Femur length in ultrasound prediction of trisomy 21 and other chromosome abnormalities. Radiology 1990; 174: 837.

Horton WA, Hall JG, Hecht JT. Achondroplasia. Lancet 2007; 370(9582): 162–172.

Hicks J. 2003. Achondroplasia family of skeletal dysplasias. In: The National Organisation for Rare Disorders, Inc., editors.NORD guide to rare disorders. Philadelphia: Lippincott Williams & Wilkins. 144 p.

Kovac CM, Brown JA, Apodaca CC, Napolitano PG, Pierce B, Patience T, Hume RF, Jr, Calhoun BC. Maternal ethnicity and variation of fetal femur length calculations when screening for Down syndrome. *J Ultrasound Med* 2002; 21: 719–722.

Kovac CM, Brown JA, Apodaca CC, Napolitano PG, Pierce B, Patience T, Hume RF Jr, Calhoun BC. Maternal ethnicity and variation of fetal femur length calculations when screening for Down syndrome. J Ultrasound Med 2002; 21(7):724-5.

Krakow D, Williams J, Poehl M, Rimoin DL, Platt LD. Use of three-dimensional ultrasound imaging in the diagnosis of prenatal-onset skeletal dysplasias. Ultrasound Obstet Gynecol 2003;21:467–72.

Krakow D, Alanay Y, Rimoin LP, Lin V, Wilcox WR, Lachman RS, Rimoin DL. Evaluation of Prenatal Onset Osteochondrodysplasias by Ultrasonography: A Retrospective and Prospective Analysis. Am J Med Genet A 2008; 146A(15): 1917-1924.

Kurtz AB, Needleman L, Wapner RJ, et al. Usefulness of a short femur in the in utero detection of skeletal dysplasias. Radiology 1990; 177:197- 200.

Kwok, C., Weller, P. A., Guioli, S., Foster, J. W., Mansour, S., Zuffardi, O., Punnett, H. H., Dominguez-Steglich, M. A., Brook, J. D., Young, I. D., Goodfellow, P. N., Schafer, A. J. Mutations in SOX9, the gene responsible for campomelic dysplasia and autosomal sex reversal. Am J Hum Genet 1995; 57: 1028-1036.

LaFollette L, Filly RA, Anderson R et al. Fetal femur length to detect trisomy 21. J Ultrasound Med 1989; 8: 657.

Lees C, Homfray T, Nicolaides KH: Prenatal ultrasound diagnosis of Leroy I cell disease. Ultrasound Obstet Gynecol 2001; 18: 275–276.

Lejeune J, Gautier M, Turpin R. Etude des chromosomes somatiques de neuf enfants mongoliens. C R Acad Sci 1959; 248: 1721-1722.

Leroy JG, Demars RI, Opitz JMI: Cell disease. Birth Defects Orig Artic Ser 1969; 5:174–184.

Lockwood C, Benacerraf B, Krinsky A, et al. A sonographic screening method for Down syndrome. Am J Obstet Gynecol 1987; 157:803.

Macpherson, R. I., Skinner, S. A., Donnenfeld, A. E. Acampomelic campomelic dysplasia. Pediat Radiol 1989; 20: 90-93.

Modaff P, Horton VK, Pauli RM. Errors in the prenatal diagnosis of children with achondroplasia. Prenat Diagn 1996;16: 525–530.

Nowaczyk, M. J., Huggins, M. J., Fleming, A., Mohide, P. T. Femoral-facial syndrome: prenatal diagnosis and clinical features. Report of three cases. Am J Med Genet 2010. 152A: 2029-2033.

Nyberg DA, Resta RG, Hickok DE et al. Femur length shortening in the detection of Down syndrome: Is prenatal screening feasible? Am J Obstet Gynecol 1990; 162: 1247.

Nyberg DA, McGahan JP, Pretorius DH, Pilu G. Diagnostic imaging of fetal anomalies. Lippincott Williams& Wilkins, Philadelphia 2003.

O'Brien GD, Queenan JT. Ultrasound fetal femur length in relation to intrauterine growth retardation. Part II. Am J Obstet Gynecol 1982; 144: 35–39.

Orioli IM, Castilla EE, Barbosa-Neto JG. The birth prevalence rates for the skeletal dysplasias. J Med Genet 1986;23:328–332.

Papageorghiou AT, Fratelli N, Leslie K, Bhide A, Thilaganathan B. Outcome of fetuses with antenatally diagnosed short femur. Ultrasound Obstet Gynecol 2008; 31(5):507.

Papp C, Beke A, Mezei G, et al. Prenatal diagnosis of Turner syndrome: report on 69 cases. J Ultrasound Med 2006;25:711–7.

Parilla BV, Leeth EA, Kambich MP, Chilis P, MacGregor SN. Antenatal detection of skeletal dysplasias. J Ultrasound Med 2003;22:255–258.

Perella R, Duerinckx AJ, Grant EG et al. Second-trimester sonographic diagnosis of Down syndrome: Role of femur-length shortening and nuchal fold thickening. AJR Am J Roentgenol 1988; 151: 981

Pierce BT, Hancock EG, Kovac CM, Napolitano PG, Hume RF Jr, Calhoun BC. Influence of gestational age and maternal height on fetal femur length calculations. Obstet Gynecol 2001; 97(5 Pt 1):742-6.

Qin X, Wergedal JE, Rehage M, Tran K, Newton J, Lam P, Baylink DJ, Mohan S. Pregnancy-associated plasma protein-A increases osteoblast proliferation in vitro and bone formation in vivo. Endocrinology 2006; 147: 5653–5661.

Rodriguez, J. I. Vascular anomalies in campomelic syndrome. Am J Med Genet 1993; 46: 185-192.

Ruano R, Molho M, Roume J, Ville Y. Prenatal diagnosis of fetal skeletal dysplasias by combining two-dimensional and three-dimensional ultrasound and intrauterine three-dimensional helical computer tomography. *Ultrasound Obstet Gynecol.* 2004; 24:134–40.

Russell, A. A syndrome of intra-uterine-dwarfism recognizable at birth with cranio-facial dysostosis, disproportionate short arms, and other anomalies (5 examples). Proc Roy Soc Med 1954; 47: 1040-1044.

Shipp TD, Bromley B, Mascola M, Benacerraf B. Variation in fetal femur length with respect to maternal race. *J Ultrasound Med* 2001; 20: 141–144. 11.

Silver, H. K., Kiyasu, W., George, J., Deamer, W. C. Syndrome of congenital hemihypertrophy, shortness of stature, and elevated urinary gonadotropins. Pediatrics 1953; 12: 368-376.

Spranger J. Bone dysplasia families. Pathol Immunpathol Res.1988;7:76–80.

Superti-Furga A, Unger S. Nosology and classification of genetic skeletal disorders: 2006 revision. Am J Med Genet A 2007; 143(1):1–18.

Sybert VP, McCauley E. Turner's syndrome. N Engl J Med 2004; 351:1227.

Todros T, Plazzotta C, Pastorin L. Body proportionality of the smallfor- date fetus: is it related to aetiological factors? Early Hum Dev 1996; 45:1– 9.

Todros T, Massarenti I, Gaglioti P, Biolcati M, Botta G, De Felice C. Fetal short femur length in the second trimester and the outcome of pregnancy. BJOG 2004; 111: 83-85.

Turner HH. A syndrome of infantilism, congenital webbed neck, and cubitus valgus. Endocrinology 1938; 23:566–74.

Vergani P, Locatelli A, Piccoli MG, et al. Critical reappraisal of the utility of sonographic fetal femur length in the prediction of trisomy 21. Prenat Diagn 2000;20:210– 214.

Wenger DA, et al: Lysosomal storage disorders:diagnostic dilemmas and prospects for therapy. Genet Med 2002; 4: 412–419

Weisz B, David AL, Chitty L, Peebles D, Pandya P, Patel P, Rodeck CH. Association of isolated short femur in the midtrimester fetus with perinatal outcome. Ultrasound Obstet Gynecol 2008; 31: 512–516.

Wiedemann HR, Glatzl J. Follow-up of Ullrich's original patient with "Ullrich-Turner" syndrome. Am J Med Genet 1991;41:134–6.

Wynne-Davies R, Walsh WK, Gormley J. 1981. Achondroplasia and hypochondroplasia. Clinical variation and spinal stenosis.J Bone Joint Surg Br 63B:508–515.

Woo JS, Wan CW, Fang A, Au KL, Tang LC, Ghosh A. Is fetal femur length a better indicator of gestational age in the growth-retarded fetus as compared with biparietal diameter? J Ultrasound Med 1985; 4: 139–142.

Yuksel A, Kayserili H, Gungor F. Short femurs detected at 25 and 31 weeks of gestation diagnosed as Leroy I-cell Disease in the Postnatal Period: A Report of Two Cases. Fetal Diagn Ther 2007; 22: 198-202.

Zalel Y, Lehavi O, Schiff E, et al. Shortened fetal long bones: a possible in utero manifestation of placental function. Prenat Diagn 2002; 22:553– 557.

6

Normal and Abnormal Fetal Face

Israel Goldstein and Zeev Wiener
Rambam Health Care Campus, Haifa
Israel

1. Introduction

During the early stages of embryogenesis, genetic factors play the predominant role in the development of the fetal face. In later stages, environmental influences increase in importance. Facial malformation may be the result of chromosomal aberrations as well as teratogenic factors. Therefore, facial dysmorphism can provide important clues that suggest chromosomal or genetic abnormalities. The post-natal diagnosis of facial dysmorphism is a well-known pediatric diagnosis, primarily based on pattern diagnosis related to the appearance of one or a combination of facial features, such as low-set ears, hypo-hypertelorism, small orbits, micrognathia, retrognatia, and more. Some of these features are detectable prenatally (Benacerraf, 1998). More than 250 syndromes are associated with disproportional growth of abnormal features of the fetal face (Smith & Jones, 1988).

Indication	**N**	%
Other fetal anomalies detected by US	118	52.8
Familial history of craniofacial malformations	72	32.2
Maternal drug intake	25	11.2
Fetal chromosomal aberrations	8	3.6
Total	**223**	

Table 1. Indications for ultrasound examination of the fetal face (Pilu et al., 1986)

Sonographic assessment of the fetal face is part of the routine anatomic survey. Recently, three-dimensional ultrasound (3D) images of the fetus can be also obtained. However, two-dimensional ultrasonographic images are more easily, rapidly, efficiently, and accurately obtained. Imaging of the fetal face is possible in most ultrasound examinations beyond 12 weeks of gestation.

This chapter describes normal structural development and the sonographic approach to evaluation of the fetal face. Clinical applications are discussed in relation to perinatal management.

2. Fetal face profile

Sonographic imaging of the fetal face can provide information for the antenatal diagnosis of fetuses with various congenital syndromes and chromosomal aberrations, many of which are known to be associated with facial malformations. Deviation from the normal proportions of the fetal face profile might be one of the 'soft sonographic signs' that can provide important clues that suggests congenital syndromes (Benacerraf, 1998).

Visualization of the curvature of the forehead is important to rule out a flat forehead, such as microcephaly, or bossing of the forehead, such as craniosynostosis (Goldstein et al., 1988). Visualization of the bridge of the nose could rule out Apert or Carpenter syndromes (Smith & Jones, 1988). Visualization of normal prominent lips can rule out cleft lip (Benacerraf, 1998). Finally, a normal jaw appearance is important to rule out microganthia or prognathia (Sivan et al., 1997).

Evaluation of the fetal face structures is suggested on the coronal and mid-sagittal views. The fetal face profile appearance should be obtained, while an imaginary line is passed through the nasion (bridge of the nose) and the gnathion (lower protrusion of the chin). This imaginary line is vertical to the maxillary bone. In this view, the following structures can be identified: the bridge and tip of the nose, the philtrum (area between the nose and the upper lip), upper and lower lips, and chin (Goldstein et al., 2010).

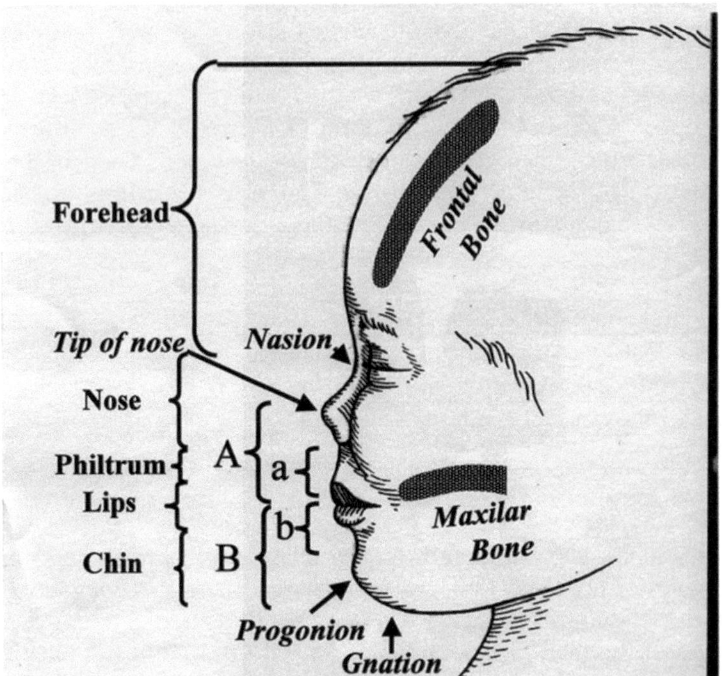

Fig. 1. **A** describes the distance from the tip of the nose to the mouth (line between the lips), **B** from the mouth to the chin, **a** describes the distances from the upper philtrum and the mouth, **b** from the mouth and the upper concavity of the chin.

The ratios between the following distances are independent of the gestational age and are almost constant: the distances between the tip of the nose and the mouth, and the distance from the mouth to the gnathion. In addition, a constant ratio was found between the upper philtrum and the mouth and from the mouth to the upper concavity of the chin (Goldstein et al., 2010).

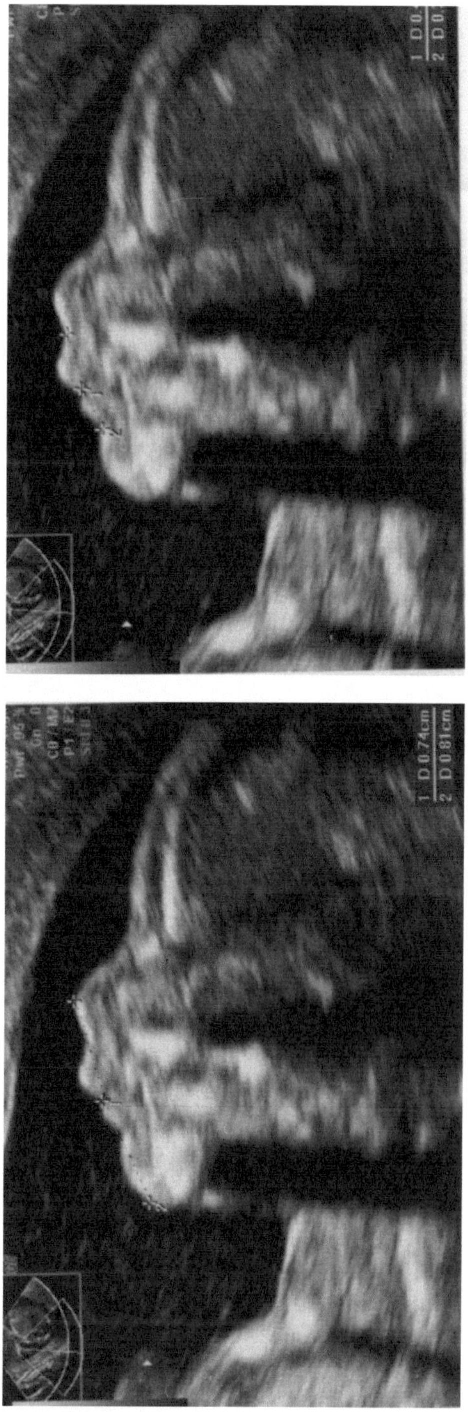

Fig. 2. Sonographic picture of the fetal face. Typical facial concavities and protrusions are presented. The calipers measured between the upper philtrum to the mouth (upper picture), and between the mouth to the chin (lower picture).

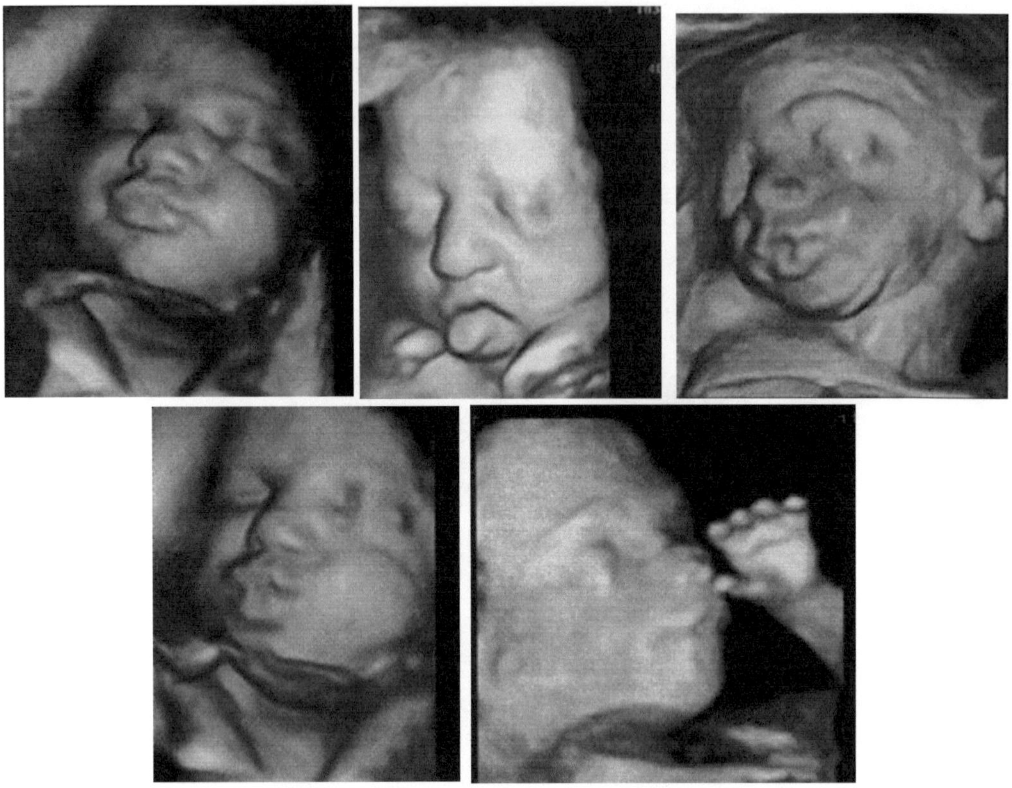

Fig. 3. 3D pictures of the fetal face. Mimics of face: a. kiss, b: open mouth and tongue, c: whistling, d: whistling, e: bye-bye

3. The forehead

Visualization of the curvature of the forehead is important to rule out a flat forehead (Figure 4). Investigators agree that microcephaly is associated with a decreased size of the frontal fossa and flattening of the frontal bone. Therefore, determination of the normal dimensions of the anterior cranial fossa and the frontal lobe of the fetal brain can provide normative

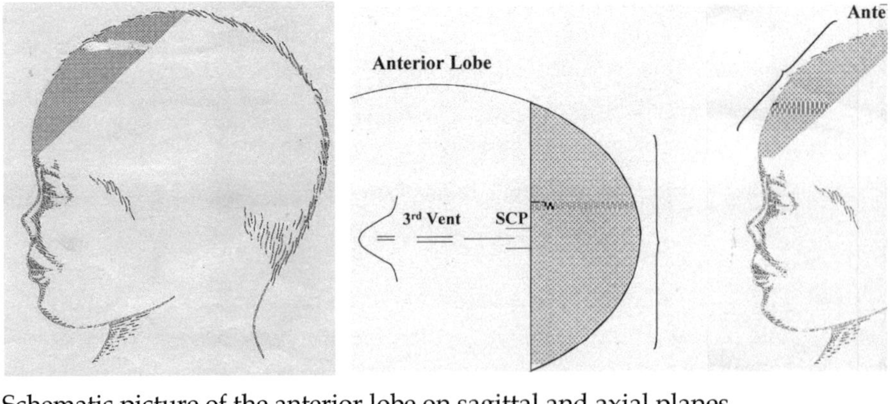

Fig. 4. Schematic picture of the anterior lobe on sagittal and axial planes

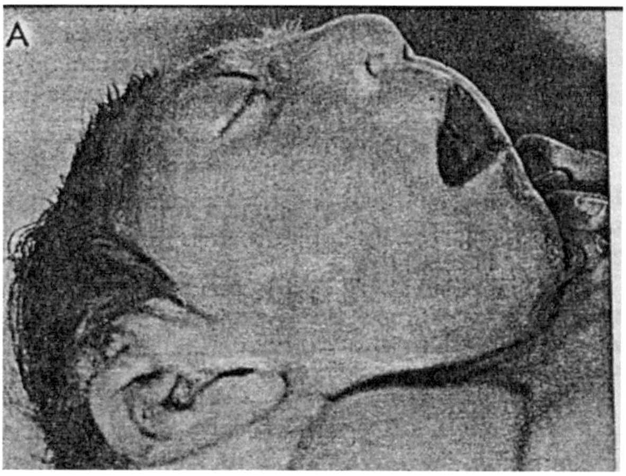

Fig. 5. A flat forehead in neonates with microcephaly

GA [weeks]	FLD [cm] mean±2SD		TFLD [cm] mean±2SD	
15	1.4	0.4	3.2	0.4
16	1.4	0.4	3.2	0.4
17	1.6	0.2	3.6	0.6
18	1.6	0.2	3.7	0.6
19	1.7	0.2	3.8	0.4
20	1.7	0.2	4.1	0.4
21	1.8	0.4	4.1	0.4
22	1.8	0.4	4.6	0.4
23	1.8	0.4	4.6	0.4
24	1.9	0.2	4.7	0.4
25	2.2	0.4	5.1	0.6
26	2.3	0.4	5.2	0.6
27	2.5	0.6	5.6	0.8
28	2.8	0.2	5.7	0.4
29	2.7	0.2	6.1	0.4
30	2.8	0.6	6.2	1.2
31	2.9	0.4	6.2	0.8
32	3.0	0.6	6.4	0.8
33	3.1	0.6	6.5	0.6
34	3.2	0.2	6.7	0.6
35	3.2	0.4	6.9	0.6
36	3.2	0.4	7.0	0.4
37	3.4	0.4	7.2	0.6
38	3.5	0.4	7.3	0.8
39	3.7	0.6	7.5	0.8
40	4.0	0.6	7.7	0.8

Table 2. Measurements of the mean±2SD of the frontal lobe distance and thalamic frontal lobe distance versus gestational age (Goldstein et al., 1988) (GA = gestational age, FLD = frontal lobe distance, TFLD = thalamic frontal lobe distance)

data against which fetuses suspected to have microcephaly or any other lesion affecting the anterior fossa can be evaluated. A dysmorphic sign with a high frequency appears to be a flat facial profile in neonates with trisomy 21 (Smith & Jones, 1988). Table 2 describes the normal dimensions of the frontal lobe of the fetal brain (Goldstein et al., 1988).

4. The nasal bone

Smallness of the nose is a common finding at postnatal examination of fetuses or neonates with trisomy 21, but also with more than 40 other genetic conditions. Measurements of the nasal bone were performed on a mid-sagittal profile in normal singleton fetuses at 14-34 weeks' gestation. It was found that the length of the nasal bones increased from 4 mm at 14 weeks to 12 mm at 35 weeks' gestation (Guis et al., 1995). Investigators examined the

Gestation [weeks]	Mean	SD
14	4.183	0.431
16	5.213	1.062
18	6.308	0.654
20	7.621	0.953
22	8.239	1.102
24	9.362	1.300
26	9.744	1.277
28	10.72	1.459
30	11.348	1.513
32	11.580	1.795
34	12.285	2.372

Table 3. Mean, standard deviation (SD), mean+2SD and mean-2SD for length of the nasal bones (mm) throughout gestation (Guis et al., 1995)

Gestation [weeks]	Mean [mm]	SD [mm]
11-11.9	1.7	0.5
12-12.9	2.0	0.5
13-13.9	2.3	0.5
14-14.9	3.4	0.7
15-15.9	3.3	0.8
16-16.9	4.4	0.7
17-17.9	5.0	0.7
18-18.9	5.5	0.9
19-19.9	5.7	0.1
20-20.9	6.2	0.1

Table 4. Fetal nasal bone length (mm), 11-20 weeks' gestation (Cuick et al., 2004)

Gestation [weeks]	Mean [mm]	SD [mm]
11-11+6	1.69	0.26
12-12+6	2.11	0.37
13-13+6	2.34	0.39
14-14+6	2.94	0.48

Table 5. Nomogram of fetal nasal bone length at 11-13 gestational weeks in fetuses (Sivri et al., 2006)

possible improvement in screening for trisomy 21 by examining the fetal nasal bone with ultrasound at 11-14 weeks of gestation (Cicero et al., 2001). The nasal bone was absent in 43 of 59 (73%) trisomy 21 fetuses, and in three of 603 (0.5%) chromosomally normal fetuses.

5. The nostrils

Smallness of fetal nose, often attributed to hypoplasia, is a common finding during postnatal examination of fetuses or neonates with trisomy 21 (Smith & Jones, 1988)

GA [weeks]	Centiles				
	10	25	50	75	90
14-15	5.5	7.2	7.6	8.3	10.2
16-17	6.5	7.3	7.9	8.5	10.5
18-19	8.5	8.9	10.0	10.5	11.0
20-21	10.2	11.0	12.0	12.0	13.0
22	13.0	13.0	14.0	15.0	15.0
23	13.0	13.0	14.0	15.0	15.0
24	13.0	14.1	15.0	16.0	16.0
25	14.2	15.0	16.3	17.0	17.0
26	14.1	15.0	16.3	17.4	18.4
27	13.4	15.4	17.2	18.4	19.0
28	15.1	16.9	17.6	18.2	20.2
29-30	16.5	17.4	18.1	19.2	20.6
31-32	16.6	17.9	19.6	20.7	21.4
33-34	17.4	19.1	20.5	21.4	23.1
35-37	17.6	20.0	20.5	22.0	23.3
38-40	17.4	17.9	18.9	20.5	23.4

Table 6. The fetal nose width (mm) (Goldstein et al., 1997)

GA [weeks]	Centiles				
	10	25	50	75	90
14-15	3.3	3.6	4.2	4.7	5.4
16-17	3.5	3.9	4.4	4.8	5.9
18-19	4.0	4.4	.6	5.0	5.8
20-21	4.2	5.0	5.0	5.7	6.0
22	5.0	5.0	6.0	6.4	7.0
23	5.0	5.6	6.0	7.0	7.0
24	5.8	6.0	6.2	7.3	7.9
25	5.9	6.0	6.4	7.0	7.7
26	5.1	6.2	7.7	8.0	9.0
27	6.4	6.8	7.8	8.4	9.4
28	6.4	7.0	7.9	8.6	9.4
29-30	5.4	7.0	7.0	8.2	9.6
31-32	4.6	7.4	7.9	9.2	10.7
33-34	5.4	6.4	8.1	9.0	9.7
35-37	5.8	6.6	8.5	9.6	10.2
38-40	6.0	6.8	8.5	9.5	10.5

Table 7. The fetal nostril distance (mm) (Goldstein et al., 1997)

6. The fetal eyes

The earliest sonographic visualization of the fetal orbit and lens has been considered to be in the beginning of the second trimester of pregnancy. On ultrasound, the orbits appear as echolucent circles in the face of the fetus, and the lens can be easily identified inside these structures. Imaging of these structures, which is possible on virtually all ultrasound examinations beyond the first trimester, is important because deviation in the relative size of the orbit and the lens can be associated with congenital malformations. The fetal orbits and lens eyes are best visualized by scanning the fetal face in coronal and axial planes. The fetal orbits should appear as two symmetrical structures on both sides of the fetal nose. Both lenses are depicted on the coronal or axial plane of the eye as circular hyperechogenic rings and with hypoechogenic areas inside the ring.

The coronal planes of the fetal face are the most important in the evaluation of the fetal orbits. Figure 6a shows the the outer orbital distance small hands, and Fig 6b the inner orbital distace the small arrows. The calipers measuring the outer orbital from the lateral mid-echogenicity to the lateral mid-echogenicity, and the calipers measuring the inner orbital distace from the middle mid-echogenicity to the middle mid-echogenicity of the orbits.

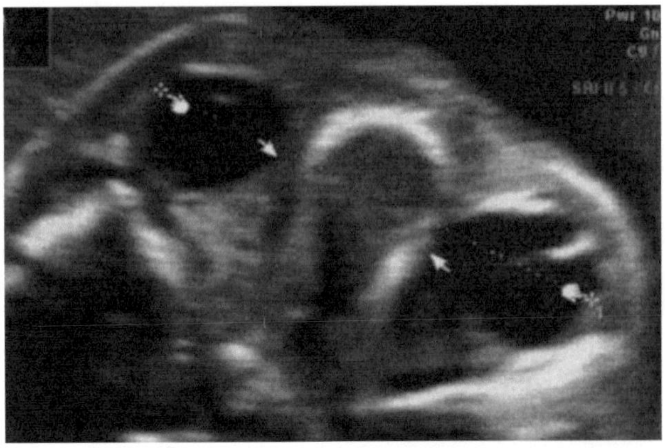

Fig. 6a. Coronal plane of the fetal orbits - small hands showing the outer orbital diameter measurement

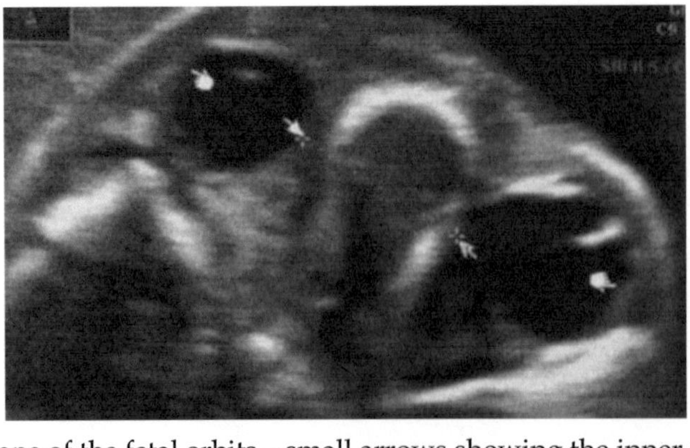

Fig. 6b. Coronal plane of the fetal orbits - small arrows showing the inner orbital diameter measurement

GA [weeks]	N	Mean	95% CI	Centiles				
				10	25	50	75	90
14	10	5.2	4.8-5.7	4.5	5.0	5.3	5.7	90
15	26	6.1	5.9-6.3	5.4	5.5	6.2	6.5	6.7
16	25	6.6	6.3-6.9	5.8	6.2	6.5	7.0	7.6
17-18	19	7.3	6.7-7.8	6.2	6.5	6.7	9.0	9.0
19-20	23	9.8	9.3-10.2	8.6	9.0	10.0	10.1	11.3
21	19	10.5	10.0-10.9	9.4	9.9	10.0	11.0	12.0
22	26	10.4	10.0-10.7	9.5	9.6	10.5	11.0	11.3
23	21	10.7	10.4-11.1	9.6	10.0	10.5	11.4	11.5
24	19	11.6	11.3-11.8	10.7	11.0	11.5	12.0	12.5.
25	13	11.2	11.4-12.4	10.3	11.0	12.2	12.5	12.8
26	16	12.7	12.0-13.4	11.0	11.0	12.7	13.8	14.5
27	14	13.0	12.4-13.5	11.9	12.0	12.9	13.4	14.8
28	21	13.0	12.7-13.3	21.1	12.0	13.1	13.3	14.1
29	23	13.9	13.4-14.4	12.6	13.0	13.7	14.6	15.7
30-31	24	14.2	13.8-14.5	13.3	13.0	13.9	14.7	15.4
32-33	24	14.4	13.7-15.1	12.2	13.0	14.1	14.8	17.5
34-36	26	15.8	15.4-16.2	14.6	15.0	15.7	16.5	16.9

Table 8. The fetal orbital diameter (mm) (Goldstein et al., 1998) GA = gestational age; CI = confidence interval

GA [weeks]	n	Mean	95% CI	Centiles				
				10	25	50	75	90
14	10	2.5	23.3-2.7	2.1	2.4	2.5	2.7	2.9
15	26	2.9	2.9-3.0	2.7	2.8	2.9	3.1	3.2
16	25	2.9	2.8-3.0	2.7	2.8	2.9	3.1	3.2
17-18	19	3.3	3.0-3.6	2.8	2.9	3.0	3.3	5.0
19-20	23	4.1	4.0-4.3	3.6	4.0	4.0	4.3	5.0
21	19	4.4	4.1-4.6	3.7	3.9	4.0	5.0	5.0
22	26	4.4	4.2-4.7	3.9	4.0	4.3	5.0	5.0
23	21	4.6	4.3-4.8	3.8	4.0	5.0	5.0	5.0
24	19	4.6	4.4-4.8	4.0	4.3	4.6	5.0	5.0
25	13	4.8	4.6-5.0	4.2	4.6	5.0	5.1	5.2
26	16	5.0	4.8-5.2	4.4	4.8	5.1	5.2	5.5
27	14	5.0	5.0-5.2	4.5	5.0	5.2	5.2	5.5
28	21	5.1	5.0-5.2	4.5	5.0	5.2	5.2	5.5
29	23	5.3	5.1-5.5	4.6	5.2	5.2	5.5	5.9
30-31	24	5.3	5.2-5.5	4.8	5.1	5.5	5.5	5.7
32-33	24	5.6	5.4-5.8	4.8	5.2	5.5	5.9	6.2
34-36	26	5.8	5.6-6.0	5.4	5.5	5.7	6.0	6.5

Table 9. Diameter of orbital lens (mm) (Goldstein et al., 1998) GA = gestational age; CI = confidence interval)

6.1 Hypotelorism

Hypotelorism is a condition pertaining to abnormally close eyes.

GA [weeks]	OOD [mm]			IOD [mm]		
	5th	50th	95th	5th	50th	95th
12	8	15	23	4	9	13
13	10	18	25	5	9	14
14	13	20	28	5	10	14
15	15	22	30	6	10	14
16	17	25	32	6	10	15
17	19	27	34	6	11	15
18	22	29	37	7	11	16
19	24	31	39	7	12	16
20	26	33	41	8	12	17
21	28	35	43	8	13	17
22	30	37	44	9	13	18
23	31	39	46	9	14	18
24	33	41	48	10	14	19
25	35	42	50	10	15	19
26	36	44	51	11	15	20
27	38	45	53	11	16	20
28	39	47	54	12	16	21
29	41	48	56	12	17	21
30	42	50	57	13	17	22
31	43	51	56	13	18	22
32	45	52	60	14	18	23
33	46	53	61	14	19	23
34	47	54	62	15	19	24
35	48	55	63	15	20	24
36	49	56	64	16	20	25
37	50	57	65	16	21	25
38	50	58	65	17	21	21
39	51	58	66	17	22	26
40	52	59	67	18	22	26

Table 10. The outer orbital diameter (OOD) and inner orbital diameter (IOD), GA = gestational age (Jeanty et al., 1984)

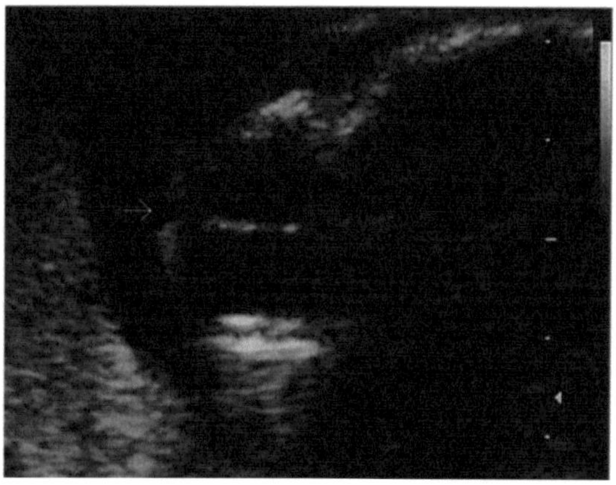

Fig. 7. Axial scan of a fetus at 25.3 weeks of gestation showing severe hypotelorism

BPD [cm]	Weeks' gestation	IOD [cm]	OOD [cm]
1.9	11.6	0.5	1.3
2.0	11.6	0.5	1.4
2.1	12.1	0.6	1.5
2.2	12.6	0.6	1.6
2.3	12.6	0.6	1.7
2.4	13.1	0.7	1.7
2.5	13.6	0.7	1.8
2.6	13.6	0.7	1.9
2.7	14.1	0.8	2.0
2.8	14.6	0.8	2.1
2.9	14.6	0.8	2.1
3.0	15.0	0.9	2.2
3.1	15.5	0.9	2.3
3.2	15.5	0.9	2.4
3.3	16.0	1.0	2.5
3.4	16.5	1.0	2.5
3.5	16.5	1.0	2.6
3.6	17.0	1.0	2.7
3.7	17.5	1.1	2.7
3.8	17.9	1.1	2.8
4.0	18.4	1.2	3.0
4.2	18.9	1.2	3.1
4.3	19.4	1.2	3.2
4.4	19.4	1.3	3.2
4.5	19.9	1.3	3.3
4.6	20.4	1.3	3.4
4.7	20.4	1.3	3.4
4.8	20.9	1.4	3.5
4.9	21.3	1.4	3.6
5.0	21.3	1.4	3.6

BPD [cm]	Weeks' gestation	IOD [cm]	OOD [cm]
5.1	21.8	1.4	3.7
5.2	22.3	1.4	3.8
5.3	22.3	1.5	3.8
5.4	22.8	1.5	3.9
5.5	23.9	1.5	4.0
5.6	23.3	1.5	4.0
5.7	23.8	1.5	4.1
5.8	24.3	1.6	4.1
5.9	24.3	1.6	4.2
6.0	24.7	1.6	4.3
6.1	25.2	1.6	4.3
6.2	25.2	1.6	4.4
6.3	25.7	1.7	4.4
6.4	26.2	1.7	4.5
6.5	26.2	1.7	4.5
6.6	26.7	1.7	4.6
6.7	27.2	1.7	4.6
6.8	27.6	1.7	4.7
6.9	28.1	1.7	4.7
7.0	28.6	1.8	4.8
7.1	29.1	1.8	4.8
7.3	29.6	1.8	4.9
7.4	30.0	1.8	5.0
7.5	30.6	1..8	5.0
7.6	31.0	1.8	5.1
7.7	31.5	1.8	5.1
7.8	32.0	1.8	5.2
7.9	32.5	1.9	5.2
8.0	33.0	1.9	5.3
8.2	33.5	1.9	5.4
8.3	34.0	1.9	5.4
8.4	34.4	1.9	5.4
8.5	35.0	1.9	5.5
8.6	35.4	1.9	5.5
8.8	35.9	1.9	5.6
8.9	36.4	1.9	5.6
9.0	36.9	1.9	5.7
9.1	37.3	1.9	5.7
9.2	37.8	1.9	5.8
9.3	38.3	1.9	5.8
9.4	38.8	1.9	5.8
9.6	39.3	1.9	5.8
9.7	39.8	1.9	5.9

Table 11. Predicted BPD and weeks' gestation from the inner orbital diameter (IOD) and outer orbital diameter (OOD) (Mayden et al., 1982)

6.2 Hypertelorism

Hypertelorism is an abnormally increased distance between two organs or body parts, usually referring to an increased distance between the eyes (orbital hypertelorism), seen in a variety of syndromes (Table 12).

Malformation	Syndromes
Anophthalmus	Trisomy 13 Vilaret, Weyers-Tier, ocular vertebral syndrome
Microphthalmus	Autosomal recessive or autosomal dominant Intrauterine infection Radiation Chromosomal aberration X-linked Associated with gingival fibromatosis Depigmentation
Ocular hypotelorism	Chromosome 5 p-syndrome Chromosome 15-p-proximal partial trisomy syndrome Chromosome 13 trisomy Craniosynostosis-medical aplasia syndrome Holoprosencephaly Meckel syndrome
Ocular hypetelorism	Aarshog syndrome Acrocephalosyndactyly Acrodystasis Auditory canal atresia Basal nevus syndrome Branchio-skeleto-genital syndrome Broad thumb-hallux syndrome Campomelic dysplasia Cerebro-hepato-renal syndrome Chromosome 18 p- syndrome Chromosome 5 p- syndrome Chromosome 4 p- syndrome Chromosome 14 p-proximal partial trisomy syndrome Coffin-Lowry syndrome Cranio-carpo tarsal dysplasia Cranio-facial dysostosis

Malformation	Syndromes
	Cranio-metaphyseal dysplasia Cranio-oculodental syndrome Deafness myopia cataract and saddle nose Ehlers-Danlos syndrome Fetal hydantoin syndrome Fetal warfarin syndrome G syndrome Hypertelorism–hypospadias syndrome Hypertelorism microtia facial clefting and conductive deafness Iris coloboma and canal atresia syndrome Larsen syndrome Multiple lentigines syndrome Cleft lip Marden-Walker syndrome Meckel syndrome Median cleft syndrome Noonan syndrome Nose and nasal septum defects Bifid nose Glioma of the nose Posterior atresia of the nose Ocular and facial anomalies with proteinuria and deafness Oculo-dento osseous dysplasia Opitz-Kaveggia FG syndrome Oto-palatodigital syndrome Bilateral renal agenesis Roberts syndrome Robinow syndrome Sclerosteosis Thymic agenesis Apert syndrome LEOPARD syndrome Crouzon syndrome Wolf-Hirschhorn syndrome Waardenburg syndrome Cri du chat syndrome DiGeorge syndrome Loeys-Dietz syndrome Morquio syndrome Hurler's syndrome Deafness

Table 12. Syndromes associated with fetal ocular malformation (Bergsma, 1979)

6.3 Cyclopia

Cyclopia is an anomaly characterized by a single orbital fossa, with fusion of bulbs, eyelids and lacrimal apparatus to a variable degree. Usually there is a single eye or partially divided eye in a single orbit and arhinia with proboscis. A normal nose is absent and a proboscis structure originating from the nasal root may be seen (Bergsma, 1979). The differential diagnosis in these cases includes ethmocephaly (extreme hypotelorism, arhinia and blinded proboscis located between the eyes) and ceboephaly (hypotelorism and a single nostril nose, without midline cleft). In ethmocephaly, the nasal bones, maxilla and nasal septum and turbinate are missing and lacrimal and palatine bones are united (Goldstein et al., 2003; McGahan et al., 1990).

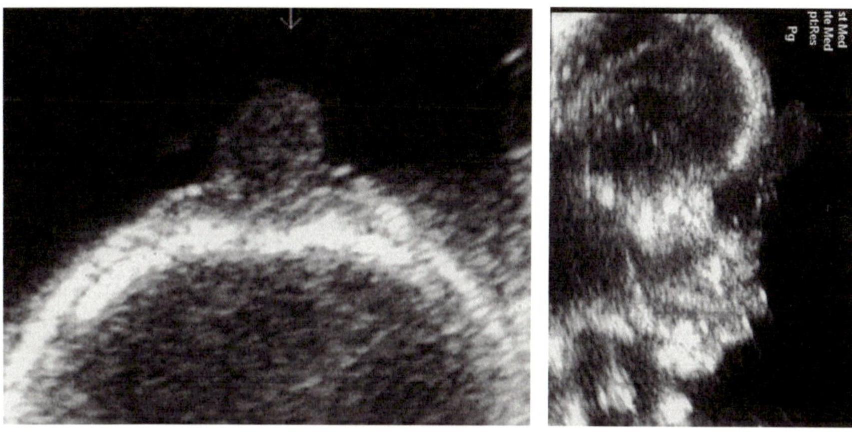

Fig. 8. Axial and sagittal scans of a fetus at 25.3 weeks of gestation show prominent forehead and proboscis

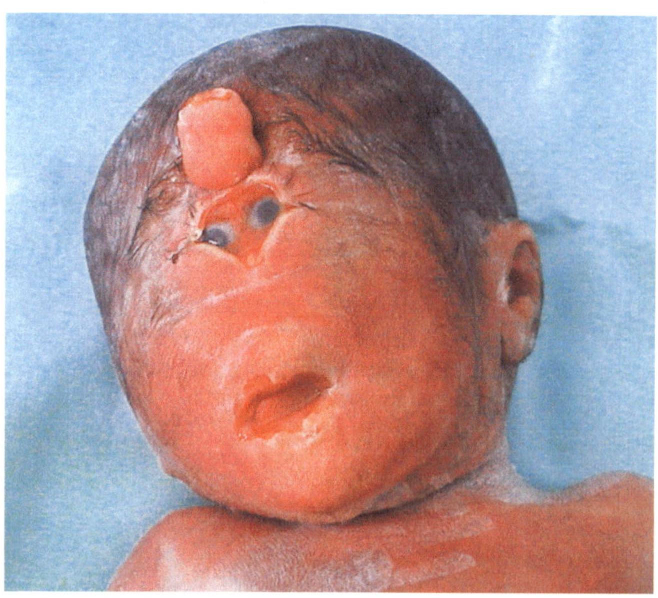

Fig. 9. Ethmocephaly – postmortem demonstrating hypotelorism and proboscis

6.4 Cataracts

A cataract is an opacity of the lens and accounts for 10% of the blindness seen in preschool age children in Western countries. Fetal cataracts may occur in association with infectious diseases, chromosomal anomalies or systemic syndromes.

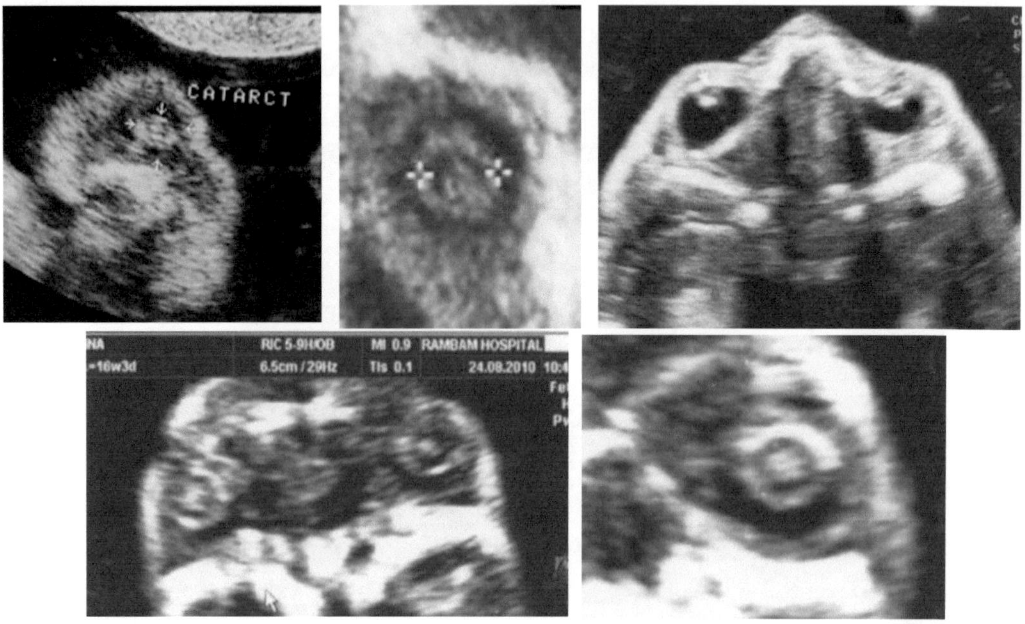

Fig. 10. Sonographic pictures of fetal cataracts at 15 weeks of gestation. Coronal views of echogenic lens.

7. The ear

Abnormally small ears have been noted to be one of the findings in newborn and infants with trisomy 21 and other aneuploidies. Ears in these infants are often described as small, low-set, and malformed. Short ear length has been found to be the most consistent clinical characteristic in making the diagnosis of Downs' syndrome (Aase et al., 1973). Sonographically, a short fetal ear length may be a parameter in predicting fetal aneouploidy (Chitkara et al., 2002). Sonographic studies have suggested that short ear length measurements might be a useful predictor of fetal anomalies (Awwad et al., 1994; Lettieri et al., 1993; Shimizu et al., 1997; Yeo et al., 1998).

Investigators had suggested that the fetal ear length may be a useful measurement in prediction of aneuploidy in patients at high risk for fetal chromosomal abnormalities (Awwad et al., 1994; Lettieri et al., 1993; Shimizu et al., 1997; Yeo et al., 1998). However, it remains to be determined whether this measurement alone, or in combination with other aneuploidy markers, will prove to be a useful predictor of aneuploidy in a population of women at low risk for fetal chromosomal abnormalty.

GA (Weeks)	Mean [mm]	SD [mm]
14	8	0.7
15	9	1.8
16	10	0.9
17	11	1.0
18	13	0.7
19	14	1.1
20	15	1.1
21	17	1.0
22	18	1.5
23	19	1.4
24	20	1.1
25	22	1.7
26	23	2.1
27	25	1.7
28	26	1.8
29	26	1.6
30	27	2.3
31	29	2.6
32	29	1.9
33	30	1.8
34	31	1.6
35	31	2.1
36	33	2.6
37	33	2.0
38	33	4.1
39	34	4.3
40	37	2.1
41	38	1.9

Table 13. Fetal ear length (Yeo et al., 1998)

8. The maxillary bone

Imaging of the maxillary bone is possible in most ultrasound examinations and is important, because deviations in maxillary bone development can also be associated with a malformed face. The relationship between the maxillary, zygomatic and palatine bones provides a capacity for rapid movement of the fetal face. The etiology of hypoplasia of the maxillary bone may, in some cases, form part of well-established structural abnormalities in the fetus such as choanal atresia, or genetic syndromes such as Marfan's syndrome. Sonographically, early prenatal detection of the maxillary bone is possible at 14 week of gestation. Hypoplasia of the maxillary bone can appear as an incidental finding. Table 14 depicts nomograms of the maxillary bone length.

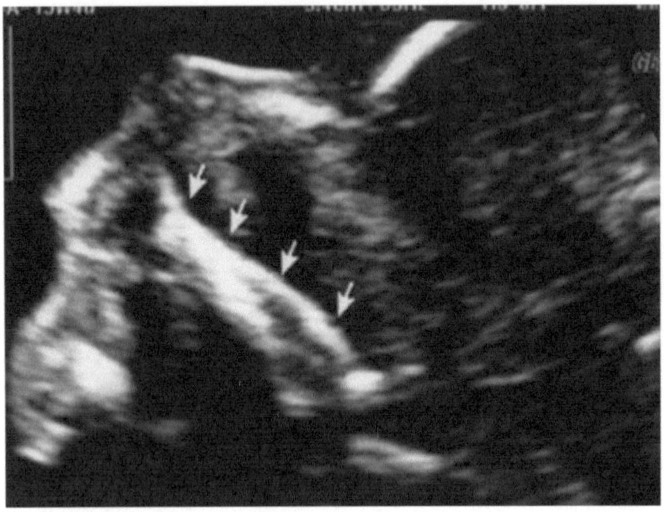

Fig. 11. Sonographic picture of the maxillary bone

GA (Weeks)	Mean	SD	Centiles………… 10	50	90
14	9.97	1.12	8.32	10	11.52
15	10.64	1.07	9.4	10.6	11.8
16	10.6	1.73	7.6	10.4	12.98
17-19	10.07	2.75	7.0	10.9	13
20-22	11.48	3.42	7.0	11.0	17.35
23-24	13.19	3.34	8.60	13	16.76
25-26	12.85	1.74	10.2	13.0	15.92
27-28	12.61	2.11	10.0	12.0	16.2
29-30	13.63	1.67	11.67	13.50	16.23
31	13.16	1.25	11	13.0	15.48
32	13.49	1.25	11.9	13.45	15.0
33	13.7	1.37	11.11	14.0	15.95
34	13.87	1.72	11.96	14.0	16.15
35	14.15	1.27	12.54	14.0	16.0
36	14.31	1.4	12.63	14.35	16.15
37	14.08	1.26	12.93	14.0	16.73
38-39	14.84	1.77	11.74	14.8	17.47

Table 14. Maxillary bone length across gestational age (Goldstein et al., 2005)

The frontomaxillary facial (FMF) angle was studied in the first trimester in a Chinese population, demonstrating that the FMF angle decreases with fetal CRL increases. Similarity in the normal values of the FMF angle was found between the Chinese and Caucasian populations (Chen et al., 2011). These authors previously studied the FMF angle in fetuses with trisomy 21 in the first trimester and found significant differences in the FMF angle between normal fetuses and fetuses with trisomy 21 in the Chinese population (Chen et al., 2009).

9. The tongue

Fetal macroglossia and microglossia are associated with several chromosomal defects. Table 15 describes the tongue circumference between 14 and 26 weeks of gestation.

GA (weeks)	Lower 95% CI	Mean	Upper 95% CI
14	24	28	31
15	26	33	36
16	33	36	38
17	37	37	38
18	40	43	46
19	47	48	51
20	47	51	56
21	51	55	61
22	52	58	62
23	58	62	68
24	60	64	67
25	68	70	73
26	71	73	76

Table 15. Tongue circumference (mm) by gestational age (weeks) and the 95% confidence interval (Achiron et al., 1997)

10. Cleft lips & palate

Cleft lip and palate is a common facial anomaly, with an incidence of 1 in 1000 live births. The incidence in fetuses is much higher, and many of these also have other malformations. Cleft palate alone occurs in about 1 of 2,500 white births. Cleft lip is more common in males, and cleft palate is more common in females. Cleft lip is one or more splits (clefts) in the upper lip. Cleft lip can range from a small indentation in the lip to a split in the lip that may extend up into one or both nostrils. Cleft lip develops in about the sixth to eighth week of gestation, when structures in the upper jaw do not fuse properly and the upper lip does not completely merge. Sometimes the nasal cavity, palate, and upper teeth are also affected in an opening in the roof of the mouth that develops when the cleft palate bones and tissues do not completely join during fetal growth, sometime between the 7th and 12th weeks of gestation. The severity and type of cleft palate vary according to where the cleft occurs on the palate and whether all the layers of the palate are affected. A mild form of cleft palate may not be visible because tissue covers the cleft. A complete cleft palate involves all layers of tissue of the soft palate, extends to and includes the hard palate, and may continue to the lip and nose. Sometimes problems associated with cleft palate also include deformities of the nasal cavities and/or the partition separating them (septum).

An ultrasound detection of cleft lip and palate may be seen as early as 14 to 16 weeks of gestation. Cleft palate and cleft lip may occur independent of each other or at the same time. The hard palate is the front part of the roof of the mouth, and the soft palate is the back part of the roof of the mouth. This description may include whether the uvulais affected. The latter is impossible to detect prenatally. Cleft lip is classified according to its location and severity. Unilateral cleft lip affects one side of the mouth; bilateral cleft lip affects both sides of the mouth. A complete cleft lip is a deep split in the upper lip extending into one or both sides of the nose; an incomplete cleft lip affects only one side of the upper lip. It may appear as a slight indentation or as a deep notch.

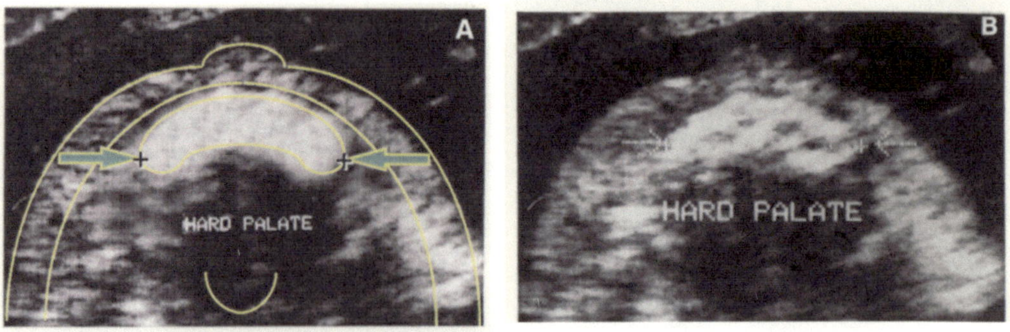

Fig. 12. Sonographic picture of normal primary palate (The alveolar ridge)

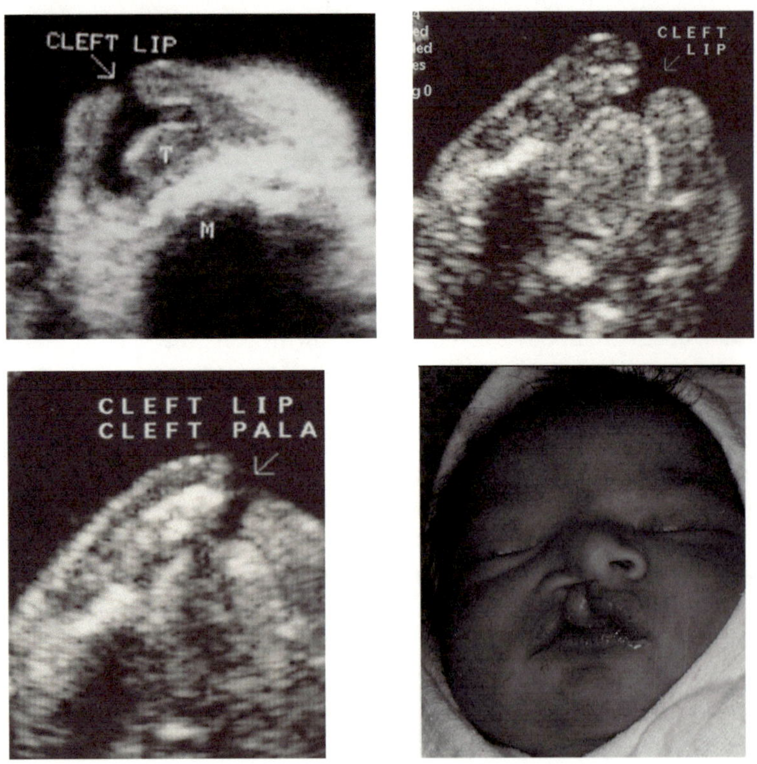

Fig. 13. Sonographic pictures of cleft lip

Ultrasonography can be used to identify clefting in the lip and primary palate (alveolar ridge). The ultrasound detecting rates of facial clefting have been reported as low as 21-30% using two-dimensional ultrasound (Crane et al., 1994). Accurate characterization of the fetal clefting is an important aspect of ultrasound diagnosis. Three-dimensional ultrasound may be useful in defining the location and extent of facial clefting *in utero* (Johnson et al., 2000). Although three-dimensional images of the fetal alveolar ridge can be obtained, two-dimensional sonographic images are obtained more easily, rapidly and accurately (Goldstein et al., 1999).

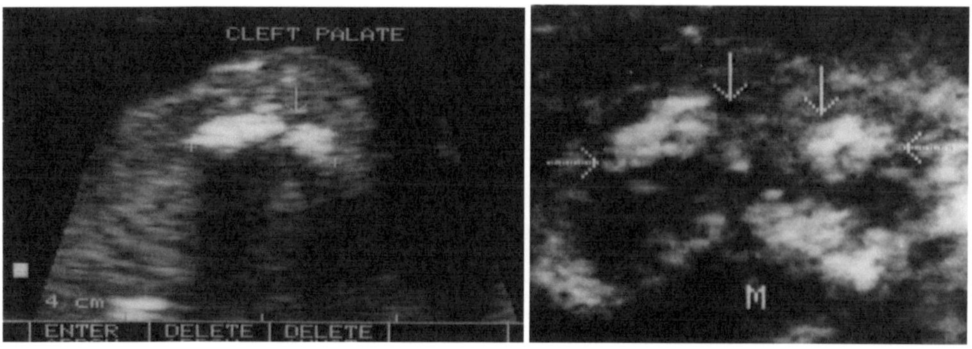

Fig. 14. Sonographic pictures of cleft palate (15 & 23 weeks of gestation)

Gestation [weeks]	Mean [mm]	±SD [mm]
14 -15	10.5	1.3
16	11.7	1.1
17	16.6	2.5
18	17.5	1.1
19	18.0	1.1
20	18.5	1.1
21	18.5	2.1
22	19.9	1.7
23	20.5	1.9
24	21.3	2.7
25	22.8	1.9
26	23.6	2.6
27-28	23.6	2.1
29	25.5	2.2
30	26.3	2.5
31	26.5	2.1
32	26.7	2.0

Table 16. Normal values of the fetal alveolar ridge width (Goldstein et al., 1999)

11. The chin: Microganthia-retroganthia or prognathia

Abnormal size of the chin, micrognathia and macrognathia, and abnormal length of the philtrum (short or long) are morphological features in numerous syndromes. Micrognathia is a common finding in many chromosome aberrations and dysmorphic syndromes (Gulla et al., 2005). Investigators have reported a series with subjective micrognathia, 66% of whom had chromosomal abnormalities (Nicolaides et al., 1993). Others reported that micrognathia was associated with aneuploidy in 25% and 38% of cases (Benacerraf et al., 1984; Turner & Twining, 1993). Sivan et al. (1997) established normative dimensions for objective chin length. Measurements of the chin length, was performed between the lower lip and the apex of the chin in mid-sagittal plane.

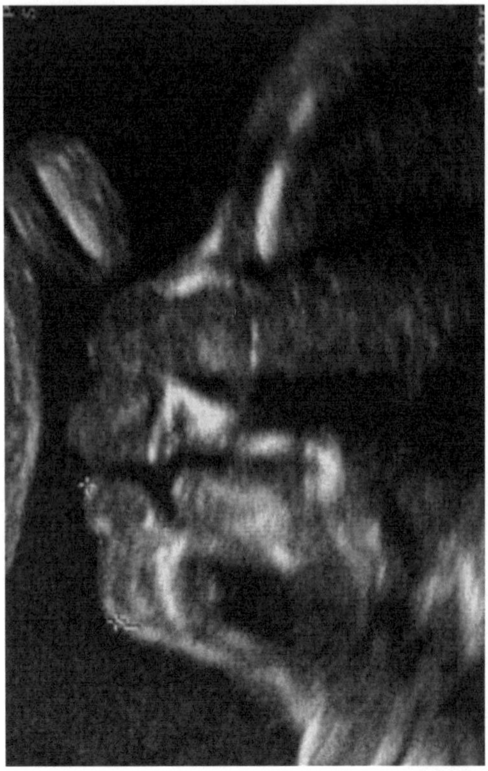

Fig. 15. Chin length measured between the lower lip and the apex of the chin (Sivan et al., 1977)

GA	Mean	SD	Range
Age (weeks)	**(mm)**		
16-17.9	5	1	3-6
18-19.9	7	1	6-9
20-21.9	8	2	7-10
22-23.9	10	1	9-11
24-25.9	11	2	8-13
26-27.9	11	2	9-12
28-29.9	13	2	11-15
30-31.9	15	2	13-17
32-33.9	18	2	16-20
34.35.9	17	2	15-19
36-37.9 23	1	22-24	

Table 17. Chin length (Sivan et al., 1997)

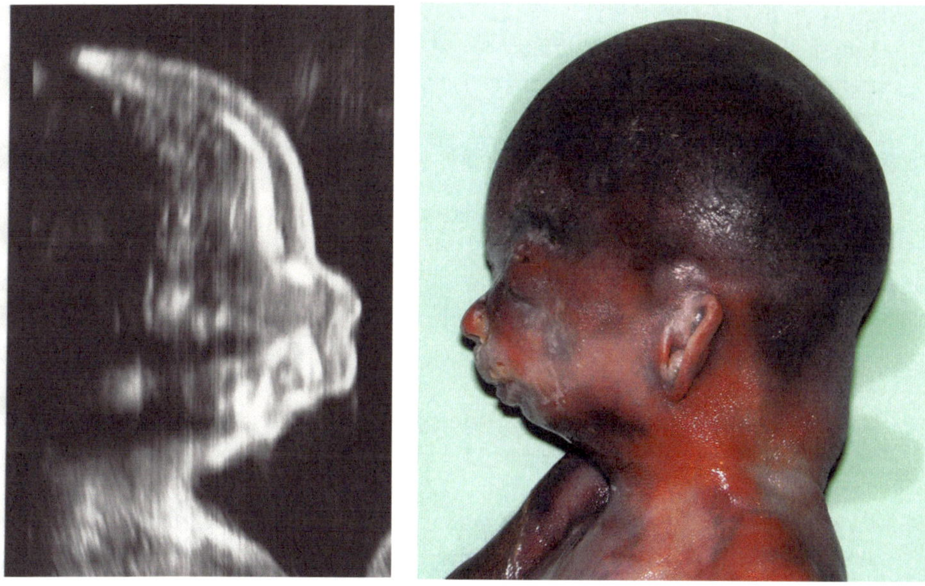

Fig. 16. Sagittal scan and postmortem of a fetus at 16 weeks of gestation shows prominent forehead and retrognathia

12. References

Arai, T. & Kragic, D. (1999). Variability of Wind and Wind Power, In: *Wind Power,* S.M. Muyeen, (Ed.), 289-321, Scyio, ISBN 978-953-7619-81-7, Vukovar, Croatia

Lima, P.; Bonarini, A. & Mataric, M. (2004). *Application of Machine Learning,* InTech, ISBN 978-953-7619-34-3, Vienna, Austria

Li, B.; Xu, Y. & Choi, J. (1996). Applying Machine Learning Techniques, *Proceedings of ASME 2010 4th International Conference on Energy Sustainability*, pp. 14-17, ISBN 842-6508-23-3, Phoenix, Arizona, USA, May 17-22, 2010

Aase, J.M.; Wilson, A.C. & Smith, D.W. (1973). Small ear in Downs' syndrome: a helpful diagnosis aid. *Journal of Pediatrics*, Vol.82, No.5, (May), pp. 845-847.

Achiron, R.; Ben Arie, A.; Gabbay, U.; Mashiach, S.; Rotstein, Z. & Lipitz, S. (1997) Development of the fetal tongue between 14 and 26 weeks of gestation: in utero ultrasonographic measurements. *Ultrasound in Obstetrics & Gynecology*, Vol. 9, No.1, (January), pp. 39-41.

Awwad, J.T.; Azar, G.B.; Karam, K.S. & Nicolaides KH. (1994). Ear length: a potential sonographic marker for Down syndrome. *International Journal of Gynaecology and Obstetrics*, Vol.44, No. 3, (March), pp. 233-238.

Benacerraf, B.R. (1998). *Ultrasound of fetal syndromes*. Churchill Livingstone: New York, London, Philadelphia, San Francisco, pp. 83-223.

Benacerraf, B.R.; Frigoletto, F.D. Jr. & Bieber, F.R. (1984). The fetal face: ultrasound examination. *Radiology*, Vol.153, No.2, (November), pp. 495-497.

Bergsma, D. (1979). *Birth defects compendium*. 2nd ed., Macmillan.

Chen, M.; Wang, H.F.; Leung, T.Y.; Sahota, D.S.; Borenstein, M.; Nicolaides, K.; Lao, T.T. & Lau, T.K. (2011). Frontomaxillary facial angle at 11 + 0 to 13 + 6 weeks in Chinese population. *Journal of Maternal-Fetal and Neonatal Medicine*, Vol.24, No.3 (March), pp. 498-501.

Chen, M.; Yang, X.; Leung, T.Y.; Sahota, D.S.; Fung, T.Y.; Chan, L.W.; Lao, T.T. & Lau, T.K. (2009). Study on the applicability of frontomaxillary facial angle in the first-trimester trisomy 21 fetuses in Chinese population. *Prenatal Diagnosis*, Vol.29, No.12, (December), pp. 1141-1144.

Chitkara, U.; Lee, L.; Oehlert, J.W.; Bloch, D.A.; Holbrook, R.H.; El-Sayed, Y.Y. & Druzin, M.L. (2002). Fetal ear length measurement: a useful predictor of aneuploidy? Ultrasound in Obstetrics & Gynecology, Vol.19, No.2, (February), pp. 131-135.

Cicero, S.; Curcio, P.; Papageorghiou, A.; Sonek, J. & Nicolaides, K. (2001). Absence of nasal bone in fetuses with trisomy 21 at 11-14 weeks of gestation: an observational study. Lancet, Vol.358, No.9294, (November 17), pp. 1665-1667.

Crane, J.P.; LeFevre, M.L.; Winborn, R.C.; Evans, J.K.; Ewigman, B.G.; Bain, R.P.; Frigoletto, F.D. & McNellis, D. (1994). A randomized trial of prenatal ultrasonographic screening: impact on the detection, management, and outcome of anomalous fetuses. The RADIUS Study Group. *American Journal of Obstetrics and Gynecology*, Vol.171, No.2 (August), pp. 392-399.

Cuick, W.; Provenzano, L.; Sullvan, C.A.; Gallousis, F.M. & Rodis, J. (2004). Fetal nasal bone length in euploid and aneuploid fetuses between 11 and 20 weeks' gestation. A prospective study. *Journal of Ultrasound in Medicine*, Vol.23, No.10, (October), pp. 1327-1333.

Goldstein I., Jakobi P., Tamir A., & Goldstick O. (1999). Nomogram of the fetal alveolar ridge: a possible screening tool for the detection of primary cleft palate. *Ultrasound in Obstetrics & Gynecology*, Vol.14, No. 5, (November), pp. 333-337.

Goldstein I., Reece E.A., Gianluigi P., O'Connor T.Z., Lockwood C.J. & Hobbins J.C. (1988). Sonographic assessment of the fetal frontal lobe: A potential tool for prenatal diagnosis of microcephaly. *American Journal of Obstetrics & Gynecology*, Vol.158, No. 5, (May), pp. 1057-1062.

Goldstein I., Reiss A., Rajamim B.S. & Tamir A. (2005). Nomogram of maxillary bone length in normal pregnancies. *Journal of Ultrasound in Medicine*, Vol.24, No.9, (September), pp. 1229-1233.

Goldstein I., Tamir A., Itskovitz-Eldor J. & Zimmer E.Z. (1997). Growth of the fetal nose width and nostril distance in normal pregnancies. *Ultrasound in Obstetrics & Gynecology*, Vol. 9, No.1, (January), pp. 35-38.

Goldstein I., Tamir A., Weiner Z. & Jakobi P. (2010). Dimensions of the fetal facial profile in normal pregnancy. *Ultrasound in Obstetrics & Gynecology*, Vol.35, No.2, (February), pp. 191–194.

Goldstein I., Tamir A., Zimmer E.Z.& Itskovitz-Eldor J. (1998). Growth of the fetal orbit and lens in normal pregnancies. *Ultrasound in Obstetrics & Gynecology*, Vol. 12, No.3, pp. 175-179.

Goldstein I., Weissman A., Brill-Zamir R., Laevsky I. & Drugan A. (2003). Ethmocephaly caused by de novo translocation 18; 21 – prenatal diagnosis. *Prenatal Diagnosis*, Vol.23; No.10, (October), pp. 788-790.

Guis F., Vill Y., Vincent Y., Doumerc S., Pons J.C. & Frydman R. (1995). Ultrasound evaluation of the length of the fetal nasal bones throughout gestation. *Ultrasound in Obstetric Gynecology*, Vol.5, No.5, (May), pp. 304-307.

Gull I., Wolman I., Merlob P.,Jaffa A.J., Lessing J.B. & Yaron Y. (2005). Nomograms for the sonographic measurement of the fetal philtrum and chin. *Fetal Diagnosis and Therapy*, Vol.20, No. 2 (March-April), pp. 127–131.

Jeanty P., Cantraine F., Consaert E., Romero R. & Hobbins J.C. (1984). The binocular distance: A new way to estimate fetal age. *Journal of Ultrasound in Medicine*; Vol.3, No.6, (June), pp. 241-243.

Johnson, D.D.; Pretorius, D.H.; Budorick, N.E.; Jones, M.C.; Lou, K.V.; James, G.M. & Nelson, T.R. (2000). Fetal lip and primary palate: three-dimensional versus two-dimensional US. *Radiology*, Vol.217, No.1, (October), pp. 236-239.

Lettieri L., Rodis J.F., Vintzileos A.M., Feeney L., Ciarleglio .L & Craffey A. (1993). Ear length in second-trimester aneuploid fetuses. *Obstetrics and Gynecology*, Vol.18, No. 1, (January), pp. 57-60.

Mayden K.L., Totora M., Berkowitz R.L., Bracken M. & Hobbins J.C. (1982). Orbital diameters: a new parameter for prenatal diagnosis and dating. *American Journal of Obstetrics & Gynecology*, Vol.1;144 No.3, (October), pp. 289-297.

McGahan J.P., Nyberg D.A. & Mack L.A. (1990). Sonography of facial features of alobar and semilobar holoprosecephaly *American Journal of Roentgenol*, Vol.154, No.1, (January), pp. 143-148.

Nicolaides K.H., Salvesen D.R., Snijders R.J. & Gosden C.M. (1993). Fetal facial defects. Associated malformations and chromosomal abnormaties. *Fetal Diagnosis and Therapy*, Vol.8, No.1, (January-February) pp.1-9.

Pilu G., Reece R.A., Romero R., Bovicelli L. & Hobbis J.C. (1986). Prenatal diagnosis of craniofacial malformations with ultrasonography. *American Journal of Obstetrics & Gynecology*, Vol.155; No.1, (July), pp. 45-50.

Shimizu T., Salvador L., Hughes-Benzie R., Dawson L., Nimrod C. & Allanson J. (1977). The role of reduced ear size in the prenatal detection of chromosomal abnormalities. *Prenatal Diagnosis*, Vol.17, No.6, (June), pp. 545-549.

Sivan E., Chan L., Mallozzi-Eberle A. & Reece E.A. (1997). Sonographic imaging of the fetal face and the establishment of normative dimensions for chin length and upper lip width. *American Journal of Perinatology*, Vol.14, No. 4, (April), pp. 191-194.

Sivri D., Dane C., Dane B., Cetin A. & Yayla M. (2006) Nomogram of fetal nasal bone length at 11-13 gestational weeks in fetuses. *Perinatal Journal*, Vol.14, No.3, (September), pp.

Smith D. & Jones K.L. (1988). *Smith's recognizable patterns of human malformation*, 4th *ed.* Philadelphia, WB Saunders Company.

Turner G.M. & Twining P. (1993) The facial profile in the diagnosis of fetal abnormalities. *Clinical Radiology*, Vol.47, No.6 (June), pp. 389-95.

Yeo L., Guzman E.R., Day-Salvatore D., Vintzileos A.M. & Walters C. (1998). Prenatal detection of fetal aneuploidy using sonographic ear length. *American Journal of Obstetrics & Gynecology*, Vol.178:S141.

7

Current Issues Regarding Prenatal Diagnosis of Inborn Errors of Cholesterol Biosynthesis

Maria Luís Cardoso[1,2], Mafalda Barbosa[3,4],
Ana Maria Fortuna[3] and Franklim Marques[1,2]
[1]*Faculty of Pharmacy, University of Porto, Porto*
[2]*Institute for Molecular and Cell Biology, University of Porto, Porto*
[3]*Medical Genetics Centre Jacinto Magalhães,*
National Health Institute Ricardo Jorge Porto
[4]*Life and Health Sciences Research Institute, School of Health Sciences,*
University of Minho, Braga
Portugal

1. Introduction

It has long been established that there is a relationship between hypercholesterolemia and cardiovascular disease in adulthood. However, only in the 90s, the biological consequence of low levels of cholesterol for mitotic cells was highlighted, with the description of the devastating effect of hypocholesterolemia on fetal development. This was supported by the discovery of a group of metabolic diseases caused by mutations in genes coding for enzymes involved in endogenous synthesis of cholesterol. This group is still growing as new diseases, phenotypes and mutated genes are being described by researchers. Despite the fact that they share some common clinical features - including abnormal morphogenesis and growth retardation - these inherited metabolic diseases are still poorly recognized in daily obstetric clinical practice.

Cholesterol is an essential lipid found in all mammalian cells. It can modulate the activity of the Hedgehog proteins, which act as morphogens that regulate the precise patterning of many embryonic structures [Gofflot et al., 2003]. Furthermore, cholesterol is a key component of lipid-rafts, which have a structural role in cellular membranes and myelin sheets and it is a precursor molecule for sterol-based compounds, including bile acids, oxysterols, neurosteroids, glucocorticoids, mineralocorticoids, and sex hormones like estrogen and testosterone [Correa-Cerro et al., 2005]. Due to the panoply of biological functions of the sterols, a decrease of its availability during pregnancy has major consequences to the fetus, severely impairing his development [Cardoso et al., 2005a].

2. Intestinal cholesterol absorption, transport and metabolism

Dietary cholesterol is absorbed from bile salt micelles, with fatty acids and phospholipids, at the proximal part of the small intestine, in a process which involves Nieman-Pick C1-Like1 protein (NPC1L1). This protein contains a sterol sensing domain (SSD) and is located in the brush-border membrane of enterocytes where it plays a critical role in the intestinal uptake of cholesterol and phytosterols [Ikonen, 2006]. Once inside the enterocyte cholesterol is esterified by acyl-CoA: cholesterol acyltransferase (ACAT) whereas sterols other than cholesterol, are transported back into the intestinal lumen by an heterodimer transporter G5/G8 ATP binding cassette (*ABCG5, ABCG8*)[1]. Such mechanism prevents phytosterols molecules from passing to the blood to any significant extent [Charlton-Menys & Durrington, 2007].

In order to enter in blood circulation cholesterol from enterocytes should be incorporated in lipoproteins named chylomicron. Chylomicrons assembly begins with the formation of primordial, phospholipid-rich particles in the membrane, taking together apolipoprotein B48 (*ApoB-48*)[2] and cholesterol. Later in the lumen of the smooth endoplasmic reticulum (ER) these particles are converted into large chylomicrons. After that, they are transported (via specialized vesicles) from the ER to the Golgi[3], for secretion into the lacteals of the intestine, and then they finally pass from linfa to blood (via thoracic duct) [Hussain et al., 2005; Charlton-Menys & Durrington, 2007; Kindel, et al., 2010]. Once chilomicrons are in blood circulation they became smaller due to the action of lipoprotein lipase (LPL)[4], which is anchored to the vascular endothelium of several organs, and hydrolyses the trigliceride from chilomicrons. Subsequently the circulating cholesterol-rich chylomicron remnant particles are uptaked by the liver in a process which involves the LDL-receptor like protein (LRP) [Charlton-Menys & Durrington, 2007].

Liver, exports exogenous and endogenous cholesterol, to tisues by VLDL lipoproteins. The biosynthesis of VLDL consists of a number of distinct stages [Hebbachi & Gibbons, 2001; Shelness et al., 2001]. Briefly, the assembly of hepatic VLDL begins inside the rough ER, where, the peptide *ApoB-100* [2] is synthesized at membrane bound ribosomes and then sent through a protein channel into the cytoplasm. Additionally, microsomal triglyceride transfer protein (MTP)[5] binds the precursor peptide and joins some triglycerides, phospholipids, and cholesteryl esters, allowing *ApoB-100* to fold around a small lipid core. Then a higher amount of triglycerides are transferred into the precursor VLDL particle, and it sorts to the Golgi apparatus where additional lipids are recruited in order to form the mature VLDL lipoprotein [Daniels et al., 2009]. Finally VLDLs enter in circulation and distribute free fatty acids to muscle and adipose tissues expressing LPL and become intermediary density lipopoteins (IDLs) that can either be removed from circulation by the liver or they can lose further free fatty acids becoming low density lipoproteins (LDLs) which are important cholesterol transporters [Daniels et al., 2009].

Therefore, low density lipoprotein receptor (LDLR)[6], a transmembrane glicoprotein responsible for uptake of cholesterol-carrying lipoproteins from blood circulation, binds lipoprotein particles at the cell surface, which are internalized by endocytosis and later in the low-pH environment of the endosome, acid-induced dissociation of ligand and receptor occurs. LDLR peptide is recycled back to the membrane and LDL particles are released into the lysosomes whose enzymes degradate the lipoproteine into amino acids and lipid components. Cholesteryl esters are hydrolyzed by lysosomal acid lipase (LAL)[7] to free cholesterol [Daniels et al., 2009; Jeon & Blacklow, 2005]. Therefore cholesterol can be re-esterified by ACAT (a membrane-bound enzyme residing in the ER) and stored as lipid droplets [Zhang et al., 2003; Liu et al., 2005]. The mechanisms by which free and esterified cholesterol ingress and egress endosomes and lipid droplets, are not fully clarified.

Neverthless proteins NPC1[8] and NPC2 are involved in such process and other proteins like MLN64 (STARD3) and MENTHO (STARD3NL), are still under evaluation [Miller & Bose, 2011; Vanier, 2010].

At steady state most cholesterol is in plasma membrane, but it must move inside the cell in order to be presented to the enzymes encharged of its metabolization, and it is transported between membrane organelles (as a component of lipid bilayers) in transport vesicles, as well as by non-vesicular means [Liscum et al., 1995; Maxfield & Wüstner, 2002].

Meanwhile, the liver is consistently manufacturing high density lipoproteins (HDL) which have the critical task of removing excess cholesterol and serve as transport particles by which peripheral cell cholesterol is collected and delivered to the liver for catabolism in a process named reverse cholesterol transport [Ikonen, 2006]. The rate limiting step in this process is cholesterol efflux mediated by ABCA1[9] [Daniels et al., 2010].

Cells inside the brain are cut off from this circuit by the blood-brain barrier and must regulate their cholesterol content in a different manner [Pfrieger & Ungerer, 2011].

As cholesterol cannot be degraded by cells into noncyclic hydrocarbon products, hepatocytes excrete it into the bile, either directly, as free cholesterol, as well as transformed in bile salts. Bile salts are synthesized via two routes, the classic or neutral pathway and the alternative or acidic one [Kosters et al., 2003]. Cholesterol 7α-hydroxylase (CYP7A1) is a hepatic microsomal cytochrome P450 enzyme that catalyzes the first step of bile acid synthesis in the classical pathway, whereas sterol 27-hydroxylase (CYP27A1) is the first enzyme of the alternative one. It is a mitochondrial cytochrome P450 ubiquitous enzyme with a much broader biologic role; it is involved in the 27-hydroxylation of a variety of sterols (cholesterol included) and in the formation of potentially important regulatory sterols [Dias & Ribeiro, 2011].

All major classes of biologically active steroid hormones are also synthesized from cholesterol by a complex array of enzymes located both in the mitochondria and ER [Miller, 2011; White, 1994]. Adrenals and gonads receive cholesterol from low-density lipoproteins, store it as cholesterol esters, and transport cholesterol to mitochondria by ill-defined but critical mechanisms [Miller, 2011]. Effectively, the acute quantitative regulation of steroidogenesis is determined by cholesterol import into mitochondria by the steroidogenic acute regulatory protein (STAR) which undergoes conformational changes for accept ing and discharge cholesterol molecules [Miller & Auchus, 2011]. Then P450scc /CYP11A1 enzyme, located in the inner mitochondrial membrane catalyses the conversion of cholesterol to pregnenolone, the first step of steroidogenesis [Miller & Auchus, 2011].

Control of cholesterol homeostasis is a highly regulated process, consistent with the overall importance of this lipid for normal cellular function, with several transcription factors and functioning proteins playing important roles and regulating intracellular cholesterol levels [Tarling & Eduards, 2011]. Mutations in genes codifying for proteins involved in the above referred pathways (and signalised with small numbers), alter sterol homeostasis and results in specific diseases. Table 1 resumes the most commum phenotypes associated to deficient cholesterol intra and extracelular transport and metabolism which was construct based on OMIM (http://www.ncbi.nlm.nih.gov/omim) available data.

Disease	MIM	Gene	Phenotype
1. Sitosterolemia	#210250	*ABCG5,* *ABCG8*	AR. Characterized by unrestricted intestinal absorption of phytosterols. Patients show very high levels of plant sterols in the plasma with accumulation in tendons (tuberous xanthomas) and arteries.
2. Hypobetalipo- proteinaemia	+107730	*APOB*	Apolipoprotein B, occurs in the plasma in 2 main forms, apoB48 (synthesized exclusively by the gut) and apoB100 (synthesized by the liver) resulting from differential splicing of the same primary mRNA transcript. Heterozygous show reduced plasma concentrations of LDL cholesterol, total triglycerides, and APOB less than 50% of normal values.
3. Anderson disease (Chylomicrons retention disease)	#246700	*SAR1B*	AR. It is a disease of severe fat malabsorption and steatorrhea, associated with failure to thrive in infancy. Patients show low fasting plasma concentrations of plasma total, HDL, and LDL cholesterol. Electron microscopy studies of jejunal biopsy specimens showed severe steatosis, and an apparent block of chylomicron secretion from the ER into the Golgi apparatus.
4. Hyperlipo- proteinemia type Ia	#238600	*LPL*	AR. Massive hyperchylomicronemia occurs when the patient is on a normal diet and disappears completely in a few days on fat-free feeding. Caused by low tissue activity of lipoprotein lipase (a defect in removal of chylomicrons and of other triglyceride-rich lipoproteins). Characterized by attacks of abdominal pain, hepatosplenomegaly, eruptive xanthomas, and lactescence of the plasma.
Hyperlipo- proteinemia type Ib	#207750	*APOCII*	Deficiency of apolipoprotein C-II the activator of lipoprotein lipase. Clinically and biochemically simulates lipoprotein lipase deficiency.
5. Abetalipo- proteinaemia	#200100	*MTP*	Caused by mutations in the microsomal triglyceride transfer protein. Features are celiac syndrome, pigmentary degeneration of the retina, progressive ataxic neuropathy and acanthocytosis. Intestinal absorption of lipids is defective, serum cholesterol very low, and serum beta lipoprotein absent.

Disease	MIM	Gene	Phenotype
6. Familial hypercholesterolemia	#143890	*LDLR*	AD. Caused by mutations in the low density lipoprotein receptor gene. Heterozygotes develop tendinous xanthomas, corneal arcus, and coronary artery disease (fourth or fifth decade). Homozygotes develop these features at an accelerated rate in addition to planar xanthomas, which may be evident at birth in the web between the first 2 digits.
7. Wolman disease	#278000	*LIPA*	It is caused by lysosomal LAL deficiency. Homozygous present liver failure, hypercholesterolemia, hypertriglyceridaemia, liver fibrosis, early atherosclerosis and early death. Heterozygous show a milder phenotype named cholesteryl ester storage disease.
8. Niemann-Pick disease type C	#257220	*NPC1*	AR. Neurodegenerative lipid storage disorder characterized by a highly variable clinical phenotype. In the classic form symptoms appearing between 2 and 4 years and patients develop neurologic abnormalities (ataxia, grand mal seizures, and loss of previously learned speech). Diagnosis relies on detection of delayed LDL-derived cholesterol esterification on skin fibroblasts as well as in filipin staining.
9. Tangier disease	#205400	*ABCA1*	AR disorder characterized by markedly reduced levels of HDL resulting in tissue accumulation of cholesterol esters. Clinical features include very large, yellow-orange tonsils, enlarged liver, spleen and lymph nodes, hypocholesterolemia, and abnormal chylomicron remnants. Coronary artery disease is increased in heterozygotes for ABCA1 deficiency.
10. 7α-hydroxylase deficiency	*118455	*CYP7A1*	Hypercholesterolemia (high LDL), hypertriglyceridemia, premature gallstone disease.
11. Cerebrotendinous xanthomatosis	#213700	*CYP27A1*	AR. Characterized by progressive neurologic dysfunction, premature atherosclerosis, and cataracts. Large deposits of cholesterol and cholestanol are found in tissues, particularly the Achilles tendons, brain, and lungs.
12. Congenital lipoid adrenal hyperplasia	#201710	*CYP11A1* *STAR*	Congenital lipoid adrenal hyperplasia is the most severe form of congenital adrenal hyperplasia. Affected individuals can synthesize no steroid hormones; hence, all are phenotypic females with a severe salt-losing syndrome that is fatal if not treated in early infancy.

Legend: AR-autosomal recessive; AD-autosomal dominant; LAL-lysosomal acid lipase

Table 1. Diseases / phenotypes associated to deficient cholesterol transport and metabolism

3. The cholesterol biosynthesis pathway

Cholesterol is a 27-carbon tetracyclic compound synthesised by all nucleated mammalian cells [Kelly & Herman, 2001] by a metabolic process involving approximately 30 enzymatic reactions [Ikonen, 2006] which take place in several cellular compartments: cytoplasm, ER (or its extensions), nuclear envelope and peroxisomes [Ikonen, 2006; Thompson et al., 1987]. The substrate for cholesterol synthesis is acetyl-CoA which is derived largely from glucose in the brain, and from fatty acids and other fuels in other tissues [Clayton, 1998].

Although complex, the biosynthesis of cholesterol is only one element of the larger isoprenoid biosynthetic system, which incorporates the *de novo* synthesis of important biomolecules as diverse as dolichol, ubiquinone, heme A or farnesyl pyrophosphate [Kelly & Herman, 2001].

For simplification one can considerer five major steps on the metabolic pathway of cholesterol synthesis [Figure 1].

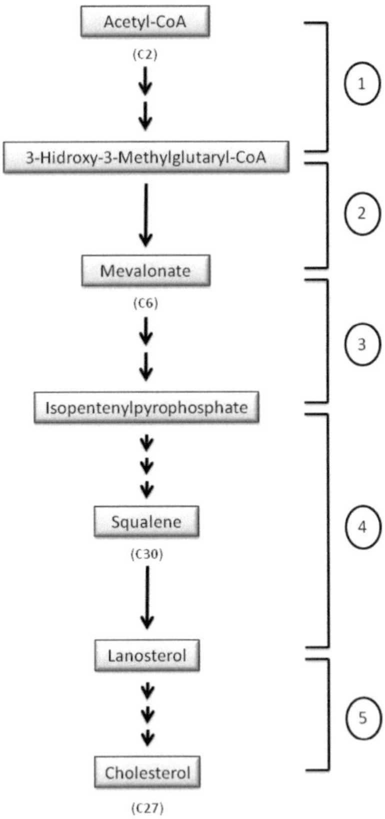

Fig. 1. Simplified schematic representation of cholesterol biosynthesis pathway.

Steps one to four catalyze the transformation of acetyl-CoA into the first sterol of the cascade: lanosterol. The fifth step includes all the reactions needed to transform this sterol into cholesterol [http://themedicalbiochemistrypage.org/cholesterol.html]. The biologically significant details of each step are:

1. Conversion of acetyl-CoAs to 3-hydroxy-3-methylglutaryl-CoA (HMG-CoA), an organic acid conjugate of intermediate metabolism that is also important for ketogenesis.
2. HMG-CoA conversion to mevalonate by HMG-CoA reductase, the limitating step of cholesterol biosynthesis. In fact, HMG-CoA reductase is subject to complex regulatory control by four distinct mechanisms (i) feed-back inhibition, (ii) control of gene expression, (iii) rate of enzyme degradation and (iv) phosphorylation-dephosphorylation (the first three are exerted by the cholesterol molecule itself).
3. 3. Mevalonate conversion to the isoprene based molecule, isopentenyl pyrophosphate with the concomitant loss of CO_2.
4. Isopentenyl pyrophosphate conversion to lanosterol. The reactions of this stage are also required for the synthesis of other important compounds as previously referred: (i) isopentenyl-tRNAs (the isopentenyl groups in tRNAs are thought to be important in stabilizing codon-anti-codon interaction, thus preventing misreading of the genetic code during protein synthesis), (ii) dolichol which is required for protein N-glycosylation, (iii) farnesyl and geranylgeranyl pyrophosphate essential for protein prenylation which is a post-translational modification required to commit proteins to cellular membranes and (iv) ubiquinone, which is an important component of mitochondrial respiratory chain [Clayton, 1998, Ikonen, 2006].
5. Lanosterol conversion to cholesterol [Figure 2].

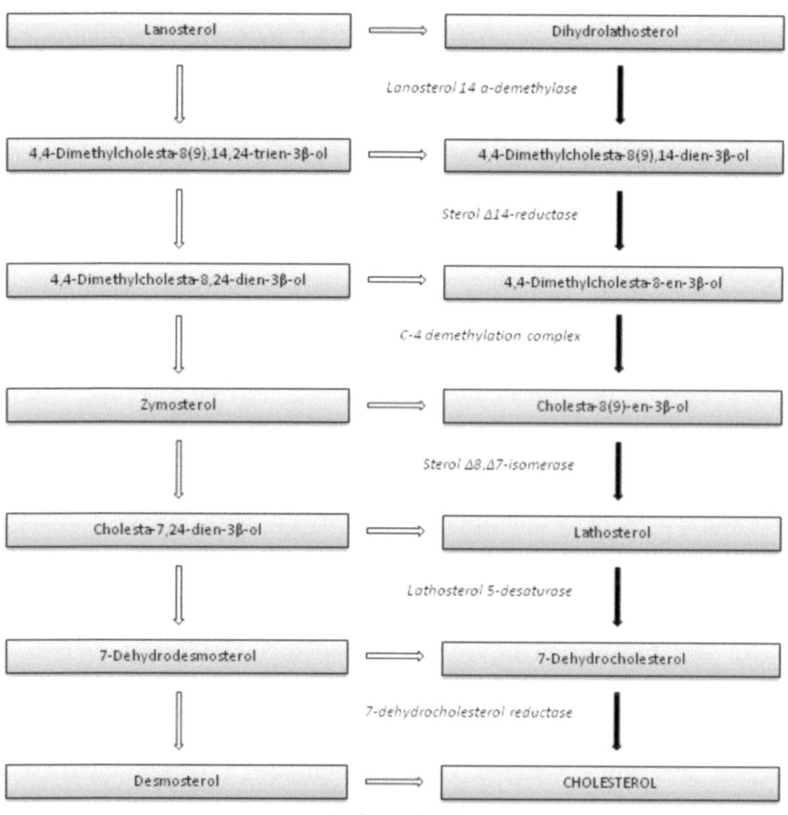

Fig. 2. The distal part of cholesterol biosyntesis pathway: from lanosterol to cholesterol

This stage constitutes the post-lanosterol part of cholesterol biosynthesis pathway. It includes a series of enzymatic reactions namely (i) three demethylations at C4α, C4β and C14, which converts the 30-carbon molecule of lanosterol into the 27-carbon cholesterol ; (ii) the isomerization of the $\Delta^{8(9)}$ double bond to Δ^7 double bond, (iii) one reaction of desaturation to form a Δ^5 double bond; (iv) and finally the reduction of three double bonds Δ^{14}, Δ^{24}, Δ^7 [Porter, 2003].

4. Sterols and development

Cholesterol is indispensable for embryogenesis and fetal development in higher vertebrates. The fetus obtains most cholesterol from *de novo* synthesis, with fetal sterols synthesis rates being greater than those observed in other extra hepatic tissues. This happens, most likely, because of the large cholesterol fetal requirements, in order to sustain the rapid intra-uterine growth [Woollett, 2005]. Nevertheless, the fetus appears to have an exogeneous source of cholesterol as well. In fact, some studies have suggested that maternal cholesterol may also contribute to the cholesterol accrued in the fetus [Lindegaard et al., 2008; McConihay et al., 2001; Yoshida & Wada, 2005]. Reinforcing this hypothesis, a strong association with preterm delivery in caucasian mothers with low serum cholesterol during pregnancy was found, and smaller birth weight in term babies from such mothers [Edison et al., 2007]. Thus, two layers of cells must be crossed by maternal cholesterol to reach the fetal circulation (i) the trophoblasts (which form the layer closest to the maternal circulation) and (ii) the endothelium (locate between the trophoblast and fetal circulation) [Woollett, 2011]. According to some experiments, the modulation of maternal-fetal cholesterol transport has potential for *in uterus* therapy of fetuses that lack the ability to synthesize cholesterol [Lindegaard et al., 2008; Woollett, 2005].

Distal inhibitors of cholesterol biosynthesis have been studied for more than 30 years as potent teratogens capable of inducing cyclopia and other birth defects. These compounds specifically block the Sonic hedgehog (Shh) signaling pathway [Cooper et al., 1998]. Hedgehog (Hh) proteins comprise a group of secreted embryonic signaling molecules that are essential for embryonic patterning [Kolejáková et al., 2010]. In higher vertebrates, including humans, they are implicated in an increasing number of different developmental processes. In fact, Shh proteins were implicated in neural tube development, lung and kidney morphogenesis and hair development, Shh and Indian hedgehog were related with skeletal morphogenesis and gastrointestinal development and Desert hedgehog with male differentiation, spermatogenesis and development of peripheral nerve sheaths [Waterman & Wanders, 2000]. Cholesterol has an important role in regulation and modification of Hedgehog proteins, what links cholesterol to early embryonic development. [Kolejáková et al., 2010]. Decreasing levels of cellular sterols correlate with diminished response of the Hh signal and sterol depletion affects the activity of Smoothened, an essential component of the Hh signal transduction apparatus [Cooper et al., 2003].

Mutations in the Sonic Hedgehog gene cause holoprosencephaly and this cerebral malformation has also been associated with perturbations of cholesterol synthesis and metabolism in mammalian embryos [Gofflot et al., 2001]. Furthermore, in rodents, triparanol treatment reproduces limb defects observed in human syndromes of cholesterol biosynthesis defects by a modification of Shh signaling in the limb resulting in an imbalance of Indian Hedgehog expression in the forming cartilage leading to reduced interdigital apoptosis and syndactyly [Gollof et al., 2003].

5. Inborn errors of post-squalene cholesterol biosynthesis

Genetic defects in enzymes responsible for cholesterol biosynthesis have recently emerged as important causes of congenital anomalies. Patients with these metabolic diseases present with complex malformation syndromes involving different organs and systems [Yu & Patel, 2005]. So far, nine polimalformative disorders due to enzymatic defects in post-squalene cholesterol biosynthesis have been identified:

a. Smith-Lemli-Opitz syndrome (SLOS),
b. X-linked dominant chondrodysplasia punctata type 2 (CDPX2),
c. Congenital hemidysplasia with ichthyosiform erythroderma and limb defects syndrome (CHILD)
d. CK syndrome
e. Greenberg dysplasia,
f. Antley-Bixler syndrome with ambiguous genitalia (POR deficiency)
g. Desmosterolosis,
h. Lathosterolosis,
i. Sterol-C4-methyloxidase–like deficiency.

6. Prenatal diagnosis of cholesterol biosynthesis disorders

For most inborn errors of metabolism, before attempting to perform prenatal diagnosis, it is essential to establish, or confirm the diagnosis of the disorder under consideration in the proband, or affected relatives. Nevertheless as inborn errors of cholesterol biosynthesis have been associated to a gestational biochemical marker (low maternal estriol) and abnormal ultrasound features, in many cases one can suspect of this spectrum of disorders in the course of a pregnancy, even without a previous index case in the family.

6.1 Smith-Lemli-Opitz syndrome

The Smith-Lemli-Opitz syndrome (SLOS, MIM #270400), is the most frequent disease of this group of inherited metabolic disorders, with a prevalence that varies between 1: 22.000 and 1: 60.000, depending on the population. Nevertheless, a higher prevalence (between 1: 2.500 and 1: 4.444) - close to that of cystic fibrosis and higher than phenylketonuria - would be expected based on carriers frequency studies [Porter et al., 2003].

SLOS is caused by a deficit of the enzyme 7-dehydrocholesterol reductase (3-β-hydroxysterol-Δ^7-reductase, E.C.1.3.1.21), encoded by the *DHCR7* gene located on 11q13. This enzyme catalyses the conversion of 7-dehydrocholesterol to cholesterol [Waterham &, Wanders, 2000].

Since most of the cholesterol required for fetal growth and development is synthesized by the fetus, enzymatic deficiency affecting endogenous cholesterol biosynthesis leads to intrauterine growth restriction and aberrant organogenesis. Surveys of large series of patients with SLOS showed a constellation of severe abnormalities including intellectual disability, microcephaly, failure to thrive, dysmorphic face, limb abnormalities and genital abnormalities in males [Cardoso et al., 2005b].

Prenatal diagnosis of SLOS has been performed in many pregnancies both retrospectively and prospectively. The prenatal diagnosis of this autosomal recessive metabolic disorder is based on a conjugation of methods that detect the dual aspects of the pathology: the polimalformative syndrome and the metabolic abnormalities [Cardoso et al., 2005a].

6.1.1 Ultrasound findings

A number of fetuses have been so far signalized as suspected of SLOS due to the identification, by ultrasound, of suggestive fetal abnormalities, such as: nuchal edema, microcephaly, cleft palate, polidactyly, cystic kidneys, ambiguous genitalia or a 46, XY karyotype in a phenotypically female fetus [Johnson et al., 1994, Kelley & Hennekam, 2001]. Nevertheless there is no pathognomonic ultrasound pattern associated with SLOS [Irons & Tint, 1998].

Concerning the detection of malformations in SLOS fetus, Goldenberg and collaborators evaluated the main abnormalities identified. Their results are as follows i) in the first trimester [11-13 weeks of gestational age]: increased nuchal translucency (26%); ii) in the second trimester [20-22 weeks of gestational age]: nuchal edema (26%), kidney malformation (26%), polydactyly (10%) [Figure 3], ambiguous genitalia (6%) [Figure 3], cerebral malformation (10%), heart malformation (10%), intrauterine growth restriction (20%); iii) in the third trimester [30-34 weeks of gestational age]: intrauterine growth restriction (46%) [Goldenberg et al., 2004]. However one should be aware that prenatal US examination of affected fetuses can also be normal [Irons & Tint, 1998].

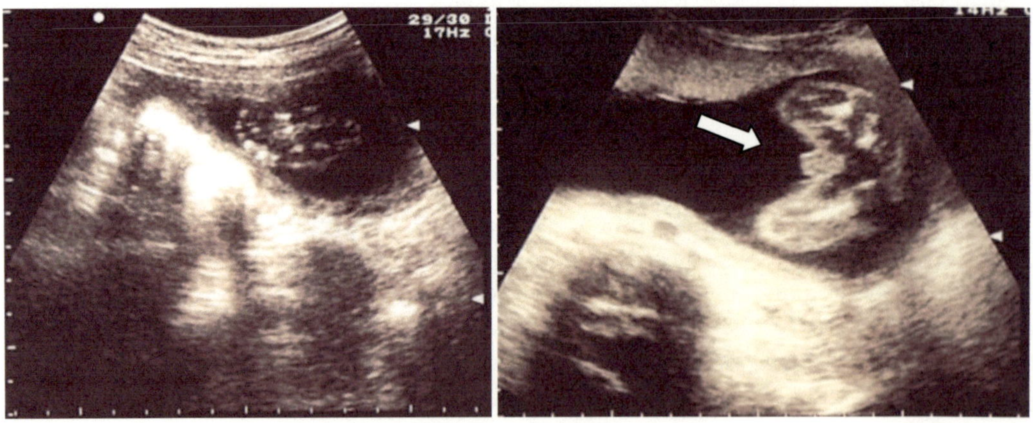

Fig. 3. Two ultrasound images of a male fetus with SLO. The white arrows are pointing a left foot with postaxial polydactyly (on the left) and a penis with large root and hypospadias (on the right).

6.1.2 Serum maternal markers

The fetoplacental biosynthesis of free estriol (μE3) requires cholesterol as substrate [Palomaki et al., 2002]. Thus unconjugated estriol is produced by the fetus and then crosses the placental barrier entering into mother's blood circulation. By consequence fetal hypocholesterolemia can be suspected, if the pregnant woman shows low levels of this compound in serum. Low or undetectable unconjugated estriol levels in maternal serum and amniotic fluid have been reported in pregnancies of fetus affected with SLO [Hyett et al., 1995; Rossiter et al., 1995; Kratz & Kelley,1999; Cardoso et al., 2005a; Craig et al., 2006].

Free estriol is not a specific marker of SLO and several other causes of low unconjugated estriol are known, namely intrauterine fetal demise and steroid sulphatase deficiency [Irons & Tint, 1998]. Meanwhile algorithms were proposed based on available values of maternal serum α-fetoprotein and human chorionic gonadotrophin together with free estriol (obtained on the second-trimester screening program, for Down syndrome and open neural tube defects) which provide a more accurate estimation of individual risk for SLOS [Palomaki et al., 2002; Craig et al., 2006; Craig et al., 2007].

According to our and others experience [Cardoso et al., 2005a; Dubuisson et al., 2008] a low level of free estriol alone is not a robust indicator for testing a pregnancy for SLOS. However the association of i) abnormal fetal US with ii) normal fetal karyotype and iii) low levels of unconjugated estriol on maternal blood are highly suggestive [Cardoso et al., 2005a; Shinawi et al., 2005; Dubuisson et al., 2008].

6.1.3 Biochemical approach

The first report concerning prenatal diagnosis SLOS based on biochemical profile of sterols in amniotic fluid was performed in 1995 by Abuelo and collaborators [Abuelo et al., 1995]. Since then several cases referring the quantification of 7-dehydrocholesterol in amniotic fluid as well as in chorionic villus either by gas chromatography or gas chromatography-mass spectrometry have been published [Irons & Tint, 1998; Chevy et al., 2005; Cardoso et al., 2005a]. The diagnosis can also be made based on the detection of low enzymatic 7-dehydrocholesterol reductase activity on cultivated amniocytes or chorionic villus [Linck et al., 2000; Ginat et al., 2004].

Nowadays liquid chromatography-tandem mass spectrometry (LC-MS-MS) is available in many clinical biochemistry laboratories and efforts have been made in order to apply this highly sensitive technology to the diagnosis of inborn errors of cholesterol biosynthesis. Recently a protocol for prenatal diagnosis of SLOS by LC-MS-MS became available [Griffiths et al., 2008]. Another promising approach concerns the non-invasive SLOS biochemical prenatal diagnosis based on identification and measurement of abnormal steroids in maternal urine [Jezela-Stanek et al., 2006; Shackleton et al., 2007].

6.1.4 Mutation analysis of *DHCR7* gene

Prenatal diagnosis of SLOS by mutation analysis of *DHCR7* gene on DNA extracted directly from amniotic fluid, chorionic villus or the respective cell cultures is widespread used at this time [Yu & Patel, 2005]. This approach is accurate and reliable [Loeffler et al., 2002]. Moreover molecular prenatal diagnosis should be considered an option: (i) in laboratories without facilities for biochemical analysis, (ii) in families with known mutations who are interested in early and rapid testing and (iii) in cases with ambiguous biochemical results [Nowaczyk et al., 2001; Löffler et al., 2009; Waye et al., 2007].

6.2 X-linked dominant chondrodysplasia punctata type 2, CHILD Syndrome and CK Syndrome

X-linked dominant chondrodysplasia punctata type 2 (CDPX2 or Conradi-Hunermann-Happle syndrome, MIM #302960) and Congenital hemidysplasia with ichthyosiform erythroderma and limb defects syndrome (CHILD syndrome, MIM #308050), are two X-linked dominant skeletal dysplasias caused by hypocholesterolemia, which affect almost exclusively females, as they are typically lethal in hemizygous males. In both diseases affected females usually present at birth with skeletal and skin abnormalities [Herman et al., 2000]. In CDPX2 these include epiphyseal stippling and asymmetric rhizomelic shortening of the limbs, follicular atrophoderma, ichthyosiform erythroderma (following the Blaschko's lines), asymmetrical cataracts and accumulation in plasma and body tissues of cholesterol precursors: 8-dehydrocholesterol and cholest-8(9)-en-3β-ol. The disorder is caused by a deficiency of the enzyme 3β-hydroxysterol-Δ^8,Δ^7-isomerase encoded by *EBP* gene [Braverman et al., 1999]. In most severe cases ultrasound during pregnancy can show polyhydramnios, intra-uterine growth restriction or both [Kelley et al., 1999].Only a few prenatal diagnosis have been reported and they were based on the identification of mutations on *EBP* gene.

Both CHILD syndrome and CK syndrome are caused by mutations in *NSDHL* gene encoding a 3β-hydroxysterol dehydrogenase [Konig et al., 2000, McLaren et al., 2010]. CHILD is associated with an inflammatory nevus with unique lateralization, ipsilateral hypoplasia of the body that affects all skeletal structures including shortness or absence of limbs and viscera such as lungs, heart or kidneys [Happle et al., 1980]. CK syndrome is an X-linked recessive intellectual disability syndrome characterized by dysmorphism, cortical brain malformations, asthenic build, increased methyl-sterol levels and it is associated to hypomorphic temperature-sensitive alleles [McLaren et al., 2010]. As far as we know, there are no reports on prenatal diagnosis of these two syndromes in literature.

6.3 Greenberg dysplasia

The Greenberg dysplasia (MIM #215140), is a rare and lethal autosomal recessive skeletal dysplasia characterized by hydrops fetalis, ectopic calcifications, "moth-eaten" skeletal dysplasia, short limbs, and abnormal chondro-osseous calcification [Madazli et al., 2001]. In 2003, Waterham and collaborators found elevated levels of a cholesterol precursor (cholesta-8,14-dien-3β-ol) in cultured skin fibroblasts of a fetus with Greenberg dysplasia, that were compatible with a deficiency of the enzyme 3-β-hydroxysterol-Δ^{14}reductase from the cholesterol biosynthesis pathway. Sequencing analysis of two candidate genes encoding putative human sterol-Δ^{14}reductases allow the identification of an homozygous mutation (resulting in a truncated protein) in *LBR* gene (which encodes a bifunctional protein - lamin B receptor - with both lamin B binding and sterol-Δ^{14}reductase domain) [Waterham et al., 2003]. After the publication of these results it was acknowledged that Greenberg dysplasia was a disorder of cholesterol biosynthesis. Nevertheless, recent studies with mice models raised some doubts about this classification and proposed that Greenberg dysplasia should be classified as a laminopathy rather than an inborn error of cholesterol synthesis [Wassif et al., 2007]. Despite this controversy i) ultrasound, ii) biochemical analysis of sterols on cultivated skin fibroblasts and iii) mutation analysis of *LBR* remain available to diagnose Greenberg dysplasia prenatally.

6.4 Antley–Bixler

Antley-Bixler syndrome (ABS) is a very rare congenital multiple malformation disorder characterized by craniofacial anomalies, skeletal defects and, in a subset of patients, ambiguous genitalia. The craniofacial anomalies include brachycephaly due to severe craniosynostosis. The typical facial dysmorphism include: depressed nasal bridge with very short upturned nose, small mouth and dysplastic ears. Skeletal features include radiohumeral or other forearm synostoses, arachnodactyly, bowing of femurs, multiple contractures and neonatal fractures. A variety of congenital heart defects and gastrointestinal malformations have also been reported. Urogenital anomalies include absent, dysplastic, ectopic, or horseshoe kidneys, abnormal ureters and abnormalities of the external genitalia, including cryptorchidism. [Porter et al., 2011]. Recently it has been considered that the minimum criteria to establish the diagnosis of ABS are the presence, from the prenatal period, of craniosynostosis and radiohumeral synostosis [McGlaughlin, et al., 2010].

ABS is genetically heterogeneous and there has been some debate about the definition of the disease: by the clinical phenotype versus according to the genetic etiology [Cragun & Hopkin, 2005; Huang et al., 2005]. In fact, some patients present ABS without disordered steroidogenesis (MIM #207410) due to one gain-of-function mutation in the *FGFR2* gene (hence following autosomal dominant inheritance) while others present ABS with disorderd steroidogenesis (MIM #201750) due to two loss of function mutations in the *POR* gene (therefore, following autosomal recessive inheritance) [Flück et al., 2004]. ABS patients with mutations in *POR* are included in the spectrum of metabolic disorders due to abnormal cholesterol pathway. The *POR* gene encodes a cytochrome P450 oxidoreductase. The POR protein is an electron donor to many cytoplasmic P450 enzymes, including the cholesterol C14-lanosterol demethylase encoded by the *CYP51* gene and several other enzymes involved in steroid hormone synthesis.

ABS patients due to POR deficiency usually present with abnormal genitalia (underdeveloped genitalia and cryptorchidism in affected 46,XY males and external virilization, with clitoromegaly and fused labia, in 46,XX females) but a much wider spectrum of the remaining phenotype (milder craniofacial and skeletal malformations and normal cognitive function). The mildest end of the *POR* spectrum presents as individual with only steroidogenesis defects (amenorrhea, polycystic ovarian syndrome and infertility) [Fukami et al., 2009].

Independently of the severity, all POR deficient patients demonstrate biochemical evidence of partial blocks at multiple steps in the conversion of cholesterol to cortisol, estrogens, and androgens and biochemical diagnosis of POR deficiency can be made by GC-MS of urinary steroids, which reveals a characteristic profile of elevated pregnenolone and 17-OH-progesterone and other progesterone metabolites, in the presence of low androgens. Mineralocorticoid synthesis and metabolism are normal. Mild abnormalities of serum steroids are often, but not always, present. The steroid metabolites that accumulate in POR deficiency are consistent with partial deficiencies of 21-hydroxylase (CYP21A2) and 17α-hydroxylase (CYP17A1). The biochemical findings are explained by the fact that the POR enzyme serves as an electron donor for all cytoplasmic P450 enzymes, including CYP17A1 and CYP21A2.

A POR deficient fetus can be referred to prenatal diagnosis due to common abnormalities such as oligohydramnios or two vessel cord, to fetus with full blown ABS (multiple craniofacial, skeletal and urogenital abnormalities as described in detail above) on the ultrasound. Moreover, the diagnosis of ABS due to POR deficiency should be considered in pregnancies with low or undetectable serum uE3, like in SLOS [Cragun et al., 2004; Williamson et al., 2006]. Likewise, maternal virilization (e.g. acne, facial edema) shouldn't be overlooked as it may comprise an important clue for the diagnosis of POR deficiency [Cragun et al., 2004].

There should be an effort towards the confirmation of the diagnosis through molecular analysis since it is clinically relevant to distinguish ABS patients with disordered steroidogenesis from ABS patients with normal steroidogenesis, not only because of differences in inheritance patterns, but also because patients with POR deficiency are vulnerable to different risk factors and require different management.

6.5 Possible approaches for prenatal diagnosis of Desmosterolosis, Lathostherolosis and Sterol-C4-methyloxidase–like deficiency

Desmosterolosis (MIM #602398) and Lathostherolosis (MIM #607330) and Sterol-C4-methyloxidase-like deficiency are additional autosomal recessive polimalformative syndromes due to defective cholesterol biosynthesis. Desmosterolosis is associated to mutations in *DHCR24* gene and 3–β-hydroxysterol-Δ^{24}-reductase deficiency [Clayton et al. 1996, Waterham et al., 2001] whereas mutations on *SC5D* gene, that encodes lathosterol-5-desaturase, cause lathostherolosis [Krakowiak et al., 2003, Brunnetti-Pierri et al., 2002]. Both diseases are still poorly characterized due to the small number of cases identified. They both share some phenotypic characteristics with SLOS and the diagnosis of new cases will contribute for a better phenotypic characterization of these metabolic disorders. In order to contribute for the recognition of these entities, we have recently established reference values for several sterols in amniotic fluid at different gestational ages (lathostherol and desmosterol included) [Amaral et al., 2010].

A patient with psoriasiform dermatitis, arthralgias, congenital cataracts, microcephaly, and developmental delay was recently identified as harboring mutations in sterol-C4-methyl oxidase–like gene (*SC4MOL*), which encodes a sterol-C4-methyl oxidase. This enzyme also belongs to the cholesterol biosynthesis pathway and catalyses the demethylation of C4-methylsterols. Sterol-C4-methyl oxidase deficiency is a novel disease of inborn errors of cholesterol biosynthesis, which clinical spectrum remains to be defined [He et al., 2011].

No prenatal diagnosis of these three disorders has so far been reported. However, in theory, it can be performed based on sterols profile of amniotic fluid or through the identification of mutations in the above mentioned genes.

7. The teratogenic effect of drugs that interfere with cholesterol biosynthesis

Many women on reproductive age take medicines on a regular basis. However, most drugs presently available on the market are not licensed for use in pregnancy. Therefore, these women may conceive on medication, leading to a large number of early pregnancies being exposed to a wide range of drugs. Moreover, fetuses have been increasingly exposed to new classes of compounds, as these compounds have been shown to be effective and well tolerated outside pregnancy [Kyle, 2006].

Drugs that block crucial steps of cholesterol biosynthesis exert a teratogenic effect on the fetus, mimicking the genetically determined enzymatic defects. These phenocopies have features that resemble the phenotype of the corresponding inherited metabolic disease. Drugs with such properties are identified among antifungal, hipocholesterolemic and some antineoplastic agents.

7.1 Antifungals

A variety of antimycotic compounds are currently available to treat systemic or mucocutaneous fungal infections and some of them are capable of penetrating the placental barrier [Moudgal & Sobel, 2003]. Azoles antifungals act by competitive inhibition of CYP51 (lanosterol 14α-demethylase) decreasing the synthesis of ergosterol, the main sterol in fungal cell membrane. Apart from ergosterol depletion, selective inhibition of CYP51 also leads to accumulation of lanosterol and other 14-methylsterols, resulting in alterations of fungal wall, cell growth, cell replication and inhibition of morphogenic transformation of yeasts into mycelia [Giavini & Menegola, 2010, Pursley et al., 1996]. The inhibitory potential of these compounds is not limited to fungi; it has also been seen in a number of mammalian cytochrom P450-dependent activities, including microsomial enzymes [Sheets & Mason, 1984] and studies carried out in pregnant animals taking high doses of azole fungicides revealed their teratogenic potential. Malformations were found at branchial apparatus (related with facial structures), axial skeleton and limbs [Giavini & Menegola, 2010, Menegola et al., 2003].

Fluconazole, a bis-triazole anti-fungal agent is commonly used to treat human mycosis. It shows excellent oral absorption, low plasma protein affinity, long half-life, high concentrations in urine and CSF, minimal adverse reactions, wide spectrum of anti-fungal activity and it has high specificity for fungal cytochrome P450 system [Agrawal et al., 1996].

Nevertheless, at least five cases reporting children with a multiple malformation syndrome due to first-trimester fluconazole exposure were published. In all cases, high doses (400-800 mg/day) of fluconazole were administrated during several weeks (in order to treat a severe systemic mycotic infection) before women were aware that they were pregnant [Aleck & Bartley, 1997; Lopez-Rangel & Van Allen, 2005; Pursley et al., 1996]. The newborns showed anomalies analogous to those seen in experimental animals [Aleck & Bartley, 1997] and the phenotype identified resembled that of Antley-Bixler syndrome (thoroughly described above) [Lopez-Rangel & Van Allen, 2005]. A possible explanation for the similarity between this embriopathy and Antley-Bixler phenotype is a compromised cytochrome P450 system in both situations.

In contrast to the above described teratogenicity of fluconazole, the use of topical azoles for treatment of superficial fungal infections in pregnancy seems safe and efficient [Moudgal & Sobel, 2003] and there are several epidemiologic reports of tens of women who took sporadically low doses (50 -150mg/day) of fluconazole during first trimester of pregnancy and did not show increased overall risk of birth defects, compared with a control group (fluconazole free during pregnancy) [Giavini & Menegola, 2010; Inman et al., 1994; Mastroiacovo et al., 1996; Nørgaard et al., 2008]. Hence, as it has been previously demonstrated for other drugs [Polifka et al., 2002], dosage seems to be a critical factor on the teratogeneticity potential of fluconzazole given that apparently the exposure is harmful only if it is chronic or exceeds a certain threshold.

7.2 Statins

Another group of compounds that strongly interferes with cholesterol biosynthesis pathway are the hypocholesterolemic drugs: statins. These compounds inhibit the enzyme 3-hydroxy-3-methylglutaryl-CoA (HMG-CoA) reductase that catalyses a limitating step of cholesterol biosynthesis: the conversion of HMG-CoA to mevalonate. Because this key compound is also required for the synthesis of several other biologically important molecules, levels of HMG-CoA reductase may regulate many cellular processes and functions in cell. In fact, knock out embryos for HMG-CoA reductase died prematurely suggesting that the loss of HMG-CoA reductase activity leads to implantation failure or to embryonic death prior to implantation [Ohashi, 2003].

The use of statins for treatment of hyperlipidemia is increasingly common [Taguchi et al., 2008] and the effectiveness of these agents in reducing mortality and morbidity associated with coronary artery disease is well established [Kusters et al., 2010]. However, when pregnancy is considered, lipid-lowering drugs are often discontinued because of the fear of teratogenic effects [Kusters et al., 2010].

There is scarce and conflicting evidence on the teratogenic potential of statins and most of the information on drug safety for the fetus is limited to animal studies, a few case reports and retrospective uncontrolled data [Avis et al., 2009]. A study focusing on the toxicity of atorvastatin in pregnant rats and rabbits has shown that only the hightest doses tested - which were also toxic for the mothers - had harmful effects in pregnancy by increasing postimplantation loss and decreasing fetal body weight [Dostal et al., 1994]. Later, studies evaluating *in vitro* effects of statins in a human placental model have demonstrated that simvastatin (i) inhibited half of the proliferative events in the villi, (ii) increased apoptosis of cytotrophoblast cells and (iii) significantly decreased secretion of progesterone from the placental explants. These effects may contribute to the failure of implantation and be deleterious to the growth of the placental tissues which could explain the higher abortion rate and teratogenicity observed in animals exposed to statins during pregnancy [Kenis et al., 2005].

Moreover, due to the occurrence of unplanned pregnancies, there are a number of cases in which statins were inadvertently taken during the first trimester of pregnancy, some of them resulting in newborns with birth defects [Edison & Muenke, 2004, 2005; Petersen et al., 2008; Trakadis et al., 2009]. Nevertheless, these studies are not conclusive due to ascertainment bias: (i) in some cases pregnant women took potentially teratogenic drugs other than statins [Trakadis et al., 2009] or (ii) previous maternal health disorders like pre-pregnancy diabetes, obesity or both [Petersen et al., 2008] or (iii) the small number of cases identified enables the validation of a stastically significant conclusion [Edison & Muenke, 2004, 2005; Petersen et al., 2008]. Furthermore, none of the studies evaluated the possibility of decreased fertility, increased pre-implantation or peri-implantation losses that could be increased as shown in animal experiments [Elkin & Yan , 1999; Lee et al., 2007; Ohashi et al., 2003; Richards & Cole, 2006; Zapata et al., 2003].

7.3 Tamoxifen

Another interesting compound is tamoxifen, a nonsteroidal selective estrogen receptor modulator, used for the treatment and prevention of breast cancer [de Medina et al., 2004]. This drug is currently used as adjuvant treatment in premenopausal women affected or at risk for breast cancer [Berger & Clericuzio, 2008]. Tamoxifen has also been reported to protect against the progression of coronary artery diseases in human and animal models [de Medina et al., 2004]. Such property can be related to the capacity of tamoxifen to inibit several enzymes related with cholesterol metabolism namely acyl-CoA cholesterol acyltransferase which catalyses cholesterol esterification [de Medina et al., 2004] as well as with its hypocholesterolemic properties. As a matter of fact, tamoxifen inibits several cholesterogenic enzymes, namely: (i) sterol Δ-8-isomerase, (ii) sterol Δ-24-reductase, (iii) sterol Δ-14-reductase, and the administration of such compound to humans and laboratory animals results in a drastic reduction in cholesterol and a marked accumulation of certain sterol intermediates in serum [Cho et al., 1998].

Despite tamoxifen long use in clinical practice, its teratogenic potential remains inconclusive. Furthermore, while the evidence of effects of tamoxifen in humans in utero is minimal, animal studies have shown evidence of teratogenicity (abnormalities of genital tract and irregulary ossified ribs in rat pups) and delayed vaginal opening in female offspring of guinea pigs [Barthelmes & Gateley, 2004; Berger & Clericuzio, 2008]. According to a review of seven papers refering tamoxifen prenatal exposure there was (i) one case of ambious genitalia after 20 weeks exposure to a diary dose of 20 mg (ii) one case of Goldenhar's syndrome after 26 weeks exposure to 20 mg/day (with simultaneous exposure to other teratogenig drugs during the first 6 weeks) [Barthelmes & Gateley, 2004]. Later, one case of Pierre Robin sequence (small mandible, cleft palate and glossoptosis) associated with first trimestre fetal exposure was also published in a pregnancy with gestational diabetes [Berger & Clericuzio, 2008].

If we put together the fact that (i) this drug was initialy developed as a contraceptive agent [Barthelmes & Gateley, 2004], (ii) it inhibits several enzymes of cholesterol biosynthesis pathway, (iii) in most cases the exposure to tamoxifen occurs very early - sometimes even before women are aware of the pregnancy - and (iv) no adverse effects were observed in 85 cases in which tamoxifen was taken as preventive drug of breast cancer (without association to other potentially teratogenic compounds exposure), we are lead to the conclusion that tamoxifen has a „all-or-none" effect. In other words, exposure to tamoxifen may cause affected embryos that are lost very early (even before women are aware of the pregnancy) or fetal survival without any malformation.

All in all, one should highlight the role of the medical appointements on the evaluation of the interation of drugs with the developing fetus. Ideally, pregnancies should be prepared in advance and, at that time, the potencially teratogenic drugs should be replaced by less harmfull medicines or, if possible, discontinued. After conception and when evaluating a fetus with malformations on the ultrasound, doctors should bear in mind the role of teratogenic drugs that can produce phenocopies of genetically determined disorders.

8. Conclusion

During the last two decades inborn errors of cholesterol biosynthesis have emerged as a group of metabolic disorders that should be included in the differential diagnosis of intrauterine growth restriction and abnormal embryogenesis as well as in the investigation of the etiology of low levels of maternal estriol in the second trimester of pregnancy.

Patients with these metabolic diseases present with complex malformation syndromes involving different organs and systems. As metabolic pathways are biological interactive networks, one specific blockage activates new routes for detoxication of accumulated products followed by excretion. For example, it was noticed that urine from pregnant women at risk for SLOS revealed abnormal steroids derived from 7-dehydrocholesterol. One can assume this as a general rule, and postulate that, in defective cholesterol biosynthesis accumulated sterols are metabolized originating "new" steroids. If quantification of abnormal steroids in maternal urine (which is non invasive and easy to perform) becomes widely available, one can envision a future in which prenatal diagnosis of inborn errors of cholesterol biosynthesis is extended to most fetuses with developmental abnormalities.

Furthermore it is possible that, as it is being developed in other fields of medical genetics, high throughput technologies might also be used in the setting of metabolic disorders: for example, a microarray chip with oligonucleotide probes targeted to all the genes involved in metabolic pathways and the application of a next generation sequencing platform to perform sequencing analysis of those genes. This would allow for the identification of both copy number variants and point mutations of the genes implicated in the inborn errors of cholesterol biosynthesis pathway, thus promoting a global and thorough approach to these diseases, a better phenotype-genotype correlation and a more accurate knowledge of the spectrum of these disorders.

9. Acknowledgment

We would like to thank Dr. Tiago Delgado and Dr. João Silva (both at the Medical Genetics Centre Jacinto Magalhães, Oporto, Portugal) and to Doctor Georgina Correia da Silva from Oporto Faculty of Pharmacy, for her critical review of this paper.

10. References

Abuelo D.N., Tint G.S., Kelley R., Batta A.K., Shefer S., Salen G. (1995). Prenatal detection of the cholesterol biosynthetic defect in the Smith-Lemli-Opitz syndrome by the analysis of amniotic fluid sterols. *Am J Med Genet*, 56(3):281-5.

Agrawal P.B., Narang A., Kumar P. (1996). Fluconazole. *Indian J Pediatr*, 63(6):775-80.

Aleck K.A. & Bartley D.L. (1997). Multiple malformation syndrome following fluconazole use in pregnancy: report of an additional patient. *Am J Med Genet*, 72(3):253-6.

Amaral C., Gallardo E., Rodrigues R., Pinto Leite R., Quelhas D., Tomaz C.L. (2010) Quantitative analysis of five sterols in amniotic fluid by GC-MS: application to the diagnosis of cholesterol biosynthesis defects. *J Chromatogr B Analyt Technol Biomed Life Sci*. 878(23):213.

Avis H.J., Hutten B.A., Twickler M.T., Kastelein J.J., van der Post J.A., Stalenhoef A.F., Vissers M.N. (2009). Pregnancy in women suffering from familial hypercholesterolemia: a harmful period for both mother and newborn? *Curr Opin Lipidol*. 20(6):484-90.

Barthelmes L. & Gateley C.A. (2004). Tamoxifen and pregnancy. *Breast*, 13(6):446-51.

Berger J.C. & Clericuzio C.L. (2008). Pierre Robin Sequence assocoated with first trimestre fetal tamoxifen exposure. *Am J Med Genet A,* 146A(16):2141-4.

Braverman N., Lin P., Moebius F.F., Obie C., Moser A., Glossmann H., Wilcox W.R., Rimoin D.L., Smith M., Kratz L., Kelley R.I., Valle D. (1999). Mutations in the gene encoding 3 beta-hydroxysteroid-delta 8, delta 7-isomerase cause X-linked dominant Conradi-Hünermann syndrome. *Nat Genet,* 22(3):291-4.

Brunetti-Pierri N., Corso G., Rossi M., Ferrari P., Balli F., Rivasi F., Annunziata I., Ballabio A., Russo A.D., Andria G., Parenti G. (2002). Lathosterolosis, a novel multiple-malformation/mental retardation syndrome due to deficiency of 3beta-hydroxysteroid-delta5-desaturase. *Am J Hum Genet.* 71(4):952-8.

Cardoso M.L., Fortuna A.M., Castedo S., Martins M., Montenegro N., Jakobs C., Clayton P., Vilarinho L. (2005a). Diagnóstico Pré-natal de Síndrome de Smith-Lemli-Opitz *ArqMed,*19(1-2) 23-27.

Cardoso M.L., Balreira A., Martins M., Nunes L., Cabral A., Marques M., Lima M.R., Marques J.S., Medeira A., Cordeiro I., Pedro S., Mota M.C., Dionisi-Vici C., Santorelli F.M., Jakobs C., Clayton P.T. and Vilarinho L. (2005b). Molecular studies in Portuguese patients with Smith-Lemli-Opitz syndrome and report of three new mutations in *DHCR7. Mol. Genet. Metab,* 85(3):228-35.

Charlton-Menys V. & Durrington P.N. (2007). Human cholesterol metabolism and therapeutic molecules. *Exp Physiol,*93(1):27-42.

Chevy F., Humbert L., Wolf C. (2005). Sterol profiling of amniotic fluid: a routine method for the detection of distal cholesterol synthesis deficit. *Prenat Diagn,* 25(11):1000-6.

Cho S.Y., Kim J.H., Paik Y.K. (1998). Cholesterol biosynthesis from lanosterol: differential inhibition of sterol delta 8-isomerase and other lanosterol-converting enzymes by tamoxifen. *Mol Cells.* 8(2):233-9.

Clayton P.T. (1998). Disorders of cholesterol biosynthesis. *Arch Dis Child,* 78: 185–189.

Clayton P., Mills K., Keeling J., FitzPatrick D. (1996). Desmosterolosis: a new inborn error of cholesterol biosynthesis. *Lancet.,* 348:404.

Cooper M.K., Porter J.A., Young K.E., Beachy P.A. (1998). Teratogen-mediated inhibition of target tissue response to Shh signaling. *Science.* 280 (5369):1603-7.

Cooper M.K., Wassif C.A., Krakowiak P.A., Taipale J., Gong R., Kelley R.I., Porter F.D., Beachy P.A .(2003). A defective response to Hedgehog signaling in disorders of cholesterol biosynthesis. *Nat Genet,* 33(4):508-13.

Correa-Cerro L.S., Porter F.D. (2005). 3β –Hydroxysterol - delta7-reductase and the Smith–Lemli–Opitz syndrome. *Mol Genet Metab,* 84 (2):112-26.

Craig W.Y., Haddow J.E., Palomaki G.E., Kelley R.I., Kratz L.E., Shackleton C.H., Marcos J., Stephen Tint G., MacRae A.R., Nowaczyk M.J., Kloza E.M., Irons M.B., Roberson M. (2006). Identifying Smith-Lemli-Opitz syndrome in conjunction with prenatal screening for Down syndrome. *Prenat Diagn,* 26(9):842-9.

Craig W.Y., Haddow J.E., Palomaki G.E., Roberson M. (2007). Major fetal abnormalities associated with positive screening tests for Smith-Lemli-Opitz syndrome (SLOS). *Prenat Diagn,* (5): 409-14.

Cragun D. & Hopkin R.J. (2005). Use of the term "Antley-Bixler syndrome": minimizing confusion. *Am J Hum Genet,* 77(2):327-8.

Cragun D.L., Trumpy S.K., Shackleton C.H., Kelley R.I., Leslie N.D., Mulrooney N.P., Hopkin R.J. (2004). Undetectable maternal serum uE3 and postnatal abnormal sterol and steroid metabolism in Antley-Bixler syndrome. *Am J Med Genet A*, 15;129A(1):1-7.

Daniels T.F., Killinger K.M., Michal J.J., Wright R.W. Jr, Jiang Z. (2009). Lipoproteins, cholesterol homeostasis and cardiac health. *Int J Biol Sci*, 5(5):474-88.

Daniels T.F., Wu X.L., Pan Z., Michal J.J., Wright R.W. Jr, Killinger K.M., MacNeil M.D., Jiang Z. (2010). The reverse cholesterol transport pathway improves understanding of genetic networks for fat deposition and muscle growth in beef cattle. *PLoS One*, 5(12):e15203.

de Medina P., Payré B.L., Bernad J., Bosser I., Pipy B., Silvente-Poirot S., Favre G., Faye J.C., Poirot M. (2004.) Tamoxifen is a potent inhibitor of cholesterol esterification and prevents the formation of foam cells. *J Pharmacol Exp Ther*, 308 (3):1165-73.

Dias V. & Ribeiro V. (2011). Ethnic differences in the prevalence of polymorphisms in CYP7A1, CYP7B1 AND CYP27A1 enzymes involved in cholesterol metabolism. *J Pharm Bioallied Sci*, 3(3):453-9.

Dostal L.A., Schardein J.L., Anderson J.A. (1994). Developmental toxicity of the HMG-CoA reductase inhibitor, atorvastatin, in rats and rabbits. *Teratolog*, 50(6):387-94.

Dubuisson J., Guibaud L., Combourieu D., Massardier J., Raudrant D. (2008). Utility of fetal ultrasonography in the prenatal diagnosis of Smith-Lemli-Opitz syndrome. *Gynecol Obstet Fertil*, 36(5):525-8.

Edison R.J. , Berg K., Remaley A., Kelley R., Rotimi C., Stevenson R.E., Muenke M. Adverse birth outcome among mothers with low serum cholesterol. (2007). *Pediatrics*, 120(4):723-33.

Edison R.J. & Muenke M. (2004). Central nervous system and limb anomalies in case reports of first-trimester statin exposure. *N Engl J Med*, 350(15):1579-82.

Edison R.J. & Muenke M. (2005). Gestational exposure to lovastatin followed by cardiac malformation misclassified as holoprosencephaly. *N Engl J Med*, 352(26):2759.

Elkin R.G. & Yan Z. (1999). Relationship between inhibition of mevalonate biosynthesis and reduced fertility in laying hens. *J Reprod Fertil*,116(2):269-75.

Flück C.E., Tajima T., Pandey A.V., Arlt W., Okuhara K., Verge C.F., Jabs E.W., Mendonça B.B., Fujieda K., Miller W.L. (2004). Mutant P450 oxidoreductase causes disordered steroidogenesis with and without Antley-Bixler syndrome. *Nat Genet*, 36(3):228-30.

Fukami M., Nishimura G., Homma K., Nagai T., Hanaki K., Uematsu A., Ishii T., Numakura C., Sawada H., Nakacho M., Kowase T., Motomura K., Haruna H., Nakamura M., Ohishi A., Adachi M., Tajima T., Hasegawa Y., Hasegawa T., Horikawa R., Fujieda K., Ogata T. (2009). Cytochrome P450 oxidoreductase deficiency: identification and characterization of biallelic mutations and genotype-phenotype correlations in 35 Japanese patients. *J Clin Endocrinol Metab*, 94(5):1723-31.

Giavini E. & Menegola E. (2010) Are azole fungicides a teratogenic risk for human conceptus? *Toxicol Lett*, 198(2):106-11.

Ginat S., Battaile K.P., Battaile B.C. Maslen C., Gibson K.M., Steiner R.D. (2004). Lowered DHCR7 activity measured by ergosterol conversion in multiple cell types in Smith-Lemli-Opitz syndrome. *Mol Genet Metab*, 83(1-2):175-83.

Gofflot F., Gaoua W., Bourguignon L., Roux C., Picard J.J. (2001). Expression of Sonic Hedgehog downstream genes is modified in rat embryos exposed in utero to a distal inhibitor of cholesterol biosynthesis. *Dev Dyn*, 220(2):99-111.

Gofflot F., Hars C., Illien F., Chevy F., Wolf C., Picard J.J., Roux C. (2003). Molecular mechanisms underlying limb anomalies associated with cholesterol deficiency during gestation: implications of Hedgehog signaling. *Human Molecular Genetics,*12 (10):1187–1198.

Goldenberg A., Wolf C., Chevy F., Benachi A., Dumez Y., Munnich A., Cormier-Daire V. (2004). Antenatal manifestations of Smith-Lemli-Opitz (RSH) syndrome: a retrospective survey of 30 cases. *Am J Med Genet A,*124A(4):423-6.

Griffiths W.J., Wang Y., Karu K., Samuel E., McDonnell S., Hornshaw M., Shackleton C. (2008). Potential of sterol analysis by liquid chromatography-tandem mass spectrometry for the prenatal diagnosis of Smith-Lemli-Opitz syndrome.*Clin Chem,* 54(8):1317-24.

Happle R., Koch H., Lenz W. (1980). The CHILD syndrome. Congenital hemidysplasia with ichthyosiform erythroderma and limb defects. *Eur J Pediatr,* 134(1):27-33.

He M., Kratz L.E., Michel J.J., Vallejo A.N., Ferris L., Kelley R.I., Hoover J.J., Jukic D., Gibson K.M., Wolfe L.A., Ramachandran D., Zwick M.E., Vockley J. (2011). Mutations in the human SC4MOL gene encoding a methyl sterol oxidase cause psoriasiform dermatitis, microcephaly, and developmental delay. *J Clin Invest,* 121(3):976-84.

Hebbachi A.M. & Gibbons G.F. (2001). Microsomal membrane-associated apoB is the direct precursor of secreted VLDL in primary cultures of rat hepatocytes. *J Lipid Res,* 42(10):1609-17.

Herman G.E. (2000) X-Linked dominant disorders of cholesterol biosynthesis in man and mouse. *Biochim Biophys Acta.* 1529(1-3):357-73.

Huang N., Pandey A.V., Agrawal V., Reardon W., Lapunzina P.D., Mowat D., Jabs E.W., Van Vliet G., Sack J., Flück C.E., Miller W.L. (2005). Diversity and function of mutations in 450 oxidoreductase in patients with Antley-Bixler syndrome and disordered steroidogenesis. *Am J Hum Genet,* 76(5):729-49.

Hussain M.M., Fatma S., Pan X., Iqbal J. (2005). Intestinal lipoprotein assembly. *Curr Opin Lipidol,* 16(3):281-5.

Hyett J.A., Clayton P.T., Moscoso G., Nicolaides K.H. (1995). Increased first trimester nuchal translucency as a prenatal manifestation of Smith-Lemli-Opitz syndrome. *Am J Med Genet,* 25;58(4):374-6.

Ikonen E. (2006). Mechanisms for cellular cholesterol transport: defects and human disease. *Physiol Rev,* 86(4):1237-61.

Inman W., Pearce G., Wilton L. (1994). Safety of fluconazole in the treatment of vaginal candidiasis. A prescription-event monitoring study, with special reference to the outcome of pregnancy. *Eur J Clin Pharmacol,* 46(2):115-8.

Irons M.B. & Tint G.S. (1998). Prenatal diagnosis of Smith-Lemli-Opitz syndrome. *Prenat Diagn,* 18(4):369-72.

Jeon H. & Blacklow S.C. (2005). Structure and physiologic function of the low-density lipoprotein receptor. *Annu Rev Biochem,* 74:535-62.

Jezela-Stanek A., Małunowicz E.M., Ciara E., Popowska E., Goryluk-Kozakiewicz B., Spodar K., Czerwiecka M., Jezuita J., Nowaczyk M.J., Krajewska-Walasek M. (2006). Maternal urinary steroid profiles in prenatal diagnosis of Smith-Lemli-Opitz syndrome: first patient series comparing biochemical and molecular studies. *Clin Genet,* 69(1):77-85.

Johnson J.A., Aughton D.J., Comstock C.H., von Oeyen P.T., Higgins J.V., Schulz R. (1994). Prenatal diagnosis of Smith-Lemli-Opitz syndrome, type II. *Am J Med Genet*, 15;49(2):240-3.

Kelley R.I. (1995). Diagnosis of Smith-Lemli-Opitz syndrome by gas chromatography/mass spectrometry of 7-dehydrocholesterol in plasma, amniotic fluid and cultured skin fibroblasts. *Clin Chim Acta*, 30;236(1):45-58.

Kelley R. & Hennekam R.C. (2001). Smith-Lemli-Opitz Syndrome, In: Metabolic and Molecular Bases of Inherited Diseases, Charles R. Scriver; Arthur L. Beaudet; William S. Sly, McGraw-Hill Education - Europe, 8 th ed, 6183-6203

Kelley R.I. & Herman G.E. (2001). Inborn errors of sterol biosynthesis. *Annu Rev Genomics Hum Genet*, 2:299-341

Kelley R.I., Wilcox W.G., Smith M., Kratz L.E., Moser A., Rimoin D.S. (1999). Abnormal sterol metabolism in patients with Conradi-Hünermann-Happle syndrome and sporadic lethal chondrodysplasia punctata. *Am J Med Genet*, 83(3):213-9.

Kenis I., Tartakover-Matalon S., Cherepnin N., Drucker L., Fishman A., Pomeranz M., Lishner M. (2005). Simvastatin has deleterious effects on human first trimester placental explants. *Hum Reprod*, 20(10):2866-72.

Kindel T., Lee D.M., Tso P. (2010). The mechanism of the formation and secretion of chylomicrons. *Atheroscler Suppl*, 11(1):11-6.

Koleјáková K., Petrovic R., Turcáni P., Böhmer D., Chandoga J. (2010). The role of cholesterol in embryogenesis and the Smith-Lemli-Opitz syndrom. *Cesk Fysiol*, 59(2):37-43.

König A., Happle R., Bornholdt D., Engel H., Grzeschik K.H. (2000). Mutations in the NSDHL gene, encoding a 3beta-hydroxysteroid dehydrogenase, cause CHILD syndrome. *Am J Med Genet*, 90(4):339-46.

Kosters A., Jirsa M., Groen A.K .(2003). Genetic background of cholesterol gallstone disease. *Biochim Biophys Acta*, 1637(1):1-19.

Krakowiak P.A., Wassif C.A., Kratz L.,Cozma D., Kovárová M., Harris G., Grinberg A., Yang Y., Hunter A.G., Tsokos M., Kelley R.I., Porter F.D. (2003). Lathosterolosis: an inborn error of human and murine cholesterol synthesis due to lathosterol 5-desaturase deficiency. *Hum Mol Genet*, 12:1631–1641.

Kratz L.E. & Kelley R.I. (1999). Prenatal diagnosis of the RSH/Smith-Lemli-Opitz syndrome. *Am J Med Genet*, 19;82(5):376-81.

Kusters D.M., Homsma S.J., Hutten B.A., Twickler M.T., Avis H.J., van der Post J.A., Stroes E.S. (2010). Dilemmas in treatment of women with familial hypercholesterolaemia during pregnancy. *Neth J Med*, 68(1):299-303.

Kyle P.M. (2006). Drugs and the fetus. *Curr Opin Obstet Gynecol*, 18(2):93-9.

Lee M.H., Cho Y.S., Han Y.M. (2007). Simvastatin suppresses self-renewal of mouse embryonic stem cells by inhibiting RhoA geranylgeranylation. *Stem Cells*, 25(7):1654-63.

Linck L.M., Hayflick S.J., Lin D.S., Battaile K.P., Ginat T., Burlingame S., Gibson K.M., Honda M., Honda A., Salen G., Tint G.S., Connor W.E., Steiner R.D. (2000).Fetal demise with Smith-Lemli-Opitz syndrome confirmed by tissue sterol analysis and the absence of measurable 7-dehydrocholesterol reductase activity in chorionic villi. *Prenat Diagn*, 20:238-40.

Lindegaard M.L., Wassif C.A., Vaisman B., Amar M., Wasmuth E.V., Shamburek R., Nielsen L.B., Remaley A.T., Porter F.D. (2008). Characterization of placental cholesterol transport: ABCA1 is a potential target for in utero therapy of Smith-Lemli-Opitz syndrome. *Hum Mol Genet,* 17(23):3806-13.

Liu J., Chang C.C., Westover E.J., Covey D.F., Chang T.Y. (2005). Investigating the allosterism of acyl-CoA:cholesterol acyltransferase (ACAT) by using various sterols: in vitro and intact cell studies. *Biochem J,* 391(Pt 2):389-97.

Liscum L., Underwood K.W. (1995). Intracellular cholesterol transport and compartmentation. *J Biol Chem,* 270(26):15443-6.

Loeffler J., Uterman G., Witsch-Baumgartner M. (2002). Molecular prenatal diagnosis of Smith-Lemli-Opitz is reliable and efficient. *Prenat Diagn,* 22(9):827-30.

Löffler J., Trojovsky A., Casati B., Kroisel P.M., Utermann G. (2009). Homozygosity for the W151X stop mutation in the delta7-sterol reductase gene (*DHCR7*) causing a lethal form of Smith-Lemli-Opitz syndrome: retrospective molecular diagnosis. *Am J Med Genet,* 95(2):174-7.

Lopez-Rangel E. & Van Allen M.I. (2005). Prenatal exposure to fluconazole: an identifiable dysmorphic phenotype. *Birth Defects Res A Clin Mol Teratol,* 73(11):919-23.

Madazli R., Aksoy F., Ocak V., Atasü T. (2001). Detailed ultrasonographic findings in Greenberg dysplasia. *Prenat Diagn,* 21(1):65.

Mastroiacovo P., Mazzone T., Botto L.D., Serafini M.A., Finardi A., Caramelli L., Fusco D. (1996). Prospective assessment of pregnancy outcomes after first-trimester exposure to fluconazole. *Am J Obstet Gynecol,* 175(6):1645-50.

Maxfield F.R. & Wüstner D. (2002). Intracellular cholesterol transport. *J Clin Invest,* 110(7):891-8.

McConihay J.A., Horn P.S., Woollett A.L. (2001). Effect of maternal hypercholesterolemia on fetal sterol metabolism in the Golden Syrian hamster. *J Lipid Res,* 42(7):1111-9.

McGlaughlin K.L., Witherow H., Dunaway D.J., David .DJ., Anderson P.J. (2010). Spectrum of Antley-Bixler syndrome. *J. Craniofac. Surg,* 21: 1560-1564.

McLarren K.W., Severson T.M., du Souich C., Stockton D.W., Kratz L.E., Cunningham D., Hendson G., Morin R.D., Wu D., Paul J.E., An J., Nelson T.N., Chou A., DeBarber A.E., Merkens L.S., Michaud J.L., Waters P.J., Yin J., McGillivray B., Demos M., Rouleau G.A., Grzeschik K.H., Smith R., Tarpey P.S., Shears D., Schwartz C.E., Gecz J., Stratton M.R., Arbour L., Hurlburt J., Van Allen M.I., Herman G.E., Zhao Y., Moore R., Kelley R.I., Jones S.J., Steiner R.D., Raymond F.L., Marra M.A., Boerkoel C.F. (2010). Hypomorphic temperature-sensitive alleles of NSDHL cause CK syndrome. *Am J Hum Genet,* 87(6):905-14.

Menegola E. Broccia M.L., Di Renzo F., Giavini E. (2003).Pathogenic pathways in fluconazole-induced branchial arch malformations. *Birth Defects Res A Clin Mol Teratol,* 67(2):116-24.

Miller W.L. (2011). Role of mitochondria in steroidogenesis. *Endocr Dev,* 20:1-19.

Miller W.L. & Auchus R.J. (2011). The molecular biology, biochemistry, and physiology of human steroidogenesis and its disorders. *Endocr Rev,* 32(1):81-151.

Miller W.L. & Bose H.S. (2011). Early steps in steroidogenesis: intracellular cholesterol trafficking. *J Lipid Res,* [Epub ahead of print]

Moudgal V.V. & Sobel J. D. (2003). Antifungal drugs in pregnancy: a review. *Expert Opin Drug Saf,* 2(5):475-83.

Nørgaard M., Pedersen L., Gislum M., Erichsen R., Søgaard K.K., Schønheyder H.C., Sørensen HT. (2008). Maternal use of fluconazole and risk of congenital malformations: a Danish population-based cohort study. *J Antimicrob Chemother,* 62(1):172-6.

Nowaczyk MJ., Garcia D.M., Eng B., Waye J.S. (2001). Rapid molecular prenatal diagnosis of Smith-Lemli-Opitz syndrome. *Am J Med Genet,* 102(4):387-8.

Ohashi K., Osuga J., Tozawa R., Kitamine T., Yagyu H., Sekiya M., Tomita S., Okazaki H., Tamura Y., Yahagi N., Iizuka Y., Harada K., Gotoda T., Shimano H., Yamada N., Ishibashi S. (2003). Early embryonic lethality caused by targeted disruption of the 3-hydroxy-3-methylglutaryl-CoA reductase gene.□*J Biol Chem,* 278(44):42936-41.

Palomaki G.E., Bradley L.A., Knight G.J., Craig W.Y., Haddow J.E. (2002). Assigning risk for Smith-Lemli-Opitz syndrome as part of 2nd trimester screening for Down's syndrome. *J Med Screen,* 9(1):43-4.

Petersen E.E., Mitchell A.A., Carey J.C., Werler M.M., Louik C., Rasmussen S.A. (2008). National Birth Defects Prevention Study Maternal exposure to statins and risk for birth defects: a case-series approach. *Am J Med Genet A,* 146A(20):2701-5.

Polifka J.E., Friedman J.M. (2002). Medical genetics: 1. Clinical teratology in the age of genomics. *CMAJ,* 167(3):265-73.

Palomaki G.E., Bradley L.A., Knight G.J., Craig W.Y., Haddow J.E. (2002). Assigning risk for Smith-Lemli-Opitz syndrome as part of 2nd trimester screening for Down's syndrome. *J Med Screen,* 9(1):43-4.

Pfrieger F.W. & Ungerer N. (2011). Cholesterol metabolism in neurons and astrocytes. *Prog Lipid Res,*50(4):357-71.

Porter F.D. (2003). Human malformation syndromes due to inborn errors of cholesterol synthesis. *Curr Opin Pediatr,* 15(6):607-13.

Porter F.D., Herman G.E. (2011). Malformation syndromes caused by disorders of cholesterol synthesis. *J Lipid Res,* 52(1)6-34.

Pursley T.J., Blomquist I.K., Abraham J., Andersen H.F., Bartley J.A. (1996). Fluconazole-induced congenital anomalies in three infants. *Clin Infect Dis,* 22(2):336-40.

Richards S.M. & Cole S.E. (2006). A toxicity and hazard assessment of fourteen pharmaceuticals to Xenopus laevis larvae. *Ecotoxicology,* 15(8):647-56.

Rossiter J.P., Hofman K.J., Kelley R.I. (1995). Smih-Lemli-Opitz Syndrome: Prenatal Diagnosis by Quantification of Cholesterol Precursors in Amniotic Fluid. *Am J Hum Genet,* 56:272-5.

Shelness G.S., Sellers J.A.(2001).Very-low-density lipoprotein assembly and secretion. *Curr Opin Lipidol,* 12(2):151-7.

Sheets J.J. & Mason J.I. (1984). Ketoconazole: a potent inhibitor of cytochrome P-450-dependent drug metabolism in rat liver. *Drug Metab Dispos,* 12(5):603-6.

Shackleton C.H., Marcos J., Palomaki G.E., Craig W.Y., Kelley R.I., Kratz L.E., Haddow J.E. (2007). Dehydrosteroid measurements in maternal urine or serum for the prenatal diagnosis of Smith-Lemli-Opitz syndrome (SLOS). *Am J Med Genet A,* 143A (18):2129-36.

Shinawi M., Szabo S., Popek E., Wassif C.A., Porter F.D., Potocki L. (2005). Recognition of Smith-Lemli-Opitz syndrome (RSH) in the fetus: utility of ultrasonography and biochemical analysis in pregnancies with low maternal serum estriol. *Am J Med Genet A,* 15;138(1):56-60.]

Taguchi N., Rubin E.T., Hosokawa A., Choi J., Ying A.Y., Moretti M.E., Koren G., Ito S. (2008). Prenatal exposure to HMG-CoA reductase inhibitors: effects on fetal and neonatal outcomes. *Reprod Toxicol*, 26(2):175-7.

Tarling E.J. & Edwards P.A. (2011). Dancing with the sterols: Critical roles for ABCG1, ABCA1, miRNAs, and nuclear and cell surface receptors in controlling cellular sterol homeostasis. *Biochim Biophys Acta.* [In press].

Thompson S.L., Burrows R., Laub R.J., Krisans S.K. (1987). Cholesterol synthesis in rat liver peroxisomes. Conversion of mevalonic acid to cholesterol. *J Biol Chem*, 262(36):17420-5.

Trakadis Y., Blaser S., Hahn C.D., Yoon G. (2009). A case report of prenatal exposure to rosuvastatin and telmisartan. *Paediatr Child Health*, 14(7):450-2.

Vanier M.T. (2010). Niemann-Pick disease type C. *Orphanet J Rare Dis*, 5:16.

Wassif C.A., Brownson K.E., Sterner A.L., Forlino A., Zerfas P.M., Wilson W.K., Starost M.F., Porter F.D. (2007). HEM dysplasia and ichthyosis are likely laminopathies and not due to 3beta-hydroxysterol Delta14- reductase deficiency. *Hum Mol Genet*, 16(10):1176-87.

Waterham H.R., Koster J., Mooyer P., Noort G.v G., Kelley R.I., Wilcox W.R., Wanders R.J., Hennekam R.C., Oosterwijk J.C. (2003). Autosomal recessive HEM/Greenberg skeletal dysplasia is caused by 3 beta-hydroxysterol delta 14-reductase deficiency due to mutations in the lamin B receptor gene. *Am J Hum Genet*, 72(4):1013-7.

Waterham H.R., Koster J., Romeijn G.J., Hennekam R.C., Vreken P., Andersson H.C., FitzPatrick D.R., Kelley R.I. & Wanders R.J. (2001). Mutations in the 3beta-hydroxysterol delta 24-reductase gene cause desmosterolosis, an autosomal recessive disorder of cholesterol biosynthesis. *Am J Hum Gene*, 69:685–694.

Waterham H.R. & Wanders R.J. (2000). Biochemical and genetic aspects of 7-dehydrocholesterol reductase and Smith-Lemli-Opitz syndrome. *Biochim Biophys Acta*, 1529(1-3):340-56.

Waye J.S., Eng B., Nowaczyk M.J. (2007). Prenatal diagnosis of Smith-Lemli-Opitz syndrome (SLOS) by DHCR7 mutation analysis. *Prenat Diagn*, 27(7):638-40.

White P.C. (1994). Genetic diseases of steroid metabolism. *Vitam Horm*, 49:131-95.

Williamson L., Arlt W., Shackleton C., Kelley R.I., Braddock S.R. (2006). Linking Antley-Bixler syndrome and congenital adrenal hyperplasia: a novel case of P450 oxidoreductase deficiency. *Am J Med Genet A*, 140A(17):1797-803.

Woollett L.A. (2005). Maternal cholesterol in fetal development: transport of cholesterol from the maternal to the fetal circulation. *Am J Clin Nutr*, 82(6):1155-61.

Woollett L.A. (2011). Transport of maternal cholesterol to the fetal circulation. *Placenta*, 32 Suppl 2:S218-21.

Yoshida S. & Wada Y. (2005). Transfer of maternal cholesterol to embryo and fetus in pregnant mice. *J Lipid Res*, 46(10):2168-74.

Yu H. & Patel S.B. (2005). Recent insights into the Smith-Lemli-Opitz syndrome. *Clin Genet*, 68(5):383-91.

Zhang Y., Yu C., Liu J., Spencer T.A., Chang C.C. & Chang T.Y. (2003). Cholesterol is superior to 7-ketocholesterol or 7 alpha-hydroxycholesterol as an allosteric activator for acyl-coenzyme A:cholesterol acyltransferase 1. *J Biol Chem*, 278(13):11642-7.

Zapata R., Piulachs M.D., Bellés X. (2003). Inhibitors of 3-hydroxy-3-methylglutaryl-CoA reductase lower fecundity in the German cockroach: correlation between the effects on fecundity in vivo with the inhibition of enzymatic activity in embryo cells. *Pest Manag Sci*, 59(10):1111-7.

8

Understanding Prenatal Iodine Deficiency

Inés Velasco[1,2], Federico Soriguer[2,3] and P. Pere Berbel[2,4]
[1]*Servicio de Ginecología y Obstetricia, Hospital de Riotinto, Huelva*
[2]*TDY Working Group of the SEEN: Sociedad Española de Endocrinología y Nutrición*
[3]*Servicio de Endocrinología y Nutrición,*
Hospital Regional Universitario Carlos Haya, Málaga
[4]*Universidad Miguel Hernández, Elche, Alicante*
Spain

1. Introduction

Iodine deficiency is a worldwide Public Health problem, mainly in pregnant women and infants, which causes permanent and irreversible sequels in the Central Nervous System (CNS) of the progeny when daily iodine intake does not reach optimal levels. Pharmacological iodine supplements have been recommended during pregnancy and lactation periods in regions with low iodine intake diet.

In recent years, maternal hypothyroxinemia has been recognized as the biochemical condition responsible for the alterations in the processes of neural development in the embryo and fetus associated to iodine deficiency.

Research Methods: The objective of this study was to review the available scientific evidence on the crucial role of iodine in early stages of neural development, to understand the international scheduling recommendations about an adequate iodine intake in vulnerable populations groups.

Iodine is a micronutrient essential for the synthesis of thyroid hormones[1]. The thyroid gland takes iodine from the diet, stores it and subsequently incorporates it into other molecules, to produce two types of thyroid hormones as a final product: triiodothyronine (T3) and thyroxine (T4) containing three and four iodine atoms respectively. Both circulate in blood bound to proteins and act on specific receptors. The free T3 is metabolically more active, but the T4 is, as we shall see, indispensable at specific developmental stages.

The thyroid hormones are involved in many metabolic and developmental processes, and they exert a broad range of actions on every tissue of the body: body temperature regulation, somatic growth. Further, it is essential for the proper development and function of the Central Nervous System.[2]

Since the first epidemiological studies conducted by Pharoah[3] and Thilly[4] in the 70's, the association between iodine deficiency in pregnant women and fetal neurological damage has been extensively reviewed and proven in scientific literature. In fact, the need to provide iodine supplementation to pregnant women in iodine-deficient regions is considered as proven by scientific evidence.[5]

Many of these studies are focused on regions where severe iodine deficiency is endemic and coexisting with mixedematous cretinism.[6] The understanding of the neurological effects of hypothyroidism on infants was partially obtained from mothers with clinically overt hypothyroidism.[7,8] All these factors have contributed to a general awareness that iodine deficiency is a problem restricted to specific geographic areas and to well-defined at-risk populations (hypothyroidism, goiter and malnutrition)[9]

For a long time, there has been a prevailing belief that the main factor responsible for alterations in fetal neurological development was maternal hypothyroidism (defined as elevated serum TSH levels) in the early stages of pregnancy.[8,10] Thus, when a pregnant woman was found to have normal thyroid function, neurodevelopmental alterations in the fetus were systematically discarded. [11]

Along history, some contradictions have arisen from mixing different concepts as endemic cretinism, congenital hypothyroidism, iodine deficiency, etc[12]. Fortunately, such contradictions have been clarified by the advances in our understanding of thyroid physiology during pregnancy[13,14] , the transfer of maternal thyroid hormones to the fetus[15,16] and the increasingly complete characterization of thyroid hormone receptors in placental and embryo tissues.[17] Nevertheless, only the most recent studies have given satisfactory explanation of the possible role of thyroid hormones (maternal and fetal) during critical stages of fetal neurological development.[18] Basing on these recent works, the relevance of an adequate balance of iodine during the early stages of life is considered proven.

2. Iodine deficiency and pregnancy

Pregnancy is accompanied by dramatic changes in the thyroid function, which are the result of a complex combination of factors specific to pregnancy that altogether stimulate the maternal thyroid machinery.[14]

During the first half of gestation the maternal thyroid undergoes some changes:

- Progressive increase of thyroglobulin, which reduces free fraction of thyroxine.
- The human chorionic gonadotropin has TSH-like effect and acts by directly stimulating the maternal thyroid.
- Meanwhile, the fetal thyroid is kept inactive and will not be functioning until 20 weeks of gestation.
- The only source of thyroid hormones in the fetus throughout the first half of pregnancy is thyroxine of maternal origin.

In healthy pregnant women with adequate iodine levels, pregnancy mainly involves a higher demand of thyroid hormones. The thyroid gland regulates the release of hormones to achieve a new balance, and maintains this balance until the end of the gestation process[19]. In general, the higher hormone need can only be met by a proportional increase in hormone release, which directly depends on the intake of iodine through the diet. At present, we know that iodine nutritional needs increase in all pregnant women due both to the higher hormone need and to the higher glomerular filtration rate[20]. This adaptation is achieved without difficulty by the thyroid machinery[21].

Conversely, when the thyroid gland fails -due, for example, to iodine deficiency-, such changes in thyroid parameters may not be adequately compensated and adaptation mechanisms fail[13, 21]

Obviously, the more severe iodine deficiency, the more serious fetal and maternal consequences are. However, it has been shown that such alterations can be found when pregnancy occurs in healthy women residing in moderately iodine-deficient areas[22].

3. Thyroid hormones and fetal brain development

3.1 Background

In 1888, the Clinical Society of London prepared a report which emphasized the key role of the thyroid gland for normal brain development[23]. The members of this committee reached this conclusion after observing that patients with both endemic and sporadic cretinism showed clear evidence of mental retardation.[24]

Initially, endemic cretinism was thought to be a congenital disease[25, 26]. However, the prenatal origin of this syndrome was confirmed when a clinical trial with iodized oil showed that it could be successfully prevented exclusively when iodine was supplied to the mother before conception.[3]

The classic works by Pharoah et al.[3,27] in Papua New Guinea in the 70's, and later by Thilly et al[4] in Ubangi (Zaire) and Malawi, provided a thorough description of the clinical symptoms of endemic cretinism (in its myxedema and neurological forms), which were characteristic of regions with severe endemic goiter.

These early studies supported the idea that severe iodine deficiency in the mother produces irreversible neurological damage in the fetus during critical development stages[12]. Cases of intrauterine deaths, miscarriages, death in childhood and the birth of cretins to women with biochemical evidence of iodine deficiency (very low free T4 levels) without clinical signs of hypothyroidism were described.[28, 29]

In 1976, *Pharoah et al*[27] pointed out that iodine deficiency was different from untreated myxedema and from congenital hypothyroidism, which are usually associated with menstrual disorders, infertility or repeated miscarriage.

Later, studies on iodine deficiency and its effects at the reproductive age and on progeny almost fell into oblivion in the scientific scene. It was believed that iodine deficiency had an impact only in certain geographic areas with severe endemic goiter, and that such dramatic consequences had been eradicated both in Europe and in the United States.[30]

Thus, a misconception of the pathophysiology of neurological deficit caused by iodine deficiency was established. The placenta was thought to prevent the transfer of thyroid hormones.[31] According to this theory, the fetal brain would develop in the absence of maternal transfer of these hormones[32] and, therefore, neurological damage could be prevented by hormone supplementation therapy at birth.[13]

In the following years in Europe, further clinical experience emphasized the significance of getting the diagnosis of congenital hypothyroidism, and initiating appropriate supplementation therapy as soon as possible after birth. The development of increasingly more precise[33, 34] screening tests of thyroid function allowed to identify congenital hypothyroidism at birth and begin treatment without delay[35].

However, clinical reports in regions with severe iodine deficiency suggested a different reality: there was a clear correlation between maternal hypothyroxinemia levels and the severity of neurological damage in the progeny. The lower the maternal FT4, the more serious the effects on the fetus, causing irreversible neurological and mental abnormalities at birth that could only be prevented by treating maternal hypothyroxinemia throughout the first half of gestation.[36] Subsequent interventions could not prevent all disorders.

But it was not until 1999 –when Haddow et al.[37] published their classic article in the *New England Journal of Medicine*– that iodine deficiency in pregnant women in developed countries was seen again as a problem also affecting populations that were so far thought to be safe from this endemic disease. Haddow et al.[37] found that infants of women with undiagnosed hypothyroidism (TSH above the 98th percentile) during pregnancy had lower scores on tests related to intelligence, attention, language, reading skills, school and visual-motor performance, and that such differences with the other infants were statistically significant in the 15 tests performed.

That same year, Pop et al [38] published an article proving that fetal neural development is not only affected when the mother has subclinical hypothyroidism, but it is just enough that

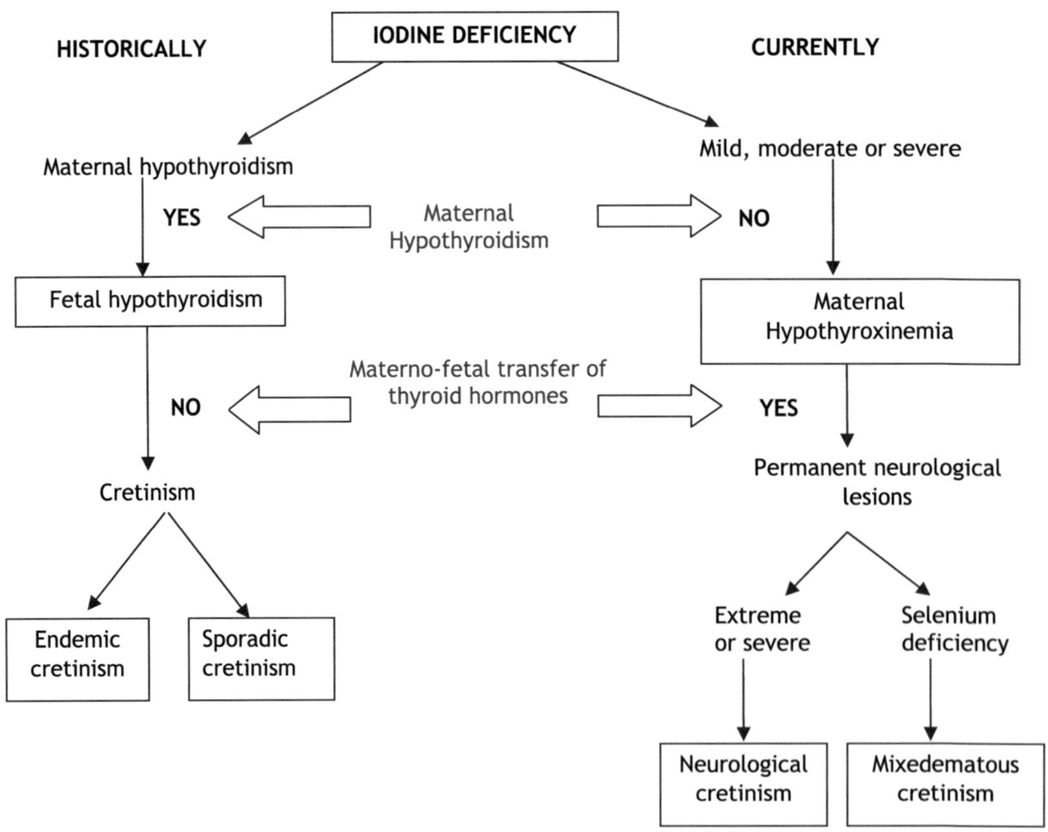

Fig. 1. Fetal and neonatal effects of iodine deficiency during pregnancy. The main advance is that maternal hormone transfer to the fetus during pregnancy has been definitely accepted, as well as the existence of damage in the progeny in absence of maternal hypothyroidism.

there is a previous stage of "maternal hypothyroxinemia" in the early stages of pregnancy. In their article, the authors showed that infants of mothers with T4 levels below the 10th percentile at the 12th week of gestation had significantly lower scores on the Bayley Psychomotor Development Scale at 10 months of age, compared with infants of mothers with higher free T4 levels.

In 2000, Morreale de Escobar et al.[36] presented epidemiological and experimental evidence strongly suggesting that first-trimester hypothyroxinemia (a low for gestational age circulating maternal free T4, whether or not TSH is increased) produces an increased risk for poor neuropsychological development of the fetus. The damage would be caused by decreased availability of maternal T4 to the developing brain.

Further, poor brain development occurs both in regions with severe iodine deficiency, and in regions with slight or moderate deficiency.[22, 28]

The identification of hypothyroxinemia as a factor which causes neurological damage in progeny -regardless whether or not the mother has hypothyroidism- is a landmark for the study of iodine deficiency in Europe.[32,36]

Figure 1 shows the differences between the classic and current understanding of the physiopathology of iodine deficiency.

4. Thyroid hormones and fetal neurological development

In humans, cerebral cortical development occurs between the 6th and the 24th week of gestation. The cortical plate begins to form around day 54 (8 weeks of gestation). Cortical neuronal migration mostly occurs between the week 8th and 24th (before the end of the second trimester), and generally before the onset of fetal thyroid hormone secretion occurs in the middle of gestation[39].

From a didactical perspective, fetal neurological development takes place in three stages relying on the thyroid hormone[40] (Figure 2):

1. The first stage takes place before the fetus starts producing thyroid hormones, and ends between the week 16th and 20th of gestation. During this period, thyroid hormone exposure comes only from maternally synthesized hormones, which influence neuronal proliferation and migration of neurons into the neocortex and hippocampus.
2. The second stage occurs during the remainder of pregnancy after the onset of the fetal thyroid function, when the developing brain derives its supply of thyroid hormones from both the fetus and the mother. At this moment, thyroid hormones will trigger neurogenesis, neuronal migration, axonal outgrowth, dendritic branching and synaptogenesis, and the onset of glial cell differentiation and migration, and myelination.
3. The third stage takes place during the neonatal and post-natal period when thyroid hormone supplies to the brain are entirely derived from the child and critical for continuing maturation. At this stage, thyroid hormones affect granule cell migration in the hippocampus and cerebellum, including the migration of cerebellar Purkinje cells. Gliogenesis and myelination continue during this stage.

Thyroid hormone receptors (TR alpha and beta) bind T3 with very high affinity, and act as ligand-induced transcription factors modulating the expression of different T3-dependent target genes[18]. Thus, although circulating levels of T4L are 4-fold higher than those of T3L, the thyroid hormone receptor has at least 15-fold more affinity for T3[40], which indicates that T4 is a prohormone that must be converted into T3 before the onset of thyroid hormone function.

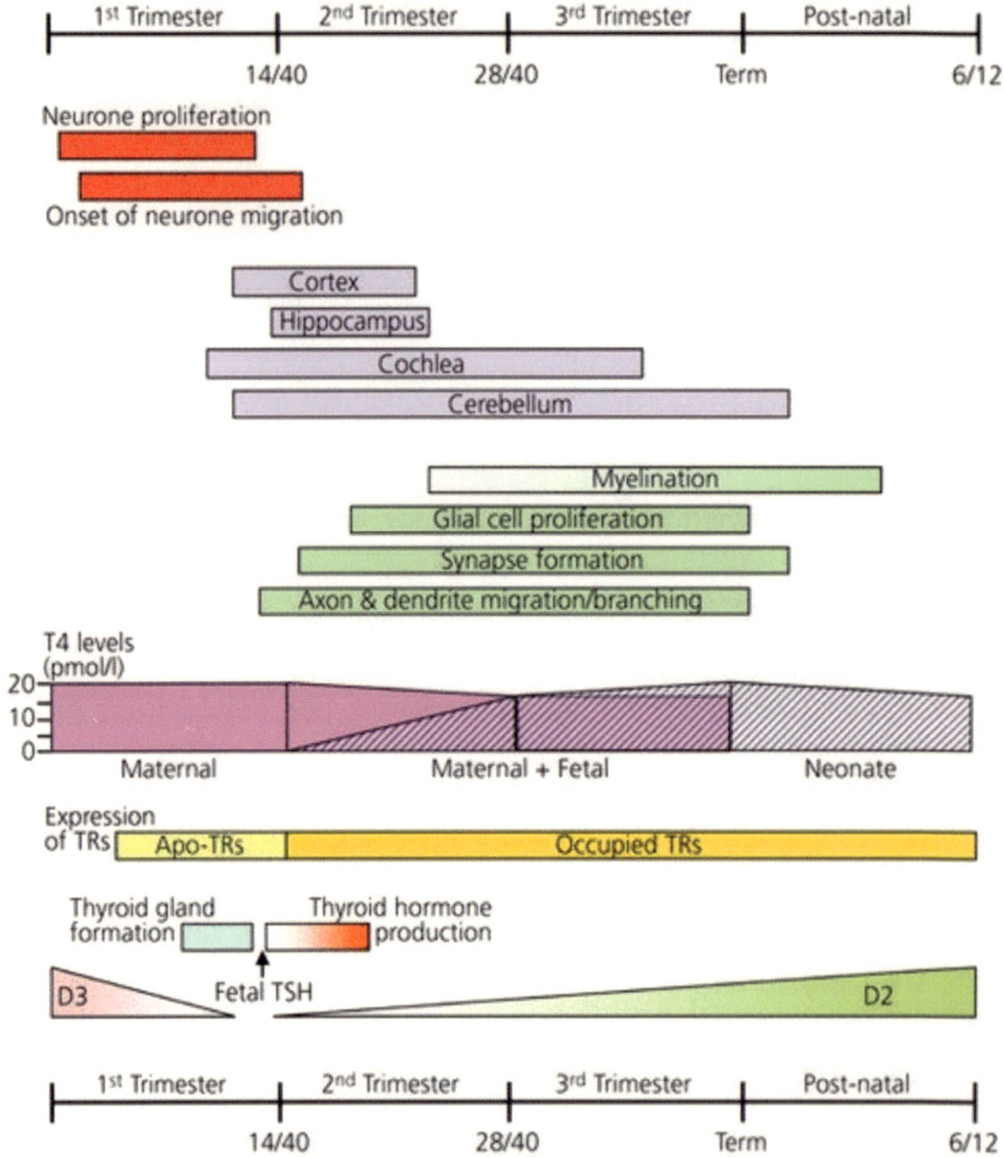

Fig. 2. Relationship between thyroid hormone action and brain development. In the first trimester of gestation, early neuronal proliferation and migration is dependent on maternal thyroxine (T4). In fetal tissues, deiodinase (ID-III, D3) enzyme expression falls and marks the onset of the fetal thyroid development. (D2: deiodinase ID-II). TRs: thyroid hormone receptors. From *Williams GR. Neurodevelopmental and Neurophysiological Actions of thyroid hormones. J Neuroendocrinol 2008; 20: 784-794.*

TR alpha and beta receptors express in most tissues, but their distribution varies from one tissue to another, which constitutes a control mechanism of T3 action that is specific in time and space.[41,42]

Towards the end of the first trimester, development of the hypothalamic-pituitary axis has occurred and causes an increase in TSH secretion that marks the onset of fetal thyroid hormone production. Then starts the activating deiodinase enzyme ID-II expression and increases the occupation of thyroid hormone receptors by T3.

Continuing development of the brain in the second and third trimesters relies increasingly on the T4 produced by both the fetus and mother. Continued post-natal development is entirely dependent on neonatal thyroid hormone secretion.

Thyroid hormones intervene directly or indirectly in most of the neurodevelopmental processes of the embryo and the fetus. This would explain that thyroid deficiency in early pregnancy causes irreversible effects[43,44].

Thyroid hormone receptors have been proven to express profusely both in neurons and in glial cells (astrocytes and oligodendrocytes)[45,46].

At neuronal level, thyroid hormones would act as "cofactors", favoring the expression of certain patterns of genes involved in axonal and dendrite outgrowth, and in the formation of synapses, myelination, cell migrations, and proliferation of specific cell populations[39].

For a proper neuronal function (synaptic transmission, laminar cytoarchitecture of the cerebral cortex) appropriate interaction with glial cells is required[47]. In this sense, thyroid hormones favor proliferation of oligodendrocyte precursor cells and their differentiation into mature oligodendrocytes (which make the myeline sheath)[46].

At the same time, thyroid hormones are involved in the maturation of radial glial cells, which are directly involved in neuronal migration into the different layers of the cerebral cortex.[48] Finally, thyroid hormones are directly involved in the development and maturation of glial cells in specific brain areas, as the hippocampus or the cerebellum.[44]

Thorough this sequence of events, it should be considered:

- That fetal neurodevelopment follows a very precise and limited sequence of events[47]. The response period of the cell is what is called competence. The same cell will not respond before or after this period.
- That the maturation sequence is not formed by a succession of independent events, but rather by cascading events where each anomaly.[49,50]

5. Thyroid hormone transfer and maternal hypothyroxinemia

In humans, maternal thyroid hormones are transferred to the fetus and the embryo during pregnancy. In fact, during the first half of gestation, the mother is the sole source of thyroid hormones[51,52].

Under normal conditions, embryonic tissues have a set of security mechanisms protecting their development. Some of these mechanisms are physical barriers (placenta and extraembryonic membranes) that avoid free transfer of maternal thyroid hormones into the fetus, and expose it to the same plasma fluctuations that occur in maternal blood serum[53,54].

Another security mechanism is the presence of deiodinase enzymes in fetal cerebral tissues[55,56]. Deiodinase enzymes take maternal free thyroxine (T4L) and subsequently convert it into T3, but do not allow direct transfer of maternal T3[57]. FNAs were made to obtain samples of fetal serum, and T4 concentrations in fetal serum were found to rely directly on maternal thyroxinemia[58].

In case of nutritional iodine deficiency, the organism activates self-regulating mechanisms where T3 is synthesized prevailingly over T4, as a way to save iodine[15] (Figure 3). This leads to a situation of maternal hypothyroxinemia, which is the fall of T4L levels in plasma, but presenting normal circulating T3L and TSH levels[36,57].

Maternal hypothyroxinemia is defined as:

- A "biochemical" status (low T4L levels with normal TSH values).
- It appears in healthy pregnant women (without any clinical sign or underlying thyroid pathology).
- It reflects a deficient nutritional status where the daily dietary intake of iodine is not adequate to meet iodine needs during pregnancy.
- It indicates maternal inability to guarantee adequate T4 transfer to the embryo, which is required for proper neurological development[36,38].

At present there is solid evidence that maternal hypothyroxinemia (low T4L) during the first half of gestation is the main cause of neurological alterations in the embryo and the fetus[57,59]. Such alterations are permanent and irreversible.

All levels of iodine deficiency (low, moderate or severe) affect the maternal and neonatal thyroid function, and infant's mental development[22].

6. Hypothyroxinemia and neurodevelopment

Animal models for iodine deficiency during pregnancy on development of the CNS have been developed for monkeys, sheep and rats.[2] These studies have shown changes in cerebellum with reductions in weight and cell number, and delayed maturation. The influence of maternal hypothyroxinemia on neocortical development has been recently studied in rats and mice.[60]

6.1 Altered migration during corticogenesis

The cerebral cortex is composed of neuronal layers with specific functions.[39] To form this cytoarchitecture, neurons undergo a Tangential migration from the basal epithelium into the upper layers of the cortex[44]. Neuronal migration is highest between the 11th and the 14th week of gestation, coinciding with the T4 peak in maternal blood serum during gestation.[32]

During this migration, neurons use glial cells like the steps of a stairway to climb into the upper layers[39,47]. This interaction between glial cells and neurons is enabled by thyroid hormones.[50,60]

Studies on radial migration during corticogenesis have revealed that in cerebral cortex of hypothyroid rats, the radial positioning of migrating neurons is altered[48,49], resulting in abnormally located Heterotopic neurons in the subcortical white matter (Figure 3)[2].

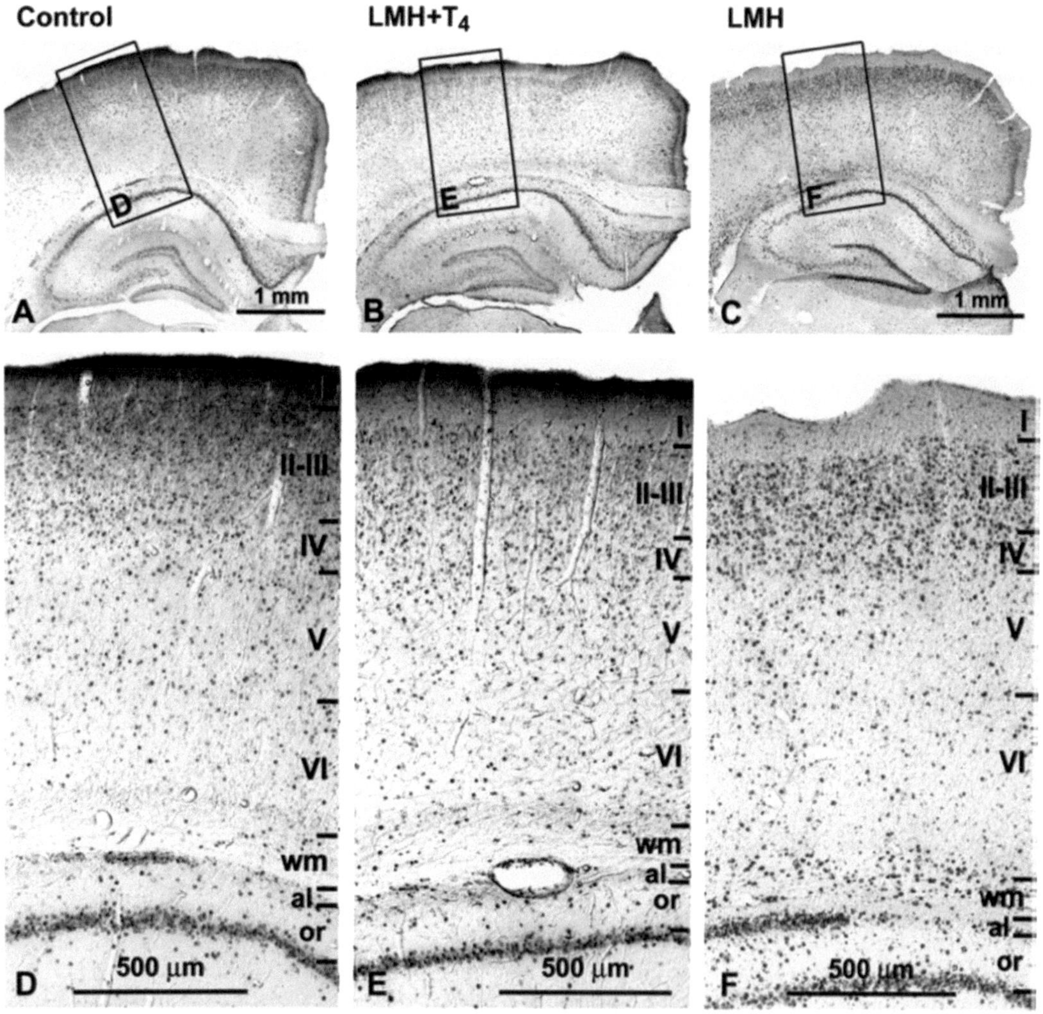

Fig. 3. (A—C) Low-magnification photomicrographs of coronal sections of the parietal cortex and hippocampus showing BrdU-immunoreactive cells after E17--20 injections in control, LMH þ T4, and LMH pups at P40. (D—F) Details (boxes in A, B, and C) showing that both in layers I—VI and white matter (wm) the neocortex and the alveus (al) and stratum oriens (or) of the hippocampus, the radial distribution of BrdU-immunoreactive cells is more widespread in LMH pups than in control and LMH þ T4 pups. Note the increased number of heterotopic BrdU-immunoreactive cells in wm, al, and or in LMH pups compared with that of control and LMH þ T4 pups. The borders between layers are indicated by horizontal lines. LMH= Late maternal hypothyroidism. *(Berbel P et al. Cerebral Cortex 2010)*[60]

6.2 Abnormal cortical cytoarchitecture and connectivity

Any situation compromising maternal thyroid hormone transfer to the fetus will disturb the neuronal migration process. As a result, neurons will not reach their final destination in the upper layers and their abnormal positioning will cause alterations in the laminar architecture of the cerebral cortex.[44]

In biopsies performed in experimental animals maternal thyroid hormone deficiency was found to cause permanent and irreversible lesions in the cerebral cortex cytoarchitecture. As in gestational hypothyroidism, hypothyroxinemia accuse neocortical layering blurred.

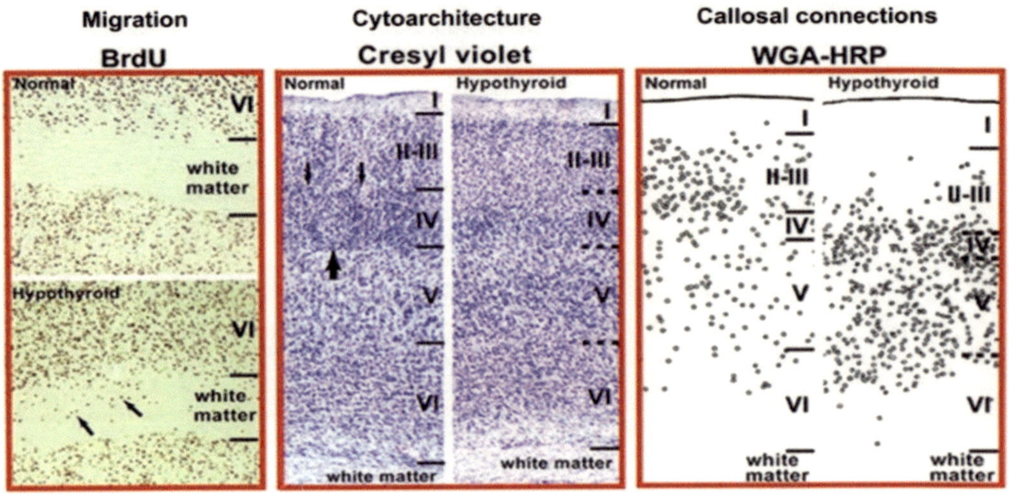

Fig. 4. **Left.** Photomicrographs of S1 coronal sections from normal and hypothyroid rats, showing the distribution of BrdU-labelled cells at P40, following injections at E15 and E17. Cells are more widely distributed in hypothyroid rats. Note the increased number of labeled cells, with respect to normal, in the white matter (wm) of hypothyroid rats. **Centre.** Photomicrographs of cresyl violet-stained coronal sections showing the PMBSF cytoarchitecture and layer borders in normal and hypothyroid rats. In normal rats, borders between layers are clear cut, while in hypothyroid rats (dashed lines) they are blurred. Note that in layer IV of hypothyroid rats, instead of normal barrels, disperse patches of high cell density can be seen. Arrowheads point to two septae adjacent to the barrel indicated by the arrow. **Right**. Plots of retrograde-labeled callosal neurons are shown in normal and hypothyroid rats. In normal rats, an important proportion of labeled neurones are in supragranular layers II and III. On the contrary, in hypothyroid rats, almost all labeled neurones are between layers IV and VI (*Berbel P. et al. Neuroscience 2001*)[62].

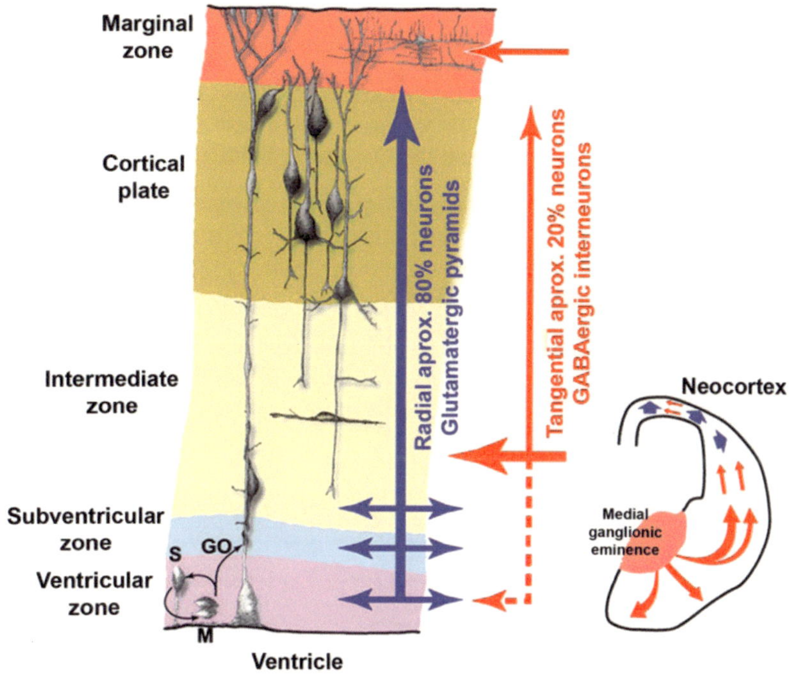

Fig. 5. Thyroid hormones play an important role in the neuronal migration process. Specifically, rats born to females with moderately low thyroid hormone levels have a disorganized cortical plate and many neurons do not migrate to their normal position. Furthermore, this action of thyroid hormones occurs during early fetal life. The figure shows the radial (blue arrow) and tangential (red arrows) migratory pathways. Both are afected by maternal hypothyroxinemia resulting in abnormal cortical lamination. (Adapted from *Berbel P. Mente y Cerebro 2003*)[63]

7. Physiopathology of fetal cerebral damage

Within this broad framework, three different situations can be found, with different results:

When maternal hormone transfer is deficient -as in cases of maternal hypothyroidism or hypothyroxinemia-, the hormone concentrations transferred to the embryo and the fetus are inadequate during early pregnancy. Later, at the onset of fetal thyroid function, there is increased secretion of T4 and T3 by the fetal thyroid gland, though it fails to meet successfully the early disruption of maternal hormone supply. Thus, T4 and T3 concentrations in fetal tissues are fairly normal when the fetus reaches term, but its intrauterine development will have suffered alterations.[38,64]

However, as the secretion of thyroid hormones increases, the fetal thyroid cannot store them. Therefore, neonates to mothers with thyroid malfunction have higher difficulty to meet the hormonal needs at birth than neonates to mother with normal thyroid function. This situation can lead to permanent neurological abnormalities[38,40].

When the maternal thyroid function is normal, but the fetal function is not -as it is the case in congenital hypothyroidism-, maternal T4 and T3 supply can partly mitigate fetal hypothyroidism. Although maternal T4 supply cannot replace completely the fetal thyroid function, it is crucial for brain development, where it does maintain normal T3 concentrations. However, such concentrations are not maintained in other tissues at normal levels.[65]

However, although maternal T3 levels are normal, this does not mitigate T3 deficiency in the fetus. The reason is that the fetal brain is totally dependent on the conversion of T4 into T3 by local action of 5'D-II, as T3 cannot be taken directly from plasma.[38,66]

Thus, these findings prove that maintaining adequate T4 levels in the mother is crucial, as it protects the brain of fetuses with congenital hypothyroidism until birth. Conversely, although the mother has normal T3 concentrations maintaining maternal euthyroid status, this hormone does not protect the fetal brain in mothers with hypothyroxinemia[38,40] .

When both the maternal and the fetal thyroid function are abnormal -as in the case of chronic iodine deficiency- mothers have very low levels of T4, though T3 concentrations are normal. In this situation, embryos and fetuses have deficient T4 levels during gestation and become increasingly deficient in T3.[64,67]

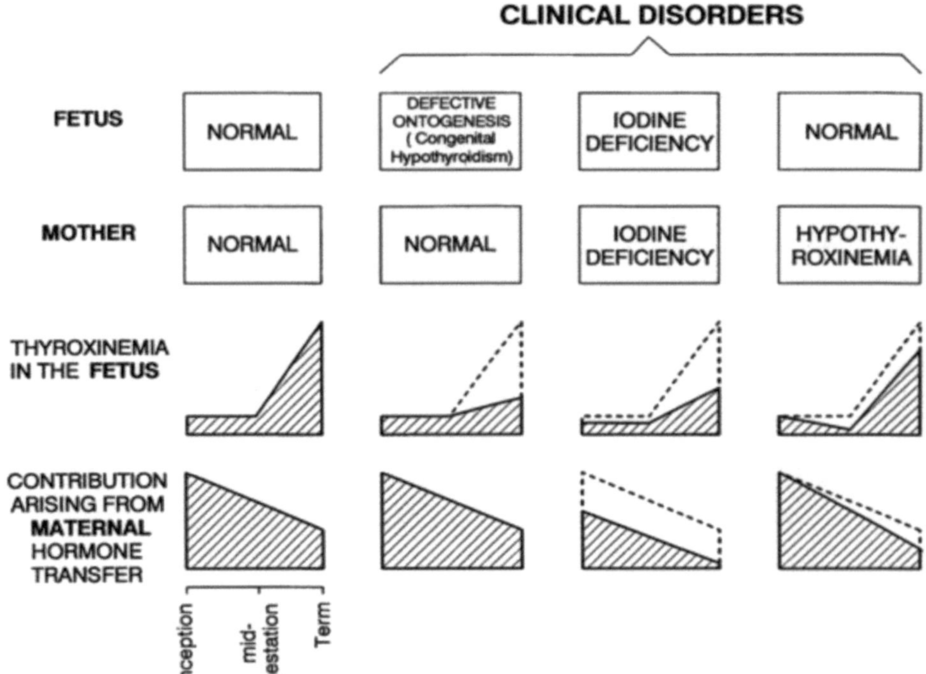

Fig. 6. In this table, the three clinical situations leading to altered maternal and/or fetal thyroid function are shown. It shows how the relative contributions of an altered maternal and/or fetal thyroid function can lead eventually to alterations in fetal thyroxine levels during intrauterine development. (From *Glinoer D, Delange F. The potential repercussions of maternal, fetal and neonatal hypothyroxinemia on the progeny. Thyroid 2000, 10 (10): 871-887)*[64].

When the fetal thyroid gland should start working, it cannot compensate for the disrupted maternal supply, since it does not have enough iodine for the synthesis and secretion of T4. At the same time, the fetal brain has not preferential protection from maternal T4, as this hormone cannot be biosynthesized due to the deficiency of iodine. As a result, fetal tissues –

including the fetal brain– are very deficient in T4 and T3 during very important stages of cerebral neurogenesis and maturation.[41,68] .

These data suggest that the pathogenic mechanisms that lead to cretinism and severe hypothyroidism are multifactorial, and the effects of severe iodine deficiency can be amplified by the deleterious effects of thiocyanate overload, selenium deficiency, and glandular destruction and fibrosis occurring gradually during childhood[69]. By contrast, when iodine supplementation is given to women in regions with endemic iodine deficiency, cretinism can be eradicated, and neonatal hypothyroidism prevented[70].

8. Clinical effects of prenatal iodine deficiency

Now that we know the "virtually universal" participation of thyroid hormones in the development and proliferation of fetal neural tissue, the complex clinical manifestations of thyroid hormone deficit in early pregnancy can be easily anticipated.

Therefore, maternal and fetal hypothyroxinemia caused by iodine deficiency determines permanent lesions in the upper cortical areas, hippocampus and cerebellum[48,64], which causes neurological abnormalities with relatively well-defined characteristics:

- Brain stem or medullar elements are not affected, so there is no direct motor dysfunction, but abnormal motor coordination function[39].
- The lesions affect the integration areas of the cerebral cortex –including “silent” areas of the association areas of the cortex– showing poorly defined anatomical alterations.
- They do not have perinatal clinical expression, although they express later during early years of life until school age.[71,72]
- Therefore, these lesions cannot be detected by modern prenatal diagnosis techniques.[30]

A number of research studies conducted in regions with moderate iodine deficiency have shown the presence of irreversible alterations in the intellectual and neuro-psycho-motor development of infants and adults that were clinically euthyroid and that did not exhibit other signs or symptoms of endemic cretinism, which is the most serious form of brain damage caused by iodine deficiency.

In follow-up studies on infants of mothers with hypothyroxinemia identified in the first trimester of pregnancy, low scores were obtained on scales measuring psychomotor development (psychometric tests used to find evidence of these abnormalities are varied and include adapted intelligence tests, regardless of the subjects' culture). Such results were especially significant in those tests that assess visual-motor coordination, object manipulation, understanding the relationship between objects, imitation and early language development[38,73]. The results showed low visual-motor performance, motor skills, perceptual and neuromotor skills, and low development and intelligence quotients (IQ)[71,76].

Bleichrodt and Born[74] conducted a meta-analysis of 19 studies on neuromotor and cognitive functions in conditions of moderate to severe iodine deficiency, and concluded that iodine deficiency leads to a loss of 13.5 IQ points, as compared with the global population. Apart from goiter, brain damage and loss of intellectual potential caused by iodine deficiency are an obstacle to the socioeconomic development of people, and must be considered as a major public health problem.

More recently, iodine deficiency –maternal hypothyroxinemia– has been identified as a causal factor of attention-deficit hyperactivity disorder[75].

9. Fetal and neonatal effects of iodine deficiency[27]

Reference	Inclusion criteria	Conclusions	Comments
Pharoah POD, Buttfield IH, Hetzel BS. Neurological damage to the fetus resulting from severe iodine deficiency during pregnancy Lancet 1971, 1: 308	*Type of participants*: Total population from 27 villages in Papua Nueva Guinea. *Type of intervention*: Administration of intramuscular iodized oil. *Type of results*: Changing incidence of endemic cretinism	Controlled clinical trial in a city of 8,000 inhabitants. Intramuscular iodized oil is effective for the prevention of endemic cretinism. To be effective, it must be administered before conception. Maternal severe iodine deficit causes neurological damage during fetal development.	Pioneer intervention study on populations with severe iodine deficit. The cohort monitored is very small, as compared with the initial group. The results obtained are expressed in terms of infant mortality and endemic cretinism incidence.
Thilly C, Delange F y cols. Fetal Hypothyroidism and maternal thyroid status in severe endemic goiter J Clin Endocrinol Metab 1978; 47: 354	*Type of participants*: A total of 109 pregnant women and 128 newborn babies from Ubangi, Zaire. *Type of intervention*: Administration of intramuscular iodized oil to a group of pregnant women. *Type of results*: Changing TSH, T4 and T3 concentrations in mothers and newborn babies.	Maternal thyroid function in regions with severe endemic goiter is a good indicator of the thyroid function in a neonate. The factors responsible for this hypothetical relationship seem to be environmental factors acting simultaneously in the mother and the fetus.	Pregnant women were grouped "randomly" into two groups. The results obtained are shown in thyroid function values of the mother and the neonate at birth.
Bleichrodt N, Born MP. A metaanalysis of research on iodine and its relationship to cognitive development. Nutr Rev 1996; 54 (4 Pt 2): S72- S78	*Type of participants*: Previous Articles *Type of intervention*: Metaanalysis of 19 studies on neuro-motor and cognitive functions under conditions of moderate to severe iodine deficiency. *Type of results*: Depending on the study reviewed.	Iodine deficiency causes a decrease of 13.5 IQ points as compared with the global population.	

Reference	Inclusion criteria	Conclusions	Comments
Haddow JE, Glenn MD y cols Maternal thyroid deficiency during pregnancy and subsequent neuropsychological development of the child N Engl J Med 1999; 341: 549.5556	*Type of participants*: 62 pregnant women with TSH above the 98th percentile, and 124 pregnant women with normal TSH levels. *Type of intervention*: Infants aged 7-9 underwent 15 tests. *Type of results*: Scores obtained in different neuropsychological performance tests.	Infants of women with high TSH concentrations scored seven points lower than the infants of 124 control women (p=0,005) in the 15 tests employed, and 19 percent scored 85 or even lower. Undiagnosed hypothyroidism in pregnant women can damage the fetus.	Retrospective study on a bank of pregnant women serum collected for a period of three years. The results are expressed in terms of the scores obtained in intelligence, attention, language, reading skills, school performance and vasomotor development tests.
Pop VJ, Kuijpens JL y cols. Low maternal free thyroxine concentrations during early pregnancy are associated with impaired psychomotor development in infancy Clin Endocr 1999; 50: 149- 155	*Type of participants*: 220 pregnant women and 220 infants at 10 months. *Type of intervention*: Study of maternal thyroid function and evaluation of the neurological development of infants at 10 months of life. *Type of results*: Scores obtained by children on the Bayley Scale of Psycho-motor development.	Low free T4 plasma concentrations during early pregnancy may be a relevant risk factor of mental retardation in the progeny. Free T4 concentrations are defined as an independent parameter for the neurological development of the progeny.	This is the first study to prove that low free TSH levels in apparently healthy women during early pregnancy increase significantly the risk of fetal neurological damage. Maternal TSH, fT and TPO antibodies are analyzed at the 12th and 32th week of gestation. Consequences at the 12th week and the rest of weeks of pregnancy.
Morreale de Escobar G, Obregón MJ y Escobar del Rey F. Is neuropsychological development related to maternal hypothyroidism or to maternal hypothyroxinemia? J Clin Endocrinol Metab 2000; 85: 3975- 3987	*Type of participants*: Previous articles *Type of intervention*: Systematic analysis of articles published on the effects of maternal hypothyroxinemia on the fetal neurological development *Type of results*: Relying on the study reviewed.	Maternal hypothyroxinemia in the first trimester increases the risk of fetal neuropsychological damage. Maternal T4 is the sole source of thyroid hormone for the fetal brain during the first trimester. Normal T3 concentrations in the mother do not prevent from potential damaged caused by a low T4 supply	Through analysis of the main findings made in regions with severe iodine deficiency, in regions without iodine deficiency and in studies with experimental animals. Development of a unifying theory on the severity and frequency of neurological damage in the progeny of mothers with hypothyroxinemia, in contrast with mothers with hypothyroidism.

10. Studies with potassium iodide supplementation

Finally, supplementation with potassium iodide (KI) from the early stages of pregnancy in pregnant women has proven to be a safe and effective method for preventing cognitive impairment associated with nutritional iodine deficiency.

Inclusion criteria	Subjects	Methods	Conclusion	Comments	Reference
Pregnant women from a moderate iodine deficiency area.	Pregnant women treated with iodized salt compared with pregnant women as control group.	Randomized Clinical Trial: 35 pregnant women of which 17 were administered 120-180 μg of iodine in form of iodized salt. Another 18 women served as the control group. Determination of TSH, Urinary iodine excretion (UIE) and thyroid volume.	Iodine Urinary Excretion in the third trimester was significantly higher in the group studied (100± 39 vs 50±37 of iodine). (p<0,0001) The thyroid volume increased significantly in the control group, mainly due to relative iodine deficiency.	Very limited sample size. The results obtained are statistically significative, although the sample size was very small. The authors suggest the use of iodine prophylaxis to prevent the increase in thyroid volume and avoid the risk of maternal and fetal hypothyroidism.	Romano R, et al, Am J Obstet Gyneol 1991.
Healthy pregnant women, recruited at early gestation. Exclusion criteria: thyroid disease or medication that could affect thyroid function	Pregnant women treated with potassium iodide (KI) solution compared with pregnant women as control group.	Randomized Clinical Trial: 28 pregnant women who received 200 μg/day of iodine from 17-18 weeks of gestation until 12 months after delivery. A total of 26 women served as the control group.	A relatively low iodine intake during pregnancy leads to thyroid stress, with increased release of TG and of thyroid volume, with little clinical effects, according to the authors. Iodine does not cause significant changes in T4, T3 or free T4 in serum.	Very small sample. The conclusions can not be considered as definitive. The same group presented seven years later a study with opposite results.	Pedersen KM, Laurberg P and cols; J Clin Endocrinol Metab 1993

Inclusion criteria	Subjects	Methods	Conclusion	Comments	Reference
Euthyroid pregnant women, selected at the end of the first trimester with biochemical criteria of excessive thyroid stimulation (thyroglobuline ↑, with a low normal free T4 index and/or increased T3/T4 ratio.	Study with a control group and two groups that received 100μg/day of iodine and the other 100 μg/day of iodine+ 100 μg/day of T4. N=60 pregnant women in each group.	Randomized clinical trial, double-blind: In both groups of women who received active treatment, alterations in thyroid function associated with pregnancy improved significantly. Maternal and neonatal parameters of thyroid function, UIE and thyroid volume were assessed by ultrasound	The administration of T4 failed to mask the beneficial effects of iodine supplementation in pregnant women, especially in the prevention of goiter.	As a starting point, the researchers selected a population at risk relying on biochemical parameters indicating thyroid overstimulation. The results can not be extrapolated to normal populations of pregnant women.	Glinoer D et al, J Clin Endocrinol Metab 1995
Healthy pregnant women at 10-12 weeks of gestation.	Clinical trial , pregnant women who received IK were compared with a control group.	Non randomized clinical trial with 108 women, of whom 38 received 300 μg of IK/day (230 μg of iodine) and 70 served as the control group. Thyroid volumen, thyroid function, UIE and TPO antibody levels were measured in the week 10-12 and after delivery.	After receiving iodine fortification, IUE increased significantly in mothers and neonate The thyroid volumen in neonates to mothers that received fortification was lower than that of the control group	Iodine supplementation during pregnancy in regions with moderate iodine deficiency causes a lower thyroid volume in neonate. This supplementation does not increase TPO antibody frequency	Liesenkötter KP et al. Eur J Endocrinol 1996

Inclusion criteria	Subjects	Methods	Conclusion	Comments	Reference
Pregnant women, entering the study at any stage of pregnancy.	Clinical trial with pregnant women treated with IK and compared with a control group.	Non randomized and comparative study in pregnant women, of whom 93 received 150 μg/day of iodine and 419 served as control group. Determination of UIE and T4L during pregnancy, anti-TPO, anti-TG, maternal and neonatal thyroid volume	Iodine supplementation enhances significantly IUE and T4L levels during the whole gestation. Lower maternal and neonatal thyroid volume was found in the group that received supplementation.	The control group consisted of a significant sample of pregnant women. In both groups UIE increases progressively during pregnancy, but the control group had normal urinary iodine excretion <100 mg / L during pregnancy.	De Santiago J, et al J Endocrinol Invest 1999
Mother/newborn pairs. All newborns were healthy and delivered at term and were breastfed.	Babies from mother treated with IK compared with babies from a control group	Randomized clinical trial in 89 mothers and their babies: 57 served as the control group, 32 received 175 μg IK/day (134 μg of iodine) during pregnancy. Identification of thyroid volumen UIE, nutritional questionnaire	UIE of neonates to supplemented mothers increased by 62 percent, while the thyroideal volume of these children decreased by 18 percent, as compared with the control group. Neonatal TSH was maintained within normal ranges.	It DOES NOT include maternal thyroid function values. In this study, the fact that the mother was a smoker was taken into account. Babies born to smoking mothers had 20 percent higher thyroid volume than those born to non smokers.	Klett M et al Acta Paediátrica Suppl 1999

Inclusion criteria	Subjects	Methods	Conclusion	Comments	Reference
Healthy pregnant women with no previous history of thyroid disease were recruited when admitted for delivery.	Pregnant women that have taken IK were compared with a control group. Babies from mother treated with IK compared with babies from a control group	Observational study 144 women and their progeny participated in the study, of which 49 received 150 µg iodine/day during pregnancy and 95 served as control subjects. Identification of maternal thyroid function (TSH, T4L, T3L, TG) and neonatal function in cord blood (TSH, T4L, T3L, thyroglobulin)	Researchers found that TSH has an opposite behavior in the mother (decreases) to that of the neonate (increases) in the group supplemented with iodine. T4L is higher in the mothers and infants of the supplemented group.	The authors attribute the rise in TSH to a transient impasse of neonatal iodine-induced thyroid.	Nøhr S, Laurberg P
TPO-Ab-positive women in early pregnancy	Three groups of study stratified by anti-TPO titers into 3 groups: 22 women received 150 mg iodine / day from conception up to 9 months postpartum (+/+), only 24 received iodine during pregnancy and 26 (+/-) did not receive iodine (-/-).	Placebo-controlled, randomized, , double blind trial. Study of thyroid function at 35 weeks of gestation and 9 months after delivery.	They found that the incidence, severity and type of thyroid dysfunction postpartum rely predominantly on anti-TPO levels (positive correlation). Supplementation with iodine during pregnancy and postpartum does not induce or worsen postpartum thyroid dysfunction.	The authors concluded that iodine supplementation during pregnancy and postpartum is safe, even in women with positive anti-TPO. Screening for anti-TPO in the first trimester can predict women at risk of developing postpartum thyroid dysfunction.	Nøhr S, et al J Clin Endocrinol Metab 2000

Inclusion criteria	Subjects	Methods	Conclusion	Comments	Reference
Pregnant women enrolled from the 10th to the 16th week of gestation.	32 pregnant women supplemented with 50 μg/day of iodine (group A) and 35 received 200 μg/day (group B) from conception to 6 months after delivery.	Randomized clinical study Determination of thyroid volume, thyroid function in all three trimesters of pregnancy.	The dose of 50 μg/day is an inexpensive and safe method to prevent goiter. The dose of 200 μg/day seems to be more effective, has not side effects and does not increase the frequency of autoimmune postpartum thyroiditis.	There were not any control group, since the Committee of Ethics and Clinical Research did not give authorization. Five cases of postpartum thyroiditis (2 in group A and 3 in group B) were detected. All these women had low circulating autoantibodies before starting the test.	Antonangeli L et al Eur J Endocrinol 2002
Children whose mothers were supplemented during pregnancy. The comparison group were children recruited at 2 years of age.	148 infants of mothers who received iodine supplementation during pregnancy were compared with 169 infants who received iodine aged from 2 years, for a period of 1 year. There were no untreated group.	Longitudinal study. Psychometric tests used: Raven Progressive Matrices, Developmental test of Visual Motor Integration (VMI) and Denver Developmental Screening Test (DDST).	Iodine before the 3rd trimester predicted higher psychomotor test scores for children relative to those provided iodine later in pregnancy or at 2 years of age.	Iodine supplementation was carried out by adding it to the irrigation water.	O'Donnell K, et al Develop Med & Child Neurol 2002
Pregnant women at the first trimester of gestation for the study group. Pregnant women at the third trimester of gestation for control group.	The study included 133 women who received 300 μg of potassium iodine and 61 women who had received no iodine supplements.	Non randomized, clinical trial. Main outcome measures: Bayley Scales of Infant Development. Maternal and infant thyroid function: TSH, free T3, free T4 and urine iodine	Infants whose mothers had received an iodine supplement had more favorable psychometric assessment and higher scores on the Psychomotor Development Index (p =0,02) and the Behavior Scale.	Given the possible presence of confounding variables no controlled for in this study, these findings should be considered as preliminary.	Velasco I et al J Clin Endocrinol Metab 2009;

Inclusion criteria	Subjects	Methods	Conclusion	Comments	Reference
Group 1 included infants of women with FT4 above the 20th percentile at 4-6 gestational weeks and at full-term. Group 2 included neonates to women with mild hypothyroxinemia diagnosed during the first 12-14 gestational weeks and with FT4 above the 20th percentile at full-term. Group 3 included infants born to women with mild hypothyroxinemia without iodine supplementation during pregnancy.	Three groups of infants were compared. Women of all groups were iodine supplemented from the day of enrolment until the end of lactation.	Clinical trial Psychometric Test: Brunet-Lézine Scale at 18 months of age.	Delayed Neuro-behavioral performance was observed in 36.8 percent and 25.0 percent of infants in groups 3 and 2, respectively, as compared with infants in group 1. A delay of 6-10 weeks in iodine Fortification of Hypothyroxine-mic mothers at the beginning of gestation increases the risk of neurodevelop mental delay in the progeny.	Women of all groups were iodine supplemented (200 μg KI per day) from the day of enrollment until the end of lactation. No women were found to be Hypothyroxine-mic at full-term after supplementation.	Berbel P, et al. Thyroid 2009

11. References

[1] Comprehensive Handbook of Iodine: Nutritional, Biochemical, Pathological and Therapeutic aspects. Watson RR, Preedy VR, Burrow GN. 2009 Elsevier Science.

[2] Berbel P, Navarro D, Ausó E, Varea E, Rodríguez AE, Ballesta JJ, Salinas M, Flores E, Faura CC, Morreale de Escobar G. Role of late maternal thyroid hormones in cerebral cortex development: an experimental model for human prematurity. Cerebral Cortex Jun 2010: 20: 1462-1475.

[3] Pharoah POD, Buttfield IH.Neurological damage to the fetus resulting from severe iodine deficiency during pregnancy. Lancet 1971:1; 308-310.

[4] Thilly CH, Delange F, Lagasse R, Bourdoux P, Ramioul L, Berquist H, Ermans AM. Fetal hypothyroidism and maternal thyroid status in severe endemic goiter. Journal of Clinical Endocrinology and Metabolism 1978: 47 (2); 354-360.

[5] Mahomed K, Gülmezoglu AM, Maternal iodine supplements in areas of deficiency. The Cochrane Database of Systematics Reviews, Issue 1, 2004.

[6] DeLong GR, Stanbury JB, Fierro-Benítez R. Neurological signs in congenital iodine-deficiency disorder (endemic cretinism). Dev Med Child Neurol 1985; 27: 317- 324.
[7] Haddow JE, Palomaki GE, Allan WC, et al. Maternal thyroid deficiency during pregnancy and subsequent neuropsychological development of the child. N EnglJ Med. 1999; 341: 549-555.
[8] Utiger RD. Maternal hypothiroidism and fetal development. N Engl J Med. 1999; 341: 601-602.
[9] Glinoer D. Maternal and fetal impact of chronic iodine deficiency. Clin Obstet Gynecol 1997; 40: 102- 116.
[10] Larsen PR, Silva JE, Kaplan MM. Relationships between circulating and intracellular thyroid hormones: physiological and clinical implications. Endocr Rev 1981; 2: 87-102.
[11] Pop VJ, Van Baar AL, Vulsma T. Should all pregnant women be screened for hypothyroidism?. Lancet 1999; 354: 1224- 1225.
[12] Morreale de Escobar G, Obregón MJ, Escobar del Rey F. Maternal thyroid hormones early in pregnancy and fetal brain development. Best Practice & Research Clinical Endocrinology & Metabolism 2004; 18 (2): 225- 248.
[13] Burrow GN, Fisher DA, Reed Larsen P. Maternal and fetal thyroid function. N England J Med 1994; 331: 1072-1078.
[14] Glinoer D. The regulation of thyroid function during normal pregnancy: importance of the iodine nutrition status. Best Practice & Research Clinical Endocrinology & Metabolism 2004; 18 (2): 133-152.
[15] Morreale de Escobar G, Escobar del Rey F: Hormonas tiroideas durante el desarrollo fetal: comienzo de la función tiroidea y transferencia maternofetal. Tratado de Endocrinología Pediátrica, Pombo y cols. 3ª Edición, 2002.
[16] Zoeller RT. Transplacental thyroxine and fetal brain development. J Clin Invest 2003; 111: 954-957.
[17] Oppenheimer JH, Schwartz HL. Molecular basis of thyroid hormone-dependent brain development. Endocr Rev 1997; 18(4): 462-475.
[18] Williams, GR. Neurodevelopmental and neurophysiological actions of thyroid hormone. Journal of neuroendocrinology 2008: 20(6):784-794.
[19] Glinoer D. Clinical and Biological consequences of iodine deficiency during pregnancy. Endocr Dev 2007:10; 62-85.
[20] Domínguez I, Reviriego S, Rojo-Martínez G, Valdés MJ, Carrasco R, Coronas I, López-Ojeda J, Pacheco M, Garriga MJ, García-Fuentes E, González Romero S, C-Soriguer Escofet FJ. Iodine deficiency and thyroid function in healthy pregnant women. Med Clin (Barc). 2004 Apr 3;122(12):449-53.
[21] Glinoer D.The importance of iodine nutrition during pregnancy. Public Health Nutr. 2007 Dec;10(12A):1542-6.
[22] Delange F. Iodine deficiency as a cause of brain damage. Postgrad Med J 2001; 77: 217-220.
[23] Ord WM. Report of a committee of the Clinical Society of London nominated December 14, 1883, to investigate the subject of mixoedema. Trans Clin Soc Lond 1888; 21 (Suppl): 1-215.
[24] Sawin CT. The invention of thyroid therapy in the late nineteenth century. Endocrinologist 2001; 11 (1): 1-3.

[25] Eggenberger H, Messerli FM. Theory and results of prophylaxis of endemic goiter in Switzerland. Transactions of the 3rd International Conference on Goitre 1938; pp 64-67.
[26] McCullagh SF. The Huon peninsula endemic. IV. Endemic goitre and congenital defect. Medical Journal of Australia 1963; 1: 884-890.
[27] Pharoah POD, Ellis SM, Ekins RP, Williams ES. Maternal thyroid function, iodine deficiency and fetal development. Clin Endocrinol 1976; 5: 159-166.
[28] Glinoer D, Delange F. The potential repercussions of maternal, fetal, and neonatal hypothyroxinemia on the progeny. Thyroid 2000; 10: 871- 877.
[29] Dunn JT, Delange F. Damaged reproduction: the most important consequence of iodine deficiency. J Clin Endocrinol Metab 2001; 86 (6): 2360-2363.
[30] Velasco López I. Anomalías prenatales asociadas a la deficiencia de yodo. Prog Diag Trat Prenat 2005; 17 (3): 123-128.
[31] Fisher DA. The unique endocrine milieu of the fetos. J Clin Invest 1986; 78: 603-611.
[32] Morreale de Escobar, G. Yodo y Embarazo. En Yodo y Salud en el Siglo XXI. Ed European Pharmaceutical Law Group. Madrid. 2005 Pags 105-144.
[33] Larsen PR, Merker A, Parlow AF. Immunoassay of human TSH using dried blood samples. J Clin Endocrinol Metab 1976; 42: 987- 990.
[34] Dussault JH, Parlow a, Letarje J, Guyda J, Laberge C. TSH measurements from blood spots on filter paper: a confirmatory screening test for neonate hypothyroidism. J Pediatr 1976; 89: 550- 552.
[35] Fisher DA, Foley BL Early treatment of congenital hypothyroidism. Pediatrics. 1989 May;83(5):785-9.
[36] Morreale de Escobar G, Obregón MJ, Escobar del Rey F. Is neuropsychological development related to maternal hypothyroidism or to maternal hypothyroxinemia?. J Endocrinol Metab 2000; 85 (11): 3975-3987.
[37] Haddow JE, Palomaki GE, Allan WC, et al. Maternal thyroid deficiency during pregnancy and subsequent neuropsychological development of the child. N EnglJ Med. 1999; 341: 549-555.
[38] Pop V, Kuipens JL, van Baar AL, et al. Low maternal free thyroxine concentrations during early pregnancy are associated with impaired psychomotor development in infancy. Clin Endocrinol (Oxf).1999; 50: 149-155.
[39] Amiel-Tison. Neurología perinatal. Barcelona, Ediciones Masson.2001.
[40] Utiger RD. Maternal hypothyroidism and fetal development. N Engl J Med 1999; 341: 601-602.
[41] Kester MHA, Martinez de Mena R, Obregón MJ, Marinkovic D, Howatson A, Visser TJ, Hume R, Morreale de Escobar G. Iodothyronine levels in the human developing brain: major regulatory roles of iodothyronine desiodinases in different areas. J Clin Endocrinol Metab 2004; 89 (7): 3117- 3128.
[42] Bianco AC, Kim BW. Deiodinases: implications of the local control of thyroid hormone action. J Clin Invest 2006; 116: 2571- 2579.
[43] Cuevas E, Ausó E, Telefont M, Morreale de Escobar G, Sotelo C, Berbel P. Transient maternal hypothyroxinemia at onset of corticogenesis alters tangential migration of medial ganglionic eminence-derived neurons. Eur J Neurosci. 2005 Aug; 22(3): 541-551.

[44] Lavado- Autric R, Ausó E, García-Velasco JV, Arufe MC, Escobar del Rey F, Berbel P, Morreale de Escobar G. Early maternal hypothyroxinemia alters histogenesis and cerebral cortex cytoarchitecture of the progeny. J Clin Invest 2003; 111: 1073- 1082.
[45] Iskaros J, Pickard M, Evans I, Sinha A, Harmidan P, Ekins R. Thyroid hormone receptor gene expression in first trimester human fetal brain. J Clin Endocrinol Metab 2000: 85 (7):2620-2623.
[46] Anderson GW. Thyroid hormones and the brain. Frontiers in Neuroendocrinology 2001; 22: 1-17.
[47] Poch ML. Neurobiologia del desarrollo temprano. Contextos educativos 2 (2001): 79-94.
[48] Martinez-Galan JR, Pedraza P, Santacana M, Escobar del Rey F, Morreale de Escobar G, Ruiz-Marcos A. Early effects of iodine deficiency on radial glial cells of the hippocampus of the rat fetus. A model of neurological cretinism. J Clin Invest 1997;99: 2701-2709.
[49] Lauffenburger DA, Horwitz AF. Cell migration: a physically integrated molecular process. Cell 1996; 84: 359- 369.
[50] Sun XZ Takahashi S, Cui C, Zhang R, Sakata-Haga H, Sawada K, Fukui Y. Normal and abnormal migration in the developing cerebral cortex. J Med Invest 2002; 49: 97-110.
[51] Morreale de Escobar G, Calvo R, Obregón MJ, Escobar del Rey F. Contribution of maternal thyroxine to fetal thyroxine pools in normal rats near term. Endocrinology 1990; 126: 2765- 2767.
[52] Calvo R, Jauniaux E, Gulbis B, Asunción M, Gervy C, Contempré B, Morreale de Escobar G. Fetal tissues are expossed to biologically relevant free thyroxine concentrations during early phases of development. J Clin Endocrinol Metab 2002; 87: 1768- 1777.
[53] Mortimer RH, Galligan JP, Cannell GR, Addison RS, Roberts MS. Maternal to fetal thyroxine transmission in the human term placenta is limited by inner ring deiodination. J Clin Endocrinol Metab 1996; 81: 2247-2249.
[54] Koopdonk-kool JM, De Vijlder J, Veenboer G, Vulsma T, Boer K, Visser TJ. Typt II and Type III deiodinase activity in human placenta as a function of gestational age. J Clin Endocrinol Metab 1996; 81: 2154-2158.
[55] Santini F, Chiovatto L, Ghirri P, Lapi P, Mammoli C, Montanelli L, Scartabelli G, Pinchera A. Serum iodothyronines in the human fetus and the newborn: Evidence for an important role of placenta in fetal thyroid hormone homeostasis. J Clin Endocrinol Metab 1999; 84: 493- 498.
[56] Carvalho DP. Modulation of uterine iodothyronine deiodinases- a critical event for fetal development? Endocrinology 2003; 144: 4250- 4252.
[57] Calvo R, Obregón MJ, Ruiz de Oña C, Escobar del Rey F, Morreale de Escobar G. Congenital hypothyroidism, as studied in rats. Crucial role of maternal thyroxine but not of 3,5,3'-triiodothyronine in the protection of the fetal brain. J Clin Invest 1990; 86: 889- 899.
[58] Contempré B, Jauniaux E, Calvo R et al. Detection of thyroid hormones in human embrionic cavities during the first trimester of pregnancy. J Clin Endocrinol Metab, 1993; 77: 1719-1722.

[59] Pop VJ, Brouwers E, Vader HL, Vulsma T, Van Baar AL, De Vijlder JJ. Maternal hypothyroxinaemia during early pregnancy and subsequent child development: a 3-year follow-up study. Clin Endocr 2003; 59: 282- 288.
[60] Berbel P, Bernal J. Hypothyroxinemia: a subclinical condition affecting neurodevelopment. Expert Review of Endocrinology & Metabolism, July 2010, Vol. 5, No. 4, Pages 563-575.
[61] Ausó, E., Lavado-Autric, R., Cuevas, E., Escobar del Rey, F., Morreale de Escobar, G. and Berbel, P., A moderate and transient deficiency of maternal thyroid function at the beginning of fetal neocorticogenesis alters neuronal migration. Endocrinology 2004:145:4037-4047.
[62] Berbel, P., Ausó, E., García-Velasco J.V., Molina, M.L. and Camacho, M., Role of thyroid hormones in the maturation and organisation of the rat barrel cortex. Neuroscience (2001) 107:383-394.
Berbel, P. Las hormonas de la inteligencia. Mente y Cerebro (2003) 2:10-20.
[63] Glinoer D, Delange F. the potential repercussions of maternal, fetal and neonatal hypothyroxinemia on the progeny. Thyroid 2000; 10: 871-877.
[64] Escobar-Morreale HF, Escobar del Rey F, Obregón MJ, Morreale de Escobar G. Replacement therapy for hypothyroidism with thyroxine alone does not ensure euthyroidism in all tissues, as studied in thyroidectomized rats. J Clin Invest 1995; 96:2828-2838.
[65] Mortimer RH, Galligan JP, Cannell GR, Addison RS, Roberts MS. Maternal to fetal thyroxine transmission in the human term placenta is limited by inner ring deiodination. J Clin Endocrinol Metab 1996; 81: 2247-2249.
[66] Zoeller RT, Rovett J. Timing of thyroid hormone action in the developing brain: clinical observations and experimental findings. J Neuroendocrinol 2004; 16: 809-818.
[67] Obregon MJ, Calvo RM, Del Rey FE, de Escobar GM. Ontogenesis of thyroid function and interactions with maternal function. Endocr Dev. 2007; 10:86-98.
[68] Contempré B, de Escobar GM, Denef JF, Dumont JE, Many MC. Thiocyanate induces cell necrosis and fibrosis in selenium- and iodine-deficient rat thyroids: a potential experimental model for myxedematous endemic cretinism in central Africa. Endocrinology. 2004 Feb;145(2):994-1002.
[69] Assessment of iodine deficiency disorders and monitoring their elimination: a guide for programme managers, 3rd Ed. WHO, Geneva, 2007.
[70] Santiago-Fernandez P, Torres-Barahona R, Muela-Martínez JA, Rojo-Martínez G, García-Fuentes E, Garriga MJ, León AG, Soriguer F.Intelligence quotient and iodine intake: a cross-sectional study in children. J Clin Endocrinol Metab. 2004 Aug;89(8):3851-3857.
[71] Soriguer F, Millón MC, Muñoz R, Mancha I, López Siguero JP, Martinez Aedo MJ, Gómez-Huelga R, Garriga MJ, Rojo-Martinez G, Esteva I, Tinahones FJ. The auditory threshold in a school-age population is related to iodine intake and thyroid function. Thyroid. 2000 Nov;10(11):991-999.
[72] Riaño Galán I, Sánchez Martínez P, Pilar Mosteiro Díaz M, Rivas Crespo MF. Psycho-intellectual development of 3 year-old children with early gestational iodine deficiency. J Pediatr Endocrinol Metab. 2005 Dec;18 Suppl 1:1265-1272.

[73] Bleichroth N, Born MP. A meta-analysis of research on iodine and its relationship to cognitive development. In: The damaged brain of iodine deficiency (Satndbury Ed) 1994; Cognizant Corporation; 195-200.

[74] Vermiglio F, Lo Presti VP, Moleti M, Sidoti M, Tortorella G, Scaffidi G, Castagna MG, Mattina F, Violi MA, Crisà A, Artemisia A, Trimarchi F. Attention deficit and hyperactivity disorders in the offspring of mothers exposed to mild-moderate iodine deficiency: a possible novel iodine deficiency disorder in developed countries. J Clin Endocrinol Metab. 2004 Dec;89(12):6054-60.

[75] Berbel P, Mestre JL, Santamaría A, Palazón I, Franco A, Graells M, González-Torga A, Morreale de Escobar G. Delayed neurobehavioral development in children born to pregnant women with mild hypothyroxinemia during the first month of gestation. Thyroid 2009; 19:511-519.

9

Real-Time Quantitative PCR for Detection Cell Free Fetal DNA

Tuba Gunel[1], Hayri Ermis[2] and Kilic Aydinli[3]
[1]*Istanbul University, Faculty of Science, Department of Molecular Biology and Genetics, Istanbul*
[2]*Istanbul University, Faculty of Medicine, Department of Obstetrics and Gynecology, Istanbul*
[3]*Medicus Health Center, Istanbul*
Turkiye

1. Introduction

Basically, diagnosis inherited diseases in gestation is very important. But amplication of the progress in early stage of pregnance is the serious and great aim for rapid application of risk assesment for both and fetus. Fetal genetic tissues collected through techniques such as amniocentesis and chorionic villus sampling (CVS) for prenatal diagnosis of fetal genetic diseases. These procedures are associated with a risk of fetal loss (1%) and two week needed for cultivation (Chiu et al., 2010). Rapid methods for prenatal diagnosis of fetal chromosomal aneuploidies have been developed. This method is multicolor fluorescence in situ hybridization (FISH). FISH is very reliable but requires intact cells and it can only be used on fresh samples (Klinger et al.,1992) The other method is quantitative fluorescent polymerase chain reaction PCR anaylsis (real-time PCR) (Lo et al., 1997). Real-time PCR is a powerful tool for quantifying gene expression combining both high sensitivity and specificity with efficient signal detection (Kubista, 2008). A major advantage of real-time PCR is that it can be used to determine the amount of initial temlates (Heidi et al., 1996). In addition, by making use of a closed whereby the samples are analyzed directly in PCR reaction vessel during the amplification. Furthermore, the assay is less prone contamination (Zimmerman, 2006). Real-time PCR has found wide spread applicability in the analysis of gene expression measurement and cell-free nucleic acids in body fluids. The assay is readily amenable to automation, and by making use of the current real-time PCR 96-384 well formats. The discovery of cff DNA in maternal plasma in 1997 has opened non-invasive prenatal diagnosis (NIPD). This research area is a rapidly developing and dynamic field. NIPD using cell-free fetal DNA (and RNA) is likely to become increasingly available within the next few years. There have been a lot of reported applications, including fetal rhesus-D genotyping (Bombard et al.,2011), fetal sexing for X-linked disorders (Costa et al., 2002), paternally inherited genetic diseases, and pregnancy-associated conditions such as preeclampsia (Zhong et al., 2001). Diagnosing by using free DNA a variety of limitations due to some of the features of this resource. CffDNA analyses would be applicable only when the involved target sequence is in the fetus but absent from mother, such as paternally inherited disorders or "de novo" mutations (Gonzales et al., 2005). In this chapter, we focused on NIPD with real-time PCR via the use of cell-free fetal DNA

2. The cell free fetal DNA

The cffDNA circulate freely in the peripheral blood during pregnancy and derived from the placenta, the fetal hematopoietic system, or the amniotic fluid, it appears to be transferred as a naked molecule or very quickly assumes that form (Robert et al., 2003). The cffDNA is most likely of placental origin (Bianchi&Lo, 2001). It rapidly disappears from the maternal circulation folowing chilbirth. Unlike fetal cells, which can persist for decades, cffNA are rapidly cleared from the maternal circulation and are undetectable 2 hours after delivery. PHG foundation group was summarized of key properties of fetal/placental elements in maternal blood, specifically cell-free fetal nucleic acids and intact fetal cells (table 1). Fetal DNA molecules are amount to just 3–6 % of the total DNA circulating in the maternal plasma (Lo et.al., 1998a). High levels of cffDNA in maternal plasma is associated with several pregnancy related disorders (Holzgre et al., 2001). The size of cffDNA have confirmed that it is of average size 300 bp or smaller than maternal free DNA (Chan et al., 2004). Fetal DNA can be detected in maternal plasma between the fifth to seventh week gestation (Gonzalez et al., 2005). The technical problem that cffDNA makes up a low proportion in maternal plasma in high background of maternal DNA.

Properties	cffNA	Fetal Cells
Earliest detection	4 weeks	~ 7 weeks
Proportion	5-10%	0.0001 - 0.01%
Persistence in maternal blood	< 24 hours	> 27 years
Relevant physical properties	Short fragments	Dense nucleus

Table 1. Differences cell-free fetal nucleic acids and intact fetal cells (phg foundation, 2009)

2.1 Isolation of cell fetal free DNA from maternal plasma

The discovery of cffDNA in maternal plasma of pregnant women in 1997 by Lo et al (Lo et al., 1998b), many laboratories have shown that several protocols for isolating this material. The nucleic acid extraction procedure is most important for the detection of fetal nucleic acids in maternal plasma. To separate plasma from whole blood, parameters including multiple centrifugations at different speed, filtration to rmove contaminating intact or apoptotic cells, and removal of protein impurities have been explored (Jorgez et. al., 2006).The critical point with techniques used is the avoidance of contamination from other blood components. The protocols for isolation of plasma were optimized to reduce cell lysis. The standard protocol for isolating plasma, which is commanly, involves two centrifugation steps. First step is high speed. This step is removal of cellular material from plasma layer. Store plasma samples in smaller aliquots (500 μL). The second step, different commercial kits have been used to isolate cell free fetal DNA. The free fetal DNA particles in maternal blood are promising as an important step for diagnosis of numerical and structural chromosome anomalies belonging to fetus without invasive procedures. The main problem is that extremely low concentration of fetal DNA is present in maternal plasma. Circulating fetal DNA concentration increases with progression of pregnancy and disappears from maternal plasma rapidly after delivery , with median half-life of 16.3 min (Lo et al., 1999, Smid et al., 2003). However, methods have been optimized for the extraction of fetal DNA from maternal plasma. Although extracted DNA is generally stable for long periods, levels of fetal DNA have been shown to decrease over long storage periods. Our laboratories use of the QIAampDSP virus kit (QIAGEN). To extract DNA, 600 μL of plasma from maternal sample for method.

3. Clinical applications of real-time PCR for non-invasive prenatal diagnosis

For many years, scientisist has focused seperation of fetal cells and fetal DNA in maternal blood. The discovery of circulating cell-free fetal nucleic acids in maternal plasma has opened up new possibilities for non invasive prenatal diagnosis. Cff DNA is detectable in maternal blood as early as 5-7 weeks of gestation (Honda et al., 2002; Galbiati et al., 2005). CffDNA present has been used succesfully for non-invasive diagnosis of the fetal sex and fetal Rhd genotype in Rh negative women (Chen et al., 2004). Recent advances in molecular methods enable other applications of fetal DNA purified from maternal plasma samples (Vlkova et al., 2010). Studies put more emphasis on this area (Purvosunu et al., 2008). The sensivity of the studies that have been recently carried out by the devoleped PCR techniques has been increased, but the greatest difficulty encountered is the isolation of pure and high scale fetal DNA. By doing this isolation, the need of invasive procedures, such as amniocentesis will largely be eliminated (Hahn et al., 2008).

3.1 Fetal RHD status

Hemolytic disease of newborn (HDN) is a clinic phenomenon, which occurs during pregnancy due to the RhD alloimmunization between Rh (-) pregnant woman, who has become sensitive with RhD antigens, and her Rh (+) fetus. Unnecessary application of Anti D Ig can be prevented for pregnant women who carry Rh - fetus, also this results in a better follow-up of pregnant women who carry Rh+ fetus with the detection of RhD genotype of fetus in maternal plasma at the first trimester of pregnancy. RHD was used as a test-bed to prove the effectiveness of detecting a paternally inherited allele carried bty circulating free fetal DNA in maternal plasma (Lo et al., 1997). Maternal plasma-based RHD genotyping has been succesfully implemented in our laboratories for use as a non-invasive prenatal diagnosis where alloimmunization has occured (Gunel et al., 2010). Real-time PCR has been the choice diagnostic test used. Fetal RhD detection can be applied routinely to Rh (-) women and the use of human anti -D can be significantly reduced (Hahn et al., 2008). A reduction in anti-D administration also has economic implications. Rh locus is composed of two homologous genes RHD and RHCE (97% homology) closely linked on chromosome 1p34-p36. Each of these genes consists of 10 exones, and they contain 69 kb of DNA. The regions of exone 7 and exone 10 within the RhD gene are the areas of focus. In all positive results, the RhD blood group has also been found positive (Huang, 1998, Wagner and Flegel, 2000). In a white population, D-negative individuals are homozygous for a deletion of RHD. The D-negative phenotype, absence of the whole RhD protein from red cell membrane. Different mechanisms may explain rare phenotypes, including gene conversion events between homologous RHD and RHCE producing hybrid genes, nonsense mutations, and deletions or insertions interrupting the reading frame of the messenger RNA (Rouillac-Le Sciellour et al., 2004. Gunel et al., 2011).

3.2 Fetal sexing

Researchers had focused on the detection of fetal-derived paternally inherited DNA because Y chromosome of male fetus, which were absent in the genome of the pregnant women (Lo YMD, 2010). Most sex-linked disease are recessive X-linked disesae such as haemophilia and and Duchenne muscular dystrophy. To determine the sex of a fetus by real-time PCR using DYS14 and SRY genes on and Y chromosome. The genotyping of these fetal loci helps preventing invasive procedures in the case of X-linked disorders (Rijinders et al., 2004). CffDNA technology has been used to identify babies at risk of congenital adrenal hyperplasia by identifying fetal sex at the requisite stage in pregnancy in 6-7 weeks (Rijinders et al., 2001).

3.3 Determination of fetal aneuploidy by real-time PCR

The free fetal DNA particles in maternal blood are promising as an important step for diagnosis of numerical and structural chromosome anomalies belonging to fetus without invasive procedures. The direct analysis of cff DNA for the NIPD of trisomies is mainly complicated. The most common chromosomal abnormalities in live births is trisomi 21 and other chromosomes 13, 18 trisomies has rapidly analysis with real-time PCR methods. The full fetal karyotype is usually determined using cultured cells and need two weeks for result. Real-time PCR has rapidly determination of template copy numbers. Tong et. al. had first demonstration of the direct detection of trisomi 18 from maternal serum (Tong et al., 2006). They were achived with use of the epigenetic allelic ratio method. Enrich et.al., had used sequence-specific taq of known chromosomal location as a quantitative representation of individual chromosomes in maternal plasma. Trisomi 21 detection by massively parallel shotgun sequencing (MPSS) in high risk women is complicated. Their overall classification showed 100% sensitivity and 99.7% specificity of detection of fetal trisomi 21 (2011). Lo et al., described a novel method for the NIPD of Down syndrome. Candidate mRNA markers shoul be encoded from genes located on chromosome 21. The PLAC4 gene on chromosome 21 and originating from fetal cells in the placenta and cleared following delivery of the fetus (Lo et al., 2007). If the fetus is euploid, that is containing two copies of the PLAC4 gene, because SNP (single nucleotide polymorphism) alleles would be 2:1. (Lo, 2009). The first large-scale noninvasive prenatal detection of trisomi 21 using multiplex sequencing to analyze fetal DNA from maternal plasma by Chiue et. al., (2011). They show that 100% sensitivity and 97.9% specificity of detection of fetal trisomi 21. They report a % 2.1 false-positive rate. This method replace invasive procedures and would be eliminated unintended procedures fetal losses as well as better targeting of pregnancy-related interventions.

3.4 Pre-eclampsia and cell free fetal nucleic acids

Preeclampsia is a potentially dangerous disorder specific to the second half of pregnancy, affecting about 2.5–3% of women (Redman & Sargent, 2005). The etiology of this disease involves the placenta. Real-time PCR, it is now possible to measure DNA/RNA content accuracy. The increased presence of cell-free fetal DNA indicates that preeclampsia is associated with damage to the placenta (Zhong et al., 2001) The cell-free fetal DNA levels in maternal blood in preeclamptic patients are significantly higher than those of normal pregnancies, and this elevation precedes the clinical occurrence of preeclampsia by approximately 1-2 weeks. The results of the studies in this area are important for pregnancy follow-up. The change of free fetal DNA levels in maternal blood in healthy pregnancies according to gestation week, was shown in various publications (Zhong et al.,2001, Ferina et al.,2004, Carty et al., 2008). By using real-time PCR technology was shown to be elevated ~ 5-fold in samples obtained from pregnant women with preeclampsia when compared with an eual-sized cohort of normotensive, pregnant women (Lo et al., 1999) All study subjects were pregnant women carrying male fetuses, and investigators amplified sequences from the SRY gene distinguish fetal from maternal DNA (Levine et al., 2004).

4. Summary

The discovery of cell-free fetal DNA (cffDNA) in maternal blood has exciting possibilities for non-invasive prenatal diagnosis (NIPD). Free fetal DNAs stemming from the destruction of fetal cells from seven weeks of gestation transport to the maternal blood via the bi-sidal flow through the placenta.The free fetal DNA particles in maternal blood are promising as an important step for diagnosis of numerical and structural chromosome anomalies belonging to fetus without invasive procedures. The detection and quantification of gene rearrangement, amplification, translocation or deletion is a significant problem, both in research and in a clinical diagnostic setting. Real-time PCR has become a well-established procedure for quantifying levels of gene expression. There are a number non-invasive prenatal diagnosis methods such as sex diagnosis or Rh blood type incompatibility and single-gene disorders have been reported. Different problems associated with placental growth and development result in changed levels of cffDNA. The cell-free fetal DNA levels in maternal blood in preeclamptic patients are significantly higher than those of normal pregnancies. It is possible the diagnostic utility of adding cffDNA concentration to the current panel of biomarkers. The test can be used very early of pregnancy, with no risk to the mother and child.

5. References

Bombard AT, Akolekar R, Farkas DH, VanAgtMael AL, Aquino F, Oeth P, Nicolaides K. (2011).

Fetal RHD genotype detection from circulating cell free- fetal DNA in maternal plasma in non-sensitized RhD negative women. *Prenat. Diagn.* 31, 802-808.

Carty DM, Delles C, Dominiczak A. (2008). Novel Biomarkers for Predicting Preeclampsia. *Trends Cardiovasc Med.* 18, 186-194.

Chan KC, Zhang J, Hui AB, Wong N, Lau TK, Leung TN, Lo KW, Huans WS, Lo YM. (2004).Size Distributions of Maternal and Fetal DNA in Maternal Plasma. *Clin Chem.*50, 88-92.

Chen JC, Lin TM, Chen YL, Wang YH, Jin YT, Yue CT.(2004). RHD 1227A is an important genetic marker for RhD(el) individuals. *Am J Clin Pathol,*122, 193-198.

Chiue RW, Ranjit Akolekar R, Zheng YWL, Leung TY,Sun H, Chan KCA, Lun FMF, Go TJI, Lau ET, William WK Leung WC, Tang RYK, Yeung SKC, Lam H, Kung YY,

Zhang X, Vugt JMG, Minekawa R, Tang MHY,Wang J, Oudejans CBM, Lau TK, Nicolaides KH, Y M Dennis LYM. (2011). Non-invasive prenatal assessment of trisomy 21 by multiplexed maternal plasma DNA sequencing: large scale validity study. BMJ, doi:10.1136/bmj.c7401, 1-9.

Costa JM, Benachi A, Gautier E. (2002). New strategy for prenatal diagnosis of X-linked disorders. *N. Engl. J Med.* 346, 1502.

Ehrich M, Deciu C, Zwiefelhofer T, Tynan JA, Cagasan L,Tim R, Lu V, McCullough R, McCarthy

E,Nygren A O.H, Dean J, Tang L, Hutchison D, Lu T, Wang H, Angkachatchai V, Oeth P, Cantor C.R, Bombard A and van den Boom D. (2011). Noninvasive detectiton of fetal trisomy 21 by sequencing of DNA in maternal blood: a study in a clinical setting. *Am J Obstet Gynecol,* 204:205.e1-11.

Farina A, Sekizawa a, Rizzo N, Concu M, Banzola I, Carinci P, Simonazzi G, Okai T. (2004). Cell-free fetal DNA (SRY locus) concentration in maternal plasma is directly correlated to the time elapsed from the onset of preeclampsia to the collection of blood. *Prenat Diagn,* 2, 293–297.

Galbiati S, Smid M, Gambini D, Ferrari A, Restagno G, Viora E, Campogrande M, Bastonero S, Pagliano M, Calza S. (2005). Fetal DNA detection in maternal plasma throughout gestation. Human Genet, 117, 243-248.

Gonzales GC, Garcia HM, Trujillo TMJ, Lorda DI, Rodriquez AM, Infantes F, Gallego J, Diaz RJ, Ayusa C, Ramos C. (2005). Application of fetal DNA detection in maternal plasma: A prenatal diagnosis unit experience. *Journal of Histochem and Cytochem.* 53, 307-314.

Gunel T , Kalelioğlu I , Ermiş H , Aydınlı K. (2010). Detection of fetal RhD gene from maternal blood. *J Turkish - German Gynecol Assoc,* 11,82-85.

Gunel T, Kalelioglu I, Gedikbasi A. Ermis, H, Aydinli K. (2011) Detection of fetal RHD pseudogene (RHDΨ) and hybrid RHD-CE-D^{s} from RHD-negative pregnant women with a free DNA fetal kit. *Genet. Mol. Res.* 10 (4), 2653 - 2657

Hahn S, Chitty L. (2008) Noninvasive prenatal diagnosis: current practice and future perspectives. *Current Opinion in Obstetrics and Gynecology,* 3, 150-157.

Heid CA, Stevans J, Livak KJ, Williams PM. (1996). Real-time quantitative PCR. *Genome Res.* 6, 986-994.

Holzgreve W, Li JC, Steinborn A, Kulz T, Sohn C, Hodel M, Hahn S. (2001). Elevation in erythroblast count in maternal blood before yhe onser of pre-eclapmsia. *Am. J.Obstet.Gynecol.* 184, 165-168.

Honda H, Miharu N, Ohashi Y, Samura O, Kinutani M, Hara T, Ohama K. (2002). Fetal gender determination in early pregnancy through qualitative and quantitative analysis of fetal DNA in maternal serum. Hum Genet.110, 75.79.

Jorgez CJ, Dang DD,, Simpson JL, Lewis DE, Bischoff FZ. (2006). Quantity versus quality: optimal methods for cell-free DNA isolation from plasma of pregnant women.Genet in Med.10, 615-619.

Klinger K, Landes G, Shook D.(1992). Rapid detection of chromosome aneuploidies in uncultured amniocytes by using fluorescence in situ hybridization (FISH). *Am.J.Hum.Genet.* 51, 55-65.

Levine RJ, Qian C, LeShane ES, Yu KF, England LJ, Schisterman EF, Wataganara T, Romero R, Bianchi DW. Two-stage elevation of cell-free fetal DNA in maternal sera before onset of preeclampsia (2004). *Am.J.Obst.Gyn.*190, 707-713.

Kubista M. Emerging real-time PCR application. (2008). *Drug Dis.*

Lo YMD, Corbetta N, Chamberlian PF, Rai V, SargentIL, Redman CW. (1997). Presence of fetal DNA in maternal plasma and serum. *Lancet,* 350, 485-487.

Lo YMD, Hjelm NM, Fidler C, Sargent IL, Murpy MF, Chamberlain PF, et.al. (1998a) Prenatal diagnosis of fetal status by molecular analysis of maternal plasma.. *N Engl J Med* .339, 1734-1738.

Lo YMD, Tenis MS, Lau MS, Haines CJ. (1998b). Quantitative analysis of fetal DNA in maternal plasma and serum: implications for noninvasive prenatal diagnosis. *Am J Hum Genet* 62, 768-75.

Lo YMD, Leung TN, Tein MS, Sargent IL, Zhang J, Lau TK, Haines CJ, Redman CW.(1999). Quantitative abnormalities of fetal DNA in maternal serum in preeclampsia. *Clin Chem.45,* 184-188.

Lo YM, Tsui NB, Chiu RW, Lau TK, Leung TN, Heung MM, et al., (2007). Plasma placental RNA allelic ratio permits noninvasive prenatal chromosomal aneuploidy detection. *Nat Med.* 13, 218-223.

Lo YM. (2009). Noninvasive prenatal detection of fetal chromosomal aneuploidies by maternal plasma nucleic acid analysis: a review of current state of the art. BJOG. 116, 152-157.

Lo YMD. (2010). Noninvasive prenatal diagnosis 2020. *Prenat Diagn,* 30, 702-703.

Lun FMF, Chiu RWK, Chan KCA, Leung TY, Lau TK, Lo YMD. (2008). Microfluidics digital PCR reveals a higher than expected fraction of fetal DNA in maternal plasma. *Clin Chem.* 54, 1664-1672.

Phg foundation (2009). Making science work for health. www.phgfoundation.org.

Purwosunu Y, Sekizawa A, Okai T. (2008), Detection and quantification of fetal DNA in maternal plasma by using LightCycler technology. *Methods Mol Biol,* 444, 231-238.

Redman CW, Sargent IL. (2005). Latest advances in understanding preeclampsia. *Science.* 308,1592–1594.

Rijnders RJ, Christiaens GC, Bossers B, van der Smagt JJ, van der Schoot CE, Haas M.(2004), Clinical applications of cell free fetal DNA from maternal plasma. *Obstet.Gynecol.* 103, 157-164.

Rijnders, R.J.P. et al (2001). Fetal Sex Determination from Maternal Plasma in Pregnancies at Risk for Congenital Adrenal Hyperplasia. *Obstet Gynecol* 98, 374-378.

Robert M. Angert, Erik S. LeShane, Y.M. Dennis Lo, Lisa Y.S. Chan, Laurent C. Delli-Bovi and Diana W. Bianchi. (2003). Fetal Cell-free Plasma DNA Concentrations in Maternal Blood Are Stable 24 Hours after Collection: Analysis of First- and Third-Trimester Samples. *Clinical Chemistry,* 49, 195-198.

Rouillac-Le Sciellour C, Puillandre P, Gillot R, Baulard C, Metral S, Le Van Kim C, Cartron JP, Colin Y, Brossard Y (2004) Large-scale pre-diagnosis study of fetal RHD genotyping by PCR on plasma DNA from RhD-negative pregnant women. *Mol. Diagn.* 8(1): 23-31

Tong YK, Ding C, Chiu RWK, Gerovassili A, Chim SSC, Leung TY, Leung TN, Lau TK, Nicolaides KH, Lo YMD. Noninvasive Prenatal Detection of Fetal Trisomy 18 by

Epigenetic Allelic Ratio Analysis in Maternal Plasma: Theoretical and Empirical Considerations. *Clin Chem.* 52, 2194-2202.

Vlkova B, Szemes T, Minarik K, Turna J, Celec P. Advances in the research of fetal DNA in maternal plasma for noninvasive prenatal diagnostics. (2010). *Med Sci Monit*, 16.4, 85-91.

Zhong XY, Holzgreve W, Hahn S.(2001), Circulatory fetal and maternal DNA in pregnancies at risk and those affected by preeclampsia. *Ann.N.Y.Acad. Sci,* 945,138-140.

Zimmermann, B., El-Sheikhah, A., Nicolaides, K., Holzgreve, W. And Hahn, S. (2005). Optimized real-time quantitative PCR measurement of male fetal DNA in maternal plasma. *Clin. Chem.* 51, 1598–1604.

Zimmermann B, Levett L, Holzgreve W, Hahn S. Use of real-time polymerase chain reaction for detection of fetal aneuploidies. (2006). *Meth of Mol Biy* , 336, 83-100.

10

The Experiences of Prenatal Diagnosis in China

Shangzhi Huang
Department of Medical Genetics, Chinese Academy of Medical Sciences and Peking Union Medical College, the WHO Collaborating Center of Community Control for Inherited Diseases, Beijing China

1. Introduction

China is situated in the south-eastern part of the Eurasian continent and has a total land area of 9.6 million square kilometers. It is composed of 23 provinces, five autonomous regions (Inner Mongolia, Ningxia Hui, Guangxi Zhuang, Xinjiang Weiwuer, and Tibet), four municipalities directly under the central authorities (Beijing, Shanghai, Tianjin and Chongqing), and two Special Administrative Region(SAR)(Hong Kong and Macao). China is a unified, multinational country (56 nationalities), with a population of about 1.37billion, of which 1.34 billion live in mainland. According to a survey carried out in 1987, the birth defects were of 4% in China. It is a big burden for the population. The government has paid attention to this situation. In order to improve the public health, China government passed the "Maternal and Child Health Law" in 1994.

Prenatal diagnosis for severe birth defects was implemented in China step by steps.

2. The outlines of the development of prenatal diagnosis in China

2.1 Prenatal diagnosis of central neural tube defects

The earliest cases of prenatal diagnosis for central neural tube defects (NTD) were performed with measuring the level of alpa-fetal protein in maternal serum in 1976. This work was awarded by the MOH of China and WHO. Ultrasoundnography was used to diagnose NTD routinely after 1980'.

2.2 Karyotyping

Fetal chromosome karyotyping was performed in 1970' on cultured amnion fluid cells to detect chromosomal diseases[1,2]. It became the major technique used for prenatal diagnosis in China in 1980'. The scale was once declined in the 1990'. After the prenatal diagnosis spreed in China, cytogenetics is the main field for prevention of hereditary diseases.

2.3 Fetoscopy

Usage of fetoscopy was reported in the late of 1980'. It was used for biopsy of the fetal material and for fetal therapy[3,4].

2.4 Maternal serum screening

Maternal serum screening for chromosomal abnormalities and other abnormalities, such as NTD, started in the early of 1990′[5]. This procedure was adopted nationwide in the 21 century. A standard operation protocol was formulated in 2010 by the National Committee of Exports on Prenatal Diagnosis.

2.5 Biochemical genetics

Electrophoresis analysis was perform on amnion fluid as the first technique in prenatal diagnosis of metabolic disease[6,7]. After the enzyme assay methods were established, prenatal diagnosis of lysosomal diseases was carried out by enzyme assay[8]. More than 20 protocols were developed for diagnosis of lysosomal storage diseases.

2.6 Techniques developed for sampling fetus material

2.6.1 Amniocentesis

Amniocentesis was the first procedure for fetal cell sampling. It was performed as early as in 1970 in China. It became the major procedure in collection fetal material nationwide now.

2.6.2 Chorionic villus sampling (CVS)

At the early stage, chorionic villus sampling via the cervix under was invented by a Chinese obstetrician[9]. Transcervical chorionic villus sampling(TC-CVS) was reintroduced into China in the early of 1980′ and got popular afterward. It was performed blindly at the very beginning, e.g. without the guidance of ultrasonography as does later, for prenatal diagnosis at early pregnancy(first trimester)[10]. It was further improved. Transabdominal chorionic vilus sampling(TA-CVS) was established in 1994[11].

2.6.3 Fetal blood sampling

Fetal blood sampling via abdominal cordocentesis was performed in the late 1980′ for cell culture or hemoglobin analysis[12]. It is used rather routinely in the area where there is a high prevalence of hemoglobinopathies, since the blood component can be analyzed with the fetal blood.

2.7 Gene diagnosis

The first prenatal gene diagnosis was performed in the early of 1980′ on thalassemia[30]. Then prenatal diagnosis was performed on more and more monogenic diseases, when the gene mutations had been characterized for the disease, such as DMD, PKU, and hemophilia A (see details in section 3).

2.8 Regulations on prenatal diagnosis

As the prenatal diagnosis was offered nationwide, there were more and more problems emerged. It was necessary to make a regulation on the practices of prenatal diagnosis. In the second national conference of prenatal diagnosis 2000, this issue was discussed and a proposal on the regulation for prenatal diagnosis was sent to the Ministry of Public Health after the meeting. A special group was organized to investigate the demands on prenatal diagnosis and the diseases needed to be put on the list for prenatal diagnosis. In the third national conference of prenatal diagnosis 2001, the draft of the regulation was discussed. After revising, "the regulations on prenatal diagnosis and diagnosis of genetic diseases" was distributed nationwide for further discussion and for modification. After one year debating, "The Regulation on Management of Techniques for Prenatal Diagnosis" was published on Dec. 22, 2002 and was implemented after May 1, 2003 [http://www.china.com.cn/policy/txt/2003-02/14/content_5276708.htm]. A National Committee of Exports on Prenatal Diagnosis was established in 2004 to assist the work of the Division of Women's Health and Community Health Care, MOH in prenatal diagnosis.

2.9 The current situation of the organizations for prenatal diagnosis

The techniques applied in the practices of prenatal diagnosis are cytogenetics, maternal serum screening, and ultrasounography. The prenatal diagnosis centers were assigned by the authorities in charge of public health of the local government. Up to year 2009, there were 511 centers carrying out maternal serum screening for chromosomal diseases and neural tube defects; 169 centers performing karyotyping for pregnancy at high risk or with a positive result of serum screening, and ultrasoundography for malformations.

A total of 93905 prenatal diagnoses were carried out for chromosomal diseases and monogenic diseases in 2009. Fetal sampling was mainly carried out via amniocentesis (80%), only a small section was by CVS (1.8%).

There were only 76 centers offering gene diagnosis, of which the most were located in the developed areas, such as Beijing , Shanghai, Hunan, Henan, Guangdong, and Guangxi.

Nineteen diseases were carried out in some of the prenatal diagnosis centers, most of which were α-thalssemia, β-thalassemia, DMD, PKU, SMA, achondroplasia, APKD, and hereditary non-syndromic deafness.

3. Prenatal gene diagnosis, the strategies and experiences in several common diseases

3.1 Thalassemias

Thalassemia is one of the most common monogenic disorders in the world. The incidence for this disease is high in tropical and subtropical areas including southern China.

In China, the carrier rate of α-thalassemia was 17.55% in Guangxi, 8.53% in Guangdong and 1% to 4.2% in other province of southern China[13,14]. The frequencies of α-thalassemic allele in Li Monority was 0.347. Fortunately, most of the thalassemic alleles were α-thal-2 ($-\alpha^{3.7}/$ or $-\alpha^{4.2}/$) , only 0.0058 for α-thal-1 allele ($--^{SEA}/$)[15]. The estimated incidence of carriers of β-thalassemia is as high as 6.43% in Guangxi, and 1% to 2.54% in populations in the endemic areas of southern China[13,16].

3.1.1 Mutation characterization

Researches on thalassemias started in the early of 1980's in China.

The organization of the α globin was analyzed with Southern blotting. Data collected in Guangxi showed the defects of α globin genes in α-thalassemia patients were mostly deletion types, $--^{SEA}/$,$-\alpha^{3.7}/$, and $-\alpha^{4.2}/$.[17] Three primers bridging the deletion breakpoints were designed to detect these three deletion mutations [18]. Abnormal hemoglobins of the α globin gene, $Hb\alpha^{CS}$ and $Hb\alpha^{QS}$, were characterized as thalassemic mutation. After sequencing the non-deletion α thalassemic mutant *HBA*, 12 mutations were revealed responsible for α-thalassemia*[http://globin.cse.psu.edu]*. Reverse dot blotting with ASO probes (RDB) for α^{CD30}(-GAG), α^{CD31}(G>A), α^{CD59}(G>A), $\alpha^{Westmead}$ (CD22, C>G), α^{QS}(CD125, T>C) and α^{CS} (CD142, T>C) were developed in detection of the non-deletion α-thalassemia alleles. [19]

The mutations causing β-thalassemia were exclusively point mutations[20]. It used to be the strategy to use the RFLP haplotype to predict mutations since there was linkage disequilibrium between the haplotypes and certain mutations [21]. The -29 A>G mutation was revealed as it was associated with a new haplotype. The mutations were identified via cloning and sequencing, the routine procedure for identifying mutations at that time. It was the first mutation of β-thalassemia characterized by the scientist from mainland China on patients collected in Guangzhou, Guagndong Province[22]. In the 1990', most of the mutations were characterized with direct sequencing the PCR products. Five mutations, CD41-42 (-CTTT), IVS2-654 (C>T), －28 (A>G), CD26 (G>A) and CD17 (A>T), account for 90% of the common mutations in south China. New mutation was revealed with the RDB and characterized by direct sequencing. To date, 46 single-nucleotide mutations and small deletions in *HBB* have been characterized in the Chinese patients with β-thalassemia [*http://globin.cse.psu.edu*]. The recently developed technique is the probe-based melting curve analysis (MeltPro HBB assay). It is a qualitative *in vitro* diagnostic method designed to genotype a panel of 24 single-nuclueotide mutations and small indels in the *HBB* gene that cause β-thalassemia or abnormal hemoglobin. The test kit is based on a proprietary, multicolored, self-quenched, probe-based melting curve analysis performed with a standard real-time PCR instrument, from which genotype information for each mutation is retrieved based on the melting temperature (Tm) or difference in Tm between wild-type and mutant DNA samples[16].

3.1.2 The strategy in thalassemia prevention

In the report on the middle term evaluation on the progress of the National Project on thalassemia during the Seventh Five-Year Developing Plan in 1988, Shangzhi Huang had made a proposal on performing a population prevention program on thalassemia by hematological screening, mutation detection, and prenatal gene diagnosis in certain areas. The trail of population screening carriers with thalassemias was carried out on the Li Minority in Hainan in 1990. It showed that it was feasible to screening thalassemias with hematological parameters [23]. In the Li Minority in Hainan the carrier rate of β-thalassemia was 8.6%, and the mutation c.124-127delTTCT accounted for 94.7% of the mutant alleles in this population [24]. In 1991, carrier screening for thalassemias was carried out for people in marriage registration in Fushan City, Guangdong Province [25]. In 1993, Xiangmin Xu et al. started the hospital-based screening program for pregnant women during their first prenatal checking up in Guangdong and Guangxi [26].

In hematological screening, quantitative test of hemoglobin, erythrocyte osmotic fragility, mean corpuscular volume (MCV), and hemoglobin electrophoresis were performed. When erythrocyte osmotic fragility <60%, MCH<27pg, and MCV <80 fl, hemoglobin electrophoresis was carried out on the positive subjects. When $HbA_2 \geq 3.5\%$ or HbA_2 normal but HbF >3%, β-thalassemia was suspected, while if $HbA_2<3.5\%$, α-thalassemia would considered. Iron deficiency anemia should be ruled out with serum iron test. The DNA were isolated later and Gap-PCR[27] and RDB[28] methods were used for α-thalassemia genotyping. β-thalassemia genotyping were carried out using RDB analysis for 18 common types of point mutation[29]. In the RDB procedure two-step hybridization was designed: the first dot strip contained ASO probes specific for seven common mutations, e.g., -28A>G, CD17A>T, CD26G>A, IVS1 nt5G>C, CD41/42 del CTTT, CD71/72 +A, IVS2 nt654C>T, and IVS2 nt652C>T; the second dot strip contained 11 less common but not rare mutations in Chinese, e.g.,-32C>A. -30T>C, -29A>G, +40_43 del AAAC, initial CD ATG>ACG, CD14/15+G, CD27/28+C, IVS1 nt1G>T, CD31-C, CD43G>T, and CD71/72+T [29]. DNA sequencing was also performed if there was an unknown allele of no-deletion α mutation remained. Four common types of α-thalassemia mutations, $-\alpha^{3.7}/$, $-\alpha^{4.2}/$, $--^{SEA}/$, and $\alpha^{CS}\alpha/$ alleles, were tested for all the subjects with β-thalassemia trait to reveal possible situation of β/α-thalassemia double heterozygote [26]. If the woman was identified as a heterzygote of thalassemia, her spouse would be tested for the same type thalassemia. If the couple were both heterozygous for the same type of thalassemias, either β- or α-thalassemia, prenatal diagnosis will be suggested to the couple.

3.1.3 Prenatal diagnosis

Thalassemia is a severe disease, and its treatment requires life-long transfusion and iron chelating. While many cities in China have facilities for diagnosis and treatment of this disease, free medical services are not provided by the government in most rural areas. Treatment is available to only a potion of patients who can afford it, although this situation is more favorable in some regions with better economical development. So, there is still a demand for prenatal diagnosis of thalassemia.

Prenatal gene diagnosis on α-thalassemia was carried out in the early stage by Southern blotting [30] or with a simple but not accurate method, dot blot hybridization with α globin probe[31]. When polymerase chain reaction (PCR) was established, gap-PCR became a major approach in prenatal diagnosis of α-thalassemia to detect the deletion mutation on fetus [32], or RDB was used to detect the point mutation of α-thalassemia [28].

Haplotypes of the RFLP sites on the β-globin cluster were used for linkage analysis in the early stage for diagnosis of β-thalassemia. Prenatal diagnosis was mainly performed with ASO probes routinely now, also there were several modifications being made, such as labeled with non-radioactive material, RDB, primer extension, and probe-based melting curve analysis (MeltPro HBB assay) [16].

The first prenatal diagnosis of β-thalassemia was carried out in 1985 with RFLP linkage analysis[33,34]. It was PCR technique that overcame the obstacle of the limited amount DNA from fetus available for RFLP analysis. Using PCR technique combined with the radioactive labeled allele specific oligonucleotide (ASO) probes, prenatal gene diagnosis for β-thalassemia become much easier, not only for less DNA was used but also for its simple and quick performance [35] . The non-radioactive labeling ASO probes and RDB made the prenatal diagnosis procedure even easier. This new techniques has been the routine approach for prenatal diagnosis of β thalassemia in China[36].

There were other techniques used in China for prenatal diagnosis, such as allele specific PCR(AS-PCR)[37], multiplex AS-PCR[38]. Another approach is RFLP analysis by introducing an artificial base substitution to create restriction sites. PCR products were cut by certain restrictive enzyme and then visualized the fragments after electrophoresis in agarose gel [39].

3.2 Duchenne muscular dystrophy (DMD)

3.2.1 Clinical aspect

Duchenne and Becker muscular dystrophy (DMD/BMD) (MIM#300377 and 300376) are allelic disorders, caused by mutations in the *DMD* gene coding for dystrophin, which locates on Xp21. The term "pseudohypertrophic muscular dystrophy" was used in the past; however, it is not used currently because pseudohypertrophy is not unique to the DMD or BMD phenotype. DMD is the severe form and usually presents in early childhood with develop delayed, including delays in sitting and standing independently. Progressive symmetrical muscular weakness, proximal severer than distal, before age 5 years, with a waddling gait and difficulty climbing, often with calf hypertrophy. Serum creatine phosphokinase (CK) concentration elevated, generally 10 times the normal range. Electromyography (EMG) is useful in distinguishing a myopathic disease from a neurogenic disorder. The characteristics were demonstrating short-duration, low-amplitude, polyphasic, rapidly recruited motor unit potentials. Muscle histology early in the disease shows nonspecific dystrophic changes, including variation in fiber size, foci of necrosis and regeneration, hyalinization, and, later in the disease, deposition of fat and connective tissue. Immunohistochemistry with antibody against dystrophin showed no signal of the dystrophin. Western blot can be used to distinguish DMD from other muscular dystrophies, such as Limb-girdle muscular dystrophy (LGMD), which are clinically similar to DMD but were autosomal recessive or autosomal dominant inheritance. LGMDs are caused by mutations in genes that encode sarcoglycans and other proteins associated with the muscle cell membrane that interact with dystrophin [40]. Testing for deficiency of proteins from the transmembrane sarcoglycans complex is indicated in individuals with dystrophin-positive dystrophies.

The affected children will loss their walking ability by age 12 years old. Few patients survive beyond the third decade, with respiratory complications and cardiomyopathy, which are the common causes of death. BMD is the mild form characterized by later-onset skeletal muscle weakness. Individuals with BMD remain ambulatory into their 20s and the lifespan is longer. Female carriers have clinical features of *DMD* were resulted in the situations either of X-Auto-chromosome crossing over involving *DMD* locus, or because of Turner syndrome or non-random X-chromosome inactivation (XCI), so called "unfortunate Lyonization".

3.2.2 Mutation analysis

The size of *DMD* gene is over 2.3 Mb, and composes 79 exons. It is the largest known human gene. The cDNA is 14kb. Large fragment deletion or duplication were the most common mutations of DMD, 60% for deletion and 6% for duplication with some were indel type, e.g., deletion with addition of several base pairs at the same site. There were cases with two deletions or deletion plus duplication scattered in the same allele[41-43]. There are two hotspots of deletion/duplication, one located on the 5′ portion, harboring exons 2 to 20, the other in the 3′ portion involving exons 44 to 53. The remaining mutations were small deletion, insertion, point mutations and splicing mutations.

There were several methods for deletion/duplication analysis. In the early stage, Southern blotting was used with either genomic probes or cDNA probes, both deletion and duplication mutations were detectable[44]. With multiplex PCR approximately 98% of deletions are detectable[45,46]. Multiplex ligation-dependent probes assay (MLPA) has been employed for deletion/duplication analysis of the *DMD* gene in probands and for carrier detection in recent years[42,43].

Array chips for deletion or duplication mutations were also developed, it had the same power in detection of large deletion/duplication as MLPA, but the strength on detection of alterations with small size is under evaluation[47].

Mutation scanning with denaturing high performance liquid chromatography (DHPLC) or high resolution melting assay (HRM) followed by direct sequence analysis was performed, but the efficiency is low [48]. It might be a good choice to perform RT-PCR and then sequencing. It would much easier to detect the size changes of the mRNA just by agarose gel electrophoresis, which were caused by large deletion/duplication or splicing abnormalities. If there is no or reduced RT-PCR products, mutations occurred on the regulatory elements would be suspected and sequence analysis would be performed then using genomic DNA to detect the sequence change. It also facilitates detection of the point mutations since the size of cDNA is much shorter than the genomic DNA.

A "one-step approach" was developed with multiplex PCR using 9 primer pairs to detect deletions and to perform linkage analysis simultaneously[49]. The primers amplified 3 exons, exon 8, 17 and 19, in the 5′ hotsport[50], and 6 short tandem repeats, 5′CA at the brain specific promoter region [51]and MP1P[52] at 3′UTR, and STR markers in introns 44, 45, 49 and 50[53]. The primers were grouped into three triplex PCR, Group A: 5′CA, MP1P and exon 8; Group B: exon 17, i44 and i49; Group C: exon 19, i45 and i50. The amplified fragments in the group can also serve as the internal control, since deletion is rarely spread all the gene, although one deletion gene had been detected, of which only one fragment was amplified with the primers for 5′CA site [Huang S, unpublished data]. The primers at both ends of the gene, 5′CA and MP1P, were used to detect the possible recombination.

3.2.3 Carrier - Testing

DMD is an X-linked recessive disease. Female carriers were at the risk to give birth to an affected male infant. Performing carrier testing offered a favorable opportunity for the carrier to get prenatal diagnosis at the first pregnancy. For deletion/duplication mutations, dosage analysis can be performed with either real-time PCR or MLPA[42,43], no mater it was a familial case or sporadic case, even the proband deceased. For point mutation, it can be carried out by direct sequencing.

For familial cases, linkage analysis can be performed[54], no mater what kind the mutation was. It would be offered with caution for the sporadic cases, especially the diagnosis of DMD was not confirmed. The markers used for linkage analysis should be highly polymorphic and informative, and lie both within and flanking the *DMD* locus[51-53].

The large size of the *DMD* gene leads to an appreciable risk of recombination. It has been estimated that the genetic distance was 12 centimorgans between the two ends of the gene[55]. Multiple recombination events may occur during meiosis and may not be detected when the marker was homozygous; thus, it might be aware in interpretation of the data generated from a linkage study.

Males with DMD usually die before reproductive age or are too debilitated to reproduce. It would be convincible that there was a plenty of de novo mutations responsible for the sporadic cases. For sporadic cases, the proband may be resulted from: 1) the mutation occurred after conception and is thus present in some but not all cells of the proband's body (somatic mosaicism), the proband's mother is not a carrier and the recurrence risk was very low; 2) germline mutation, passed from the mother. The later situation was completed, since the mutation could be one of the followings: a) a *de novo* mutation occurred in the egg, a meiosis mistake and the mother was normal; b) the mutation is resulted in mitosis in the ovary and partial of the cells carry the mutation, termed "germline mosaicism" or "gonad mosaicism", the recurrence risk depends on the proportion of the mutant cell line; c) somatic mosaicism, the mutation presented in some but not all of the mother's body including the ovary, the recurrence risk is high, up to 50%; d) a germline mutation, passed from one of grand-parents, or passed from ancestor on the grandmother side, the mother is the carrier. Put all these considerations together, carrier testing on the mother may be not informative, since the mutation could only be detectable in the last two situations. Since it is hard to tell at which level the mutations occurred, to provide carrier testing on the proband's mother in the sporadic case is controversial. There might be a misleading for the family, since the negative result of the testing may be misunderstood even misinterpreted as the mother was not a carrier at all, and the prenatal diagnosis was not necessary. It would be dangerous. For these reasons, prenatal diagnosis must be suggested to all cases especially the mutation has been identified; just in case the mother had the mutant cell line. The carrier status of the patient's sister can be performed if there was a detectable mutation in the proband. It should be aware that if the germline mutation is of the grandfather's origin, the maternal aunts would be at risk for a carrier, since there was a possibility that the grandfather is of germline mosaicism. The origin of the mutation can be revealed with linkage analysis[54,56]. This information is important in genetic counseling for determining which branches of the family are at risk for the disease. The carrier detection can be performed with either mutation detection if the proband's mutation was identified, or with linkage analysis. There is an ethics issue for carrier detection: the optimal time for determination of genetic risk, clarification of carrier status, and discussion of availability of prenatal testing, is before the person's pregnancy. It is appropriate to offer genetic counseling to young adults female relatives who are at risk of being carriers[56].

3.2.4 Prenatal diagnosis

In preventing birth of DMD fetus, prenatal test was carried out by sex selection in the early era, e.g., if the fetus was 46,XY, abortion would be induced.

The first case of prenatal diagnosis was performed in 1987 in China, via pathology analysis of the fetus muscle biopsy taken at 20 week gestation[57]. CK measurement on amnion fluid was used for prenatal diagnosis of DMD before gene analysis was available[58]. This approach is still used as the complementary or "rescue" procedure in prenatal diagnosis, when gene analysis is uninformative or linkage analysis has revealed that the fetus inherited the same haplotype as the proband in sporadic case.

Prenatal diagnosis for at-risk pregnancies requires prior identification of the disease-causing mutation in the family. It can be offered with 50% exclusive detection if the small mutation detection can not be carried out. The fetal material is obtained either by chorionic villus sampling (CVS) at approximately ten to 12 weeks' gestation or by amniocentesis usually performed at approximately 15-18 weeks' gestation.

The usual procedure in prenatal diagnosis is to determine fetal sex by PCR amplification of the male specific fragment, such as the *ZFY* gene. If the fetus is male, DNA from the fetus will be analyzed for the known causal mutation or tracking linkage established previously. If the fetus is a female, test will be stopped at this point, unless the mutation of the proband was identified. In this circumstance the carrier status of the female fetus might be tested.

Prenatal testing is possible for the first pregnancy of woman in the family whose carrier status has been recognized by mutation detection or linkage analysis.

The first gene diagnosis on DMD was carried out with restriction fragment length polymorphism (RFLP)[59]. With PCR method available, it is much easier to perform prenatal diagnosis for deletion cases using multiplex PCR[60,61], or with linkage analysis using STR markers[56,62,63], and recently MLPA method was used[56, 64].

In our center, prenatal gene diagnosis on DMD was performed mainly with "one-step approach", a linkage analysis protocol[49]. In reviewing the data of the cases analyzed with one-step approach since 1995, it was informative in almost all the families. After MLPA analysis on the remaining"non-deletion" cases screened by "one-step approach" , it revealed that 80% of the deletions were detected with linkage analysis [43,47]. For prenatal diagnosis, it was required that differentiation diagnosis and gene analysis should be performed prior to prenatal diagnosis with one-step approach. Since this approach can detect deletion and establish linkage phase simultaneously. Prenatal diagnosis was performed with the information collected from the pre-analysis. If it was uninformative with the linkage analysis, or the male fetus shared the same haplotype with the proband, or there was a chromosome recombination observed, MLPA analysis would be performed as a rescue procedure to see whether there was a deletion/duplication existed for the proband or not[56].

As for all X-linked genetic diseases, it should be aware that contamination with maternal DNA is a critical risk causing error in prenatal diagnosis. It should be incorporated the personal identification procedure in prenatal diagnosis. It was carried out with a set of multiplex PCR of unrelated markers, such as the STR markers on chromosome 21(please refer to the section of quality control, QC). We had the experiences that the material of CVS was from the mother and the amniocentesis cell grown up in the cell culture was of maternal origin. Fortunately, all these contamination events were revealed with the QC procedure.

3.3 Phenylketonuria (PKU)

3.3.1 Heterogeneity and prevalence of HPA

Phenylketonuria (PKU) (MIM 261600), an autosomal recessive inherited metabolic disease, is caused by phenylalanine hydroxylase (PAH) deficiency. It was called classical PKU in

China before, for distinguishing it from BH4 deficiency, which was called un-classic PKU or malignant PKU. In China the newborn screening data showed that the incidence of hyperphenylalaninemia (HPA) is around 1 in 11000[65], with the highest prevalence of 1 in 1666 in Gansu province[66]. Differentiated diagnosis was made by HPLC pterin analysis of the urine, measurement of RBC DHPR activity, and BH4 loading test. Classic PKU is diagnosed in individuals with plasma phenylalanine (Phe) concentrations higher than 1000 μmol/L in the untreated state. PKU accounts for 80% to 94% of HPA cases in Chinese, with the remaining as BH4 deficiency[67]. Patients with PKU are intolerance to the dietary intake of phenylalanine, one of the essential amino acids. Without dietary restriction of phenylalanine in the early life, most children with PKU will develop irreversible profound intellectual disability. Newborn screening has been launched in the early of 1980's in China [68]and free dietary treatment for the patients detected through the newborn screening program started in the early of 21 century, although the coverage of the newborn screening program varied from 100% in the developed area to 20% in developing areas, and no screening program at all in the remote areas, such as Tibetan and Qinghai province.

3.3.2 Mutation spectrum of *PAH* in China

PAH gene, located on 12q23.2, contains 13 exons and spans 90 kb, coding for a 2.4-kb mature mRNA. Mutation detection of the *PAH* gene in the PKU patients started in the late of 1987 on Chinese patients[69]. More than 100 different mutations have been identified up to date in Chinese PKU patients, accounting for 94.3% of the mutant alleles [70,71]. Mutations observed in the *PAH* gene include missense, splice site, and nonsense mutations, small deletions, and insertions. Eight mutations, c.728G>A(p.R243Q), IVS4-1G>A(rs62514907), c.611A>G (p.Y204C), c.1238G>C(p.R413P), c.331C>T(p.R111X), c.1068C>A(p.Y356X), and c.1197A>T(pV399V), accounting for 66.2% of the mutant alleles, with the proportions of 18.8%, 10%, 10%, 9.4%, 7%, 6%, and 5% of mutant alleles respectively [71].

When a panel of samples was collected in a certain area, mutation scanning was carried out with either ASO hybridization, denaturing high-performance liquid chromatography, or multiple AS-PCR. In the clinical service, we use a two-step procedure to detect the mutations of the *PAH* gene. In the first step, six exons, exon 3, 5, 6, 7, 11 and 12, and their flanking intronic sequences were amplified by PCR and then sequenced. In a panel of the patients, mutations were identified in 83% of the mutant alleles in the first step. If there was unknown allele remained in an individual, the second step of mutation scanning was carried out by sequencing the other seven exons. The total detection rate was 92.3%[71].

3.3.3 The strategy of prenatal diagnosis of PKU

Although there has been a good newborn screening program in China for decades and efficient early dietary treatment was available in the country[72], there is still a demand for prenatal diagnosis on the second pregnancy in the family. Prenatal diagnosis of PKU may be controversial if the testing is for the termination of the affected fetus. But it is the alternative choice of the families. The reasons for the parents seeking for prenatal diagnosis are: the first, the cost of the dietary treatment is high, beyond the economic capacity for the families with an average income, although there is a free treatment in some province, and the second is that in the families the parents had the bit experience already in managing the first child and would not want to risk the further baby bearing with the condition. It was not convenience in bring up the affected child and it is hard for them to make the child adhered to the dietary.

The first prenatal diagnosis on PKU was performed with RFLP linkage analysis in 1987[73]. There were other centers offering prenatal diagnosis, of which the centers at Peking Union Medical College[74,75] and Shanghai Xinhua Children's Hospital[76] played the main roles now.

In the beginning, linkage analysis with RFLP was tried. But unfortunately it was not as informative with RFLP markers as in the Caucasians, since 80% of the chromosomes were with haplotype 4 in Chinese [77]. Prenatal diagnosis got into service until mutation detection was carried out by PCR amplification and hybridized with ASO probes labeled with isotope [78]. The mutations of PAH gene could also be detected by methods of AS-PCR[79], single strand conformation polymorphism(SSCP)[80], or RFLP[81]

The limitation for all these procedures was that the two mutant alleles in the family must be characterized. But not in all of the cases the two mutant alleles could be identified, especially there was no time for detecting the mutations as the pregnant women came to clinic asking for prenatal diagnosis without any previous gene analysis. In addition, as more and more mutations being characterized in Chinese, it was hard and inconvenient for any diagnostic center to have all the probes ready for use. The quick procedure needed to be deveoped to perform prenatal diagnosis. The linkage analysis with short tandem repeats (STR), (ACAT)n in the intron 3 of *PAH* gene, emerged in 1992[82]. This marker was introduced into China in the same year [83]and a "quick approach" for prenatal diagnosis of PKU was proposed by combining this STR maker with a novel SNP (IVS3 nt-11A/C)in the *PAH* gene[84]. It was further expanded with additional STR markers incorporated. Three markers, PAH-STR, PAH-26 and PAH32, were used for haplotype analysis. They are highly informative and are both intragenic and flanking to the *PAH* locus. Linkage phase of mutant alleles and the haplotype of the markers could be established in almost all the cases[85]. For families in which only one *PAH* mutation was identified, or there is a urgent case for prenatal diagnosis, linkage analysis would be an option for prenatal diagnosis. But it should be kept in mind that the diagnosis of phenylketonuria should be confirmed (e.g. it is caused by mutation of phenylalanine hydroxylase gene). The shortage for using linkage strategy is that there is genetic heterogeneity of the HPA and not all the HPA were caused by mutation in *PAH* gene. If the differentiation diagnosis could not be made, there would be a miss management to treat all the cases as that caused by *PAH* mutation. Linkage studies are based on accurate clinical diagnosis of PAH deficiency in the affected family and accurate understanding of the genetic relationships in the family. Prenatal diagnosis should be applied with a caution and linkage analysis should be performed with combined with mutation detection.

Different families have different story: the mutation details, the linkage phase for the STR markers. So, it was required for cases asking for prenatal diagnosis, that gene analysis should be carried out prior to being pregnant, e.g., the differentiation diagnosis, especially when linkage analysis was employed, and DNA typing, either mutation detection or STR typing. In cases that probands deceased, it was still possible to perform prenatal diagnosis if the Guthrie card bloodspot was available, which might be kept in the newborn screening center. If differentiation diagnosis had been confirmed on the patient before death, linkage analysis can be done utilizing the remained genetic material. It would be better if mutations can be characterized using the DNA isolated from the bloodspots. The mutations in the family could be also identified by sequencing the parents' DNAs if the proband's DNA was not available, although the procedure was rather complicated in confirming the causal mutation.

3.4 Spinal muscular atrophy (SMA)

3.4.1 Molecular genetics of SMA

Spinal muscular atrophy (SMA) is characterized by progressive muscle weakness resulting from degeneration and loss of the anterior horn cells in the spinal cord and the brain stem nuclei. Onset ranges from before birth to adolescence or young adulthood. Electromyography (EMG) reveals denervation and diminished motor action potential amplitude.

SMA was classified into clinical subtypes according to the onset age and maximum function achieved. Infants of SMA 0, with prenatal onset and severe joint contractures, facial diplegia, and respiratory failure, died soon after birth. Children with SMA I (Werdnig-Hoffmann disease) manifest weakness before age six months and never be able to sit independently. The life expectancy for SMA I patients is less than two years. For SMA II (Dubowitz disease), with onset between age six and 12 months, the life expectancy is not known with certainty, some live into adolescence or as late as the third or fourth decade. The individuals with SMA III (Kugelberg-Welander disease) clinically manifest their weakness after age 12 months and are able to walk independently. SMA IV is the adult onset type.

SMA is inherited in an autosomal recessive manner. Two genes were considered related to SMA, *SMN1* (survival motor neuron 1) and *SMN2*, which locate on 5q12.2-q13.3 head to head with *SMN1*. *SMN1* is the primary disease-causing gene. Most people have one copy of *SMN1* on each chromosome, and there are about 4% of the chromosomes have two copies of *SMN1*. The number of *SMN2* copies ranges from zero to five in normal individuals, while there is at least one copy of *SMN2* remains in SMA patients. *SMN1* and *SMN2* differ by five single base-pair, locate in introns 6(g/a) and 7(a/g and a/g), and exons 7(C/T) and 8(G/A). The C/T SNP at position 6 of exon 7 is critical, since this change causes skipping of exon 7 in the mRNA of *SMN2* resulted in loss the function of *SMN2*, while the difference in exon 8 is a SNP in the 3'UTR of the genes.

About 95%-98% of individuals with SMA are homozygous deletion and about 2%-5% are compound heterozygotes for an *SMN1* deletion and an intragenic *SMN1* mutation. Some of the deletion of *SMN1* is caused by conversion between *SMN1* and *SMN2*, with the 3' portion of *SMN2*, not actually a real deletion.

3.4.2 Advantages in genetic testing

Prenatal gene diagnosis was carried out in China mainly on homozygous deletion cases, typically determined by lack of exon 7 of *SMN1*. Since there is at least on copy of *SMN2* remains in the SMA patients, Methods developed for deletion detection attempting to avoid amplification of the *SMN2* gene. In the beginning diagnosis of homozygous deletion of *SMN1* was carried out by SSCP analysis [86]. Since the pattern of the SSCP bands was rather complicated, a PCR-RFLP protocol was then adapted to replace SSCP procedure[87]. The difference at position 6 of exons 7 between *SMN1* and *SMN2* was considered for primer design. An artificial restriction site of Dra I (T*T*T|A|AA) was created by introducing a mismatched *T* in the primer. The exons 7 of both *SMN* genes were amplified and the PCR products were cut with Dra I. Since the products of *SMN2* has the restriction site while *SMN1* fragment doesn't, there would be no band corresponding to *SMN1* and only a smaller band for *SMN2* remained in homozygous deletion patients. For the PCR-RFLP procedure, there is a shortage of uncompleted digestion of the SMN2 fragment, which would be misinterpreted as the present of normal *SMN1* copy. It was dangerous when it occurred in prenatal diagnosis. Other methods were investigated to overcome this limitation, such as DHPLC and MLPA to detect the copy numbers of *SMN*s[88]. For the purpose for detection of homozygous deletion, a more simplified approach was developed. *SMNl* gene was amplified specifically with double allele-specific PCR(AS-PCR)(e. g. both primers for *SMN1* amplification were *SMN1* specific, utilizing SNPs at exon 7 and intron 7), coupled with a pair of primers for an irrelevant gene as internal control[89]. The products were separated by agarose gel electrophoresis or PAGE to determine whether the patients were of homozygous deletion of SMN1 gene. Comparing to PCR-RFLP and DHPLC used in the past, this approach can diagnose homozygous deletion of *SMN1* much more accurate, easier and more convenient without the interference of *SMN2*.This approach could be further modified by keeping the PCR cycles by 25 and quantitatively determining the density of the bands by densitometer, or using fluorescent labeling primer for quantitative PCR.

3.4.3 The feasibility of prenatal diagnosis for first pregnancy at risk for SMA

With all the progress, it is possible to perform prenatal diagnosis for the family in which the proband deceased, the same story as in PKU. Deletion detection could be performed by dosage analysis if there were tissue samples available from the proband, such as bloodspots from newborn screening. If there is no DNA available, *SMN1* dosage analysis may be performed on both parents to see if they were both with only one copy of *SMN1*. It is much easier to confirm the carrier status for the parents with real-time PCR or MLPA. But there might be a blind corner when the patient was a compound heterozygote or one of the parents has two *SMN1* copies on one chromosome when dosage analysis was performed. It is reasonable to offer prenatal diagnosis for these family as a 50% exclusive diagnosis, in hope that the deceased proband was really homozygous deletion no mater that one of his/her parents had two copies of *SMN1*on one chromosome or he/she was resulted in a de novo mutation of deletion. In case of intragenic mutation, the mutation might be revealed by sequencing the *SMN1* gene of the parent with two copies of *SMN1*. It is also feasible to detect carrier of deletion mutation in the population using this approach, at least for the relatives of the patient and his/her spouse. It was proposed to carry out population screening with the double AS-PCR procedure, since the rate of the carrier with deletion type was as high as 1 in 50[89]. It will make the prenatal diagnosis possible on the first pregnancy for the couples both with a single copy of *SMN1*, as doing on thalassemias in Southern China.

It may be further increase the chance of prenatal diagnosis for the patients of non-homozygous deletion by screening the possible intragenic mutation by sequence *SMN1* gene of the patient. But it should be offered with caution since the heterozygote frequency of SMN1 deletion is as high as 1 in 50, the diagnosis of SMA must be confirmed. For sequencing the *SMN1* gene, it can be achieved by a method that facilitates *SMN1*-specific amplification. Since there were more copies of *SMN2* than *SMN1* at DNA level, and only 15% of the SMN2 mRNA was full length (fl-mRNA), it may be easier to reveal the mutation by cDNA sequencing approach. Sequencing the full length mRNA of *SMN*s will increase the signal of the mutant allele since the ratio of fl-mRNA of *SMN2* to that of *SMN1* was reduced at the mRNA level. It has additional strength with cDNA sequencing strategy. The mutations affecting mRNA processing would be revealed much easier, no mater how deep it was hided within the intron. It will be able to detect the mutation responsible for transcription regulation if quantitative analysis of *SMN1* mRNA was performed. There is also an alternative approach for characterizing the intragenic mutation, e.g., by long-range PCR protocol and subcloning.

3.4.4 Be ware of contamination

Prenatal diagnosis of SMA was relied on deletion detection. If there was no amplification the fetus would be considered as affected. It would be dangerous when contamination of maternal material occurred. The amplification of SMN1 exon 7 might be from the maternal DNA, since the mother had a normal *SMN1* allele. To rule out the contamination of maternal material linkage analysis was performed routinely with STR markers on chromosome 21(section of quality control for prenatal diagnosis).

3.5 Personalized service in rare disease

Prenatal diagnosis was also offered to families with other genetic diseases as personalized services. In this case, mutation detection should be carried out in advance. There were more than 40 diseases available for this service in our center and more than 70 diseases were offered in other prenatal diagnosis center or department of medical genetics.

4. Quality control on the prenatal diagnosis

4.1 Be ware of heterogeneity

In practice of prenatal diagnosis the accuracy is very important. Since there is heterogeneity for genetic diseases, it was critical to confirm the diagnosis of the disease in the family seeking prenatal diagnosis.

4.2 Using different procedures to confirmed the output

It would be helpful to use two different protocols to carry out prenatal diagnosis, mutation detection and linkage analysis. For deletion analysis, in addition to use internal control linkage analysis should be used, which can tell if there was a contamination occurred.

4.3 Emphasis on pre-analysis in advance to prenatal diagnosis

It is always happened that the pregnant women come for prenatal diagnosis at high gestation weeks without confirmation diagnosis of the proband or with no previous gene analysis. Without genetic analysis in advance, it would be not sure if the prenatal diagnosis can be performed, since it might be uninformative with the commonly used polymorphic markers, or the mutations in the family can not be identified.

4.4 Ensure the fetal material is really from fetus

The maternal contamination was a serious risk, esprcially for deletion mutation. The mother always carried a normal allele which will give a positive amplification. We put an emphasis on sampling and sample processing: 1)CVS would be the first choice to get fetus material in our practice. When the sample received the chorionic villus would be carefully selected. 2)If amnion fluid had to be used the sample should be check for sure there was no blood contaminated. It can be told by sitting the fluid for a half hour to see if there was red cells precipitated. If it is so, cell culture will be set up. To avoid omission of the contamination, linkage analysis should be performed paralleling with mutation detection.

4.4.1 Get three birds with one stone

In our practice we performed linkage analysis first using two STRs on chromosome 21. By this procedure, we can get three answers: 1) whether the fetus was at risk for trisomy 21. If there is three alleles for the fetus or there were just two alleles but the density of one allele was nearly doubled, the fetus was affected with trisomy 21. Since we detected 2 markers, the chance for there was only one band, e. g. the parents were homozygous for two markers, was rare; 2) whether the fetal sample was taken from the fetus tissue. If the alleles were the same as the maternal ones and there is no paternal allele, it implied that the sample was not from the fetus but of maternal origin. It also showed whether there was a contamination with the maternal material, if there was an extra allele passed form the mother, and the density of the extra band was much weaker; 3) was the sample misplaced, if the genotypes of the parents and fetus were not matched.

In our practice we have confronted with the situation 2, there were maternal contamination and even worse that the sample was taken from the mother, not from the fetus. To confirm the later situation, more marker, other than markers on chromosome 21, were used for personal identification as doing in paternity testing. We called this procedure as "get three birds with one stone". If it implied the possibility for trisomy 21, markers on other chromosome would be tested. If there was no extra allele for the new markers, trisomy 21 was suspected, and AF sampling would be suggested in order to rule out the confined trisomy 21 in the CVS. If there was maternal contamination, fetus sample should be collected again. If there was a trouble in sample preparation, DNA would be extracted from the back up material, which was reserved in the original sample tube. If the polymorphic marker didn't give sufficient information, dosage analysis could be help. In our practice the contaminating band was always with a lower density, much less than 1 copy.

4.4.2 Be aware of the maternal origin of the grown cells from AF culture

When contamination of the maternal blood was suspected on AF sample, the routine way to get ride of the maternal white blood cells is to culture the amnion fluid cells. After several changes of the medium the blood cells would be washed away, leave the fetal cells grow up as fibroblast cells adhering on the culture flask. But in our practice in one case it turned to be that the grown cells were maternal origin since all the markers tested gave the same genotype as the mother's DNA did. Considering this situation, we added the STR testing procedure to all the prenatal diagnosis for monogenic diseases, such as for enzyme assay.

5. References

[1] Sun NH, et al. Intrauterine diagnosis for hereditary diseases, review on 78 cases. Chin J Ob & Gyn 1980; (1): 19-23

[2] Zhou XT, et al. Prenatal diagnosis on hereditary disease I, culturing the amnion fluid cells and prenatal diagnosis, with report on 100 cases. Acta Genetica Sinica 1980 (1):79-81

[3] Sun Nianhu, et al. Apply fetoscope in prenatal diagnosis and intrauerne therapy. Chin J Ob & Gyn (6): 356-358, 1986

[4] Guo YP, Gao SF, Dai YY, Sun NH, Wang FY, Ning Y. Pseudohypertrophic muscular dystrophy, a case report on prenatal diagnosis with fetal muscle biopsy and pathology analysis. Chin J Neurol and Psychit 1990; 23(1): 35-37

[5] Ye GL, Liao SX, Zhao XL, Xi HY, Liu Q, Cai XN. The possibility for maternal serum screening for fetal defects with AFP、β-HCG and UE3 in second trimester. J Xi'an Med. Univ. 16(4): 408-411, 1995

[6] WuWenyan, et al. Intrauterine diagnosis of mucopolysaccharidosis tye Ⅵ. Chin J Obs & Gyn. 1985; (2): 117

[7] Li Shanguo, Wang Peilan, Wu Wenyan. Two-dimentional electrophoresis of amnion fluid and its application in prenatal diagnosis of mucopolysaccharidosis. Shanghai Medicine 1989; 12(3): 153-156

[8] Shi Huiping, et al. Postnatal and prenatal diagnosis for lysosomal diseases. Natl J Med Chin. 1988; (3): 124-127

[9] Dept of Obstet & Gynocol. Fetal sex determination with chorionic villus sampling from cervix. Chin Med. J. 1(2):117-126, 1975

[10] Sun Nianhu, et al. The study on prenatal diagnosis with chorionic villus in early pregnancy. Heredity and diseases 1985; (1): 1-4

[11] Xiang Yang, Chang Xin, Wang Fengyun, Hao Na, Sun Nianhu. Prenatal diagnosis of genetic diseases at the early pregnancy by transabdominal chorionic vilus sampling. Chin J Obstet & Gynol 1997, 32(4): 253-254

[12] Ye HY, Hu YZ, et al. The study in performance of abdominal cordocentesis and its clinical application. Chin J Obstet Gynecol. 1988:23: 218-20

[13] Xu XM, Zhou YQ, Luo GX, Liao C, ZhouM, Chen PY, Lu JP, Jia SQ, Xiao GF, Shen X, Li J, Chen HP, Xia YY, Wen YX, MoQH, Li WD, Li YY, ZhuoLW, Wang ZQ, Chen YJ, Qin CH, Zhong M. et al. The prevalence and spectrum of alpha and beta thalassemia in Guangdong Province: implications for the future health burden and population screening. J Clin Pathol 57:517-522, 2004

[14] Xiong F, Sun M, Zhang X, Cai R, Zhou Y, Lou J, Zeng L, Sun Q, Xiao Q, Shang X, Wei X, Zhang T, Xhen P, Xu X. Molecular epidemiological survey of haematoblobinopathies in the Guangxi Zhuang Autonomous Region of southern China. Clin Genet 2010. 78(2):139-48

[15] Ou Caiying, Ming Jin, Xu Yunbi, Wang Chuanwen, and Huang Shangzhi. Study on the genotypes of α-thalassemia in 343 school children of the Li Nationality in Hainan. Hainan Med. J. 10(2): 112-113, 1999

[16] Fu Xiong, Qiuying Huang, Xiaoyun Chen, Yuqiu Zhou, Xinhua Zhang, Ren Cai, Yajun Chen,_Jiansheng Xie, Shanwei Feng, Xiaofeng Wei, Qizhi Xiao, Tianlang Zhang, Shiqiang Luo, Xuehuang Yang,_ Ying Hao, Yanxia Qu, Qingge Li, and Xiangmin Xu. A Melting Curve Analysis-Based PCR Assay for One-Step Genotyping of β-Thalassemia Mutations. J Mol Diagn 2011, 13:427–435

[17] Zhang Junwu, Wu Guanyun, Xu Xiaoshi, et al. The organization of the α-globin gene in Hb H patients from Guangdong Province. Actae Academiae Medicinae Sinicae 6:79-82, 1984

[18] Zhou Yuqiu, Xhang Yongliang, Li Liyan, Li Wendian, Mo Qiuhua, Zheng Qing, Xu Xiangmin. Rapid detection of three common deletional α-thalassemias in Chinese by single-tube multiplex PCR. Chin J Med Genet 2005, 22(2):180-184

[19] Li Liyan, MO Qiuhua, XU Xiangmin · Rapid diagnosis of non-deletion α-thalassemias by reverse dot blot. Chin J Med Genet 2003, 20(4):345-347

[20] Haig H. Kazazian Jr., Carol E. Dowling, Pamela G. Waber, Shangzhi Huang and Wilson H. Y. Lo: The spectrum of βthalassemia genes in Chinas and Southeast Asia. Blood 68: 964-966, 1986.

[21] Shangzhi Huang, Haig H. Kazazian Jr., Pamela G. Waber, Wilson H. Y. Lo, Ruo-lian Cai and Mei-qi Wang: βthalassemia in Chinese. Analysis of polymorphic restriction site haplotype in the β-globin gene cluster. Chin Med J 98: 881-886, 1985.

[22] Shangzhi Huang, Corinne Wong, Stylianos E. Antonarakis, Rolian Tsai, Wilson H. Y. Lo and Haig H. Kazazian Jr.: The same 'TATA' box β-thalassemia mutation in Chinese and U.S. blacks: another example of independent origins of mutation. *Hum. Genet.* 74: 162-164, 1986.

[23] Chen LC, Huang DA, Han JX, Chen LF, Huang S. The trial on population screening for β-thalassemia and mutation detection. Natural Science Journal of Hannan University 1993,11(1)：45-49;

[24] Chen Luofu, Huang Dongai, Wen Zhongping, Chen Lichang, and Huang Shangzhi. Genotyping of β-thalassemia on 95 cases of Li Minority. Natural Science Journal of Hannan University 1993,11(2)：47-49

[25] Liu Weipei, Zhang Luming, Zhang Yuhong, Ou Xiuyi, Liang Bo, Feng Shaoyan, Li Weiwen, Zhou Runtian, and Xing Tiehua. Six year practice in pre-marriage screening for thalassemia in Fushan City. Chinese J of Family Planning. 1999, 4: 187-168

[26] Xu Xiangmin, Liao Can, Liu Zhongying, Huang Yining, Zhang Jizeng, Li Jian, Peng Chaohui, Qiu Luoling, and Cai Xuheng. Antenatal screening and fetal diagnosis of β-thalassemia in the Chinese population. Chin J Med Genet 1996, 13(5):258-261

[27] Zhou Yuqiu, Xhang Yongliang, Li Liyan, Li Wendian, Mo Qiuhua, Zheng Qing, Xu Xiangmin. Rapid detection of three common deletional α-thalassemias in Chinese by single-tube multiplex PCR. Chin J Med Genet 2005, 22(2):180-184

[28] Li Liyan, MO Qiuhua, ·XU Xiangmin · Rapid diagnosis of non-deletion α-thalassemias by reverse dot blot. Chin J Med Genet 2003, 20(4):345-347

[29] Zhang JZ and Xu XM. Reverse dot blot, a quick approach for prenatal diagnosis of β-thalassemia. Chin Sci Bulletin 1993, 38(24): 2285-2287
[30] Wu Guanyun, Wang Limng, Zhang JunWu, Liang Xu, Zhou Peng, Long Guifang, Tang Zhining, Liang Rong, Fei Yongjun, Huang Youwen, Zhao Letian, Wang Rongxin, Su Jidong, Zhanlg Nijia. First-trimester fetal diagnosis for α-thalassemia. Actae Academiae Medicinae Sinicae 6(6):389-392, 1984
[31] Zeng YT and Huang SZ. Alpha-globin gene organisation and prenatal diagnosis of alpha-thalassaemia in Chinese. Lancet. 1(8424):304-7, 1985
[32] Zhang JZ, Cai SP, Huang DH, et al. Application of polymerase chain reaction in prenatal diagnosis of Bart's. Natl J Med Chin 1988, 12(3): 183-187
[33] Zhang Junwu, Zuo jin, Wu Guanyun, et al. Prenatal gene diagnosis on β-thalassemia in the first trimester(short report). Actae Academiae Medicinae Sinicae 7:180, 1985
[34] Zeng YT, Huang SZ, Qiu XK, Chen MJ, Dong JH, Ku AL, Lu FQ, and Huang YZ. Prenatal diagnosis on β-thalassemia. Natl J Med China. 1985, 65(11): 690
[35] Liu Jingzhong, Wu Guanyun, Gao Qingsheng, Jiang Zhe, Liang Zhiquan, Wilson HY Lo, Li Qi, Long Guifang, Zhang Jing, Deng Bing, Wang Rongxin, Huang Youwen, and Zeng Ruiping. Studies of β-thalassemia mutations and prenatal diagnosis in Guangxi, Guangdong and Sichuan Provinces of South China. Acta Academiae Medicinae Sinicae 1990, 12(2): 90-95
[36] Cai SP, Zhang JZ, Huang DH, Wang ZX, Liao FP, and Kan JW. Prenatal gene diagnosis on β-thalassemia with nonradioactive allele-specific oligonucleotide probes. Chin J Hematol 1989. 10(11): 567-568
[37] Liu JZ, Wu GY, Song F, and Wen XJ. Prenatal diagnosis of β-thalassemia with 3′ end specific primer PCR. Natl J Med Chin. 71(4):208-209, 1991
[38] Mao Yaohua, Sun Qiong, Li Zheng, Sheng Min, Huang Shuzhen, and Zeng Yitao. Applicfication of multipex allele-specific PCR for molecular diagnosis of β-thalassemia · J Med Genet. 1995, 12(4):209-211
[39] G Chang, PH Chen, SS Chiou, LS Lee, LI Perng and TC Liu. Rapid Diagnosis of β-Thalassemia Mutations in Chinese by Naturally and Amplified Created Restriction Sites. Blood, 180(8): pp 2092-2096, 1992
[40] Bushby KM. The limb-girdle muscular dystrophies—multiple genes, multiple mechanisms. *Hum Mol Genet*. 1999;8: 1875–82.
[41] Fanyi Zeng, Zhao-Rui Ren, Shang-Zhi Huang, Margot Kalf, Monique Mommersteeg, Maarten Smit, Stefan White, Chun-Lian Jin, Miao Xu, Da-Wen Zhou, Jing-Bin Yan, Mei-Jue Chen, Rinie van Beuningen, Shu-Zhen Huang, Johan den Dunnen, Yi-Tao Zeng, and Ying Wu. Array-MLPA: Comprehensive Detection of Deletions and Duplications and Its Application to DMD Patients. Hum Mutat. 2008 Jan;29(1):190-197
[42] Xiaozhu Wang, Zheng Wang, Ming Yan, Shangzhi Huang, Tian-Jian Chen and Nanbert Zhong. Similarity of DMD gene deletion and duplication in the Chinese patients compared to global populations. *Behavioral and Brain Functions* 2008, 4:20;
[43] Peng Yuan-yuan , Meng Yan , Yao Feng-xia , Han Juan-juan , Huang Shang-zhi. New multiplex-PCR assays for deletion detection on the Chinese DMD patients. Chin J of 中Chin J Lab Med. 2010; 33:106-110

[44] Zhang Junwu, Zhao Yanjun, Wu Guanyun, Chu Wenming, Liu Jingzhong, Wu Husheng, Zhao Shimin, and Sun Hianhu. Genetic analysis of 60 Duchenne muscular dystrophy(DMD) or Becker muscular dystrophy (BMD) patients using dystrophin cDNA. Actae Academiae Sinicae. 15(6):399-404, 1993

[45] Beggs AH, Koenig M, Boyce FM, et a1. Detection of 98% of DMD/BMD gene deletions by polymerase chain reaction[J]. Hum Genet, 1990, 86:45-48;

[46] Shenlin Ma, Guanyun Wu,Wenming Chu, et al.Two-step multiplex PCR amplification for quick detection of deletion mutations in Duchenne muscular dystrophy. Acta Academiae Medicinae Sinicae. 1993, 15:74-8.

[47] Huang S and Zhang L, unpublished results

[48] Chen Yanan, Zhou Xin, Jin Chunlian, et al. Scanning mutations of *DMD* gene in non-deletion allele by DHPLC method. Chin J Pediatrics 45(6): 2007

[49] Huang shangzhi. "Gene diagnosis and prenatal gene diagnosis", in "Medical Genetics".2ed ed. Li Pu et al eds, pp264-307 , Peking Union Medical College Press. Beijing, 2004

[50] Chamberlain JS, Gibbs RA, Ranier JE, et al. Deletion screening of the Duchenne muscular dystrophy locus via multiplex DNA amplification. Nucleic Acids Res, 16:11141-56, 1988.

[51] Xu Shunbin, Huang Shangzhi, Lu Shan, and Wilson HY Lo. Assay of two microsatellite polymorphisms at the 5' and 3' ends of the dystrophin gene and its application to DMD carrier diagnosis. Chin J Med Genet 10(6):324-327. 1993

[52] Huang Shangzh, Chu Haiying, Xu Shunbin, Zhou Yu, Wilson HY Lo. Amp-FLP analysis on MP1P site at the 3' untranslated region of dystrophin gene and its application to linkage analysis in gene diagnosis of DMD. Chin J Med. Genet 11(4):197-199, 1994

[53] Xu Shunbin, Huang Shangzhi, and Wilson HY Lo. A new approach to gene diagnosis of Duchenne/Becker muscular dystrophy, Amplified fragment length polymorphisms. Chin Med Sci. J 9(3): 137-142, 1994

[54] Chen Fan, Huang S, Pan XL,Fang B, Wu YY and Lo WHY. Molecular study of Duchenne muscular dystrophy, Carrier detection by means of RFLP linkage analysis .Natl J Med Chin 71: 339-341, 1991

[55] Abbs S, Roberts RG, Mathew CG, Bentley DR, Bobrow M. Accurate assessment of intragenic recombination frequency within the Duchenne muscular dystrophy gene. *Genomics*. 1990;7:602–6.]

[56] Huang Shangzhi.Gene diagnosis and prenatal diagnosis on Duchenne muscular dystrophy and spinal muscular atrophy. Chin J Neuroimmunol & Neurol 15(4):317-320, 2008

[57] Sun Nianhu, et al. Prenatal diagnosis on pseudohypertrophic muscular dystrophy, a case report on fetal muscle biopsy with the add of fetoscopy. Heredity and Diseases 4(2): 136-137, 1987

[58] Wu Yinyu, Pan Xiaoli, Li Shuyi, Qu Lurong, Wang Fuwei, Zhou Zhuoran, Jin Chunlian, Lin Changkun, Jiang Li, and Sun Kailai. Clinical study on prenatal diagnosis of DMD by combined assay of aminion fluid CK, LDH, and Mb. Zhong Guo You Sheng Yu Yi Chuan Za Zhi 3(1):10-13, 1995

[59] Zeng Yitao, et al. Prenatal diagnosis on Duchenne muscular dystrophy using DNA restriction fragment length polymorphism. Natl J Med of China 68(10): 565-567, 1988

[60] Wu Yuanqing and Sun Nianhu, Prenatal gene diagnosis on DMD with multiplex PCR using 9 pairs of primers. Chin J Med. Genet. 10(1):28-29, 1993

[61] Wu Yuanqing, Sun Nianhu, Wu Yuzhen, Wang Fengyun, and Ning Ynag. Prenatal gene diagnosis on psudohypertrophic muscular dystrophy with multiplex PCR using 14 pairs of primers. Natl J Med. Chin. 73(9):532-534, 1993

[62] Wu Yuanqing, Sun Nianhu, Huang Shangzhi, Xu Shunbin. Performing prenatal diagnosis and carrier detection in two families with high risk of DMD by STR markers linkage analysis. J. You Sheng You Yu. 6(1):1-4, 1995

[63] Liu Yuge, Xie Bingdi, and Dai Zhihua. The prenatal diagnosis of Duchenne /Becker muscular dystrophy using STR haploid linkage analysis. Chin J Neurol. 31(5):296-98, 1998

[64] Qing LI，Shao-ying LI，Dong-gui HU，Xiao-fang SUN，Dun-jin CHEN，Cheng ZHANG，Wei-ying JIANG. Prenatal molecular diagnosis of Duchenne and Becker muscular dystrophy. J. Peking University (health Sci.) 38(1)53-56, 2006

[65] GU Xuefan and WANG Zhiguo,Screening for phenylketonuria and congenital hypothyroidism in 518 million neonates in China. Chin J Prev Med. 2004, 38(2): 99-102

[66] Yan You-sheng, Wang Zheng, Hao Sheng-ju, et al. Mutation analysis of the PAH gene in patients with phenylketonuria in Gansu Province. Chin J Med Genet 2009, 26(4): 419-422CHN)

[67] Liu TT, Chiang SH, Wu SJ, Hsiao KJ. Tetrahydrobiopterin-deficient hyperphenylalaninemia in the Chinese. *Clin Chim Acta 2001;313:157-169*

[68] National consortium of newborn screening. The 5 years practice of newborn screening in eight cities. Chin J Pediatr, 1997, 35(12):255-256

[69] T Wang, Y Okano, R Eisensmith, S Z Huang, Y T Zeng, W H Lo, and S L Woo. Molecular genetics of phenylketonuria in Orientals: linkage disequilibrium between a termination mutation and haplotype 4 of the phenylalanine hydroxylase gene. Am J Hum Genet. 45(5): 675–680, 1989

[70] Song F, Qu YJ, Zhang T, Jin YW, Wang H, Zheng XY.Phenylketonuria mutations in Northern China. Mol Genet Metab. 86 Suppl 1:S107-18, 2005

[71] Huang Shangzhi. unpublished data

[72] Chen Ruiguan, Qian Dalong, Guo Hua, Feng Weijun, Gu Xuefan, Zhou Jiande, Zhang Yafen, Zhang Meihua, Pan Xinshi, Shen Yongnian, Lu Yongzhang. Treatment on patients of phenylketonuria with low phenylalanine dietary powder (BENTONG'AN) made in China. Chin J Pediat.. 28(5): 258-260, 1990

[73] Zeng YT, Huang SZ, Ren ZR,et al.. Prenatal diagnosis of phenylketonuria. Natl Med. J of China. 1986, 66:193-194

[74] Wang Tao, Yuan Lifang, Fang Bingliang, Huang Shangzhi, Wilson HY Luo, Sun Nianhu, Zhao Shimin, Liu Shenru, and Woo SLC. Prenatal diagnosis of phenylketonuria with polymerase chain reaction and oligonucleotide probes. Chin J Pediatrics 30(1): 30-31, 1992

[75] Wang Mei, Fang Bingliang, Yuan Lifang, Huang Shangzhi, Ye Jue, Li Jia, Lu Shan, and Wilson HY Lo. Characterization of the mutaion spectrum of phenylalanine hydroxylase and prenatal gen diagnosis. Natl J Med China 72(11):670-673, 1992

[76] Ye Jun, Gu Xuefan, zhang Yafen, Huang Xiaodong, Gao Xiaolan, Chen Ruiguan. Treatment of 769 cases with hyperphenylalanemia and gene study. Chin J of Pediatrics. 40(4):210-213, 2002

[77] Daiger SP, Reed L, Huang S-S, Zeng Y-T, Wang T, Lo WHY, Okana Y, et al (1989) Polymorphic DNA haplotypes at the phenylalanine hydroxylase (PAH) locus in Asian families with phenylketonuria (PKU). Am J Hum Genet 45: 319-324

[78] Zeng YT, Xue JR, Zhang ML, et al. Prenatal diagnosis of phenylketonuria (10 cases report). Natl Med. J of China. 1988, 68:61-64

[79] Song Fang, Wu Guanyun, Xu Guangzhi, Cai Weinian, and Ding Xiuyuan. Frequency of five point mutations of phenylalanine hydroxylase and prenatal gene diagnosis of phenylketonuria. Chin J Med Genet 12(6):321-324, 1995

[80] Yang Tao, Yuan Lifang, Huang Shangzhi, Fang Bingliang, Wang Mei, Sun Nianhu, Zhao Shimin, and Wilson HY Lo. Detectton of the mutational gene in phenylketanuria and prenatal diagnoses by using single strand conformation polymorphism methods.Chin J Obst. and Gynol 31(7):401-403, 1996

[81] Song Li, Xu Fengduo, Meng Yingtao, Shan Zhongmin. Prenatal gene diagnosis and synthetic analysis in high risk phenylketonurja. Tianjin Med J 31(2):82-84, 2003

[82] Goltsov AA, Eisensmith RC, Naughton ER, Jin L, Chakraborty R, Woo SL. A single polymorphic STR system in the human phenylalanine hydroxylase gene permits rapid prenatal diagnosis and carrier screening for phenylketonuria. Hum Mol. Genet. 1993, 2(5):577-581;

[83] Huang S, Fang BL, Chu HY, et al. Analysis of STR polymorphism in the PAH gene and its application to prenatal gene diagnosis of PKU. Natl Med. J. of China. 1995, 75(1):22-24(CHN)

[84] Huang S, Li H, Miao SR, Xu LT, Fang BL, Liu GY, and Luo HY. Analysis of the A/C polymorphic site within the phenylalanine hydroxylase gene. Acta Genetica Sinica 1996, 23(3):169-173

[85] Yao Feng-xia, Guo Hui, Han Juan-juan, Meng Yan, Sun Nian-hu, Huang Shang-zhi. The power of linkage analysis on *PAH* gene in prenatal gene diagnosis improved with three additional short tandem repeat markers. Chin J Med Genet. 2007, 24(4):382-386

[86] Yuan Lifang，Liu Tianci，Yang Tao, et a1. Gene diagnosis and prenatal diagnosis of spinal muscular atrophy in children. 1997.12.16; 35(12): 631-634

[87] Zhang YJ，Ma HW，Wang Y，et al．Prenatal gene diagnosis of infantile spinal muscular atrophy．J Shanghai Tiedao Univ(Nat Sci ed.), 2000, 21: 319-320

[88] Long Mei-juan, Wang Hong, Jin Yu-wei, et al. Quantitatice analysis of SMN1 and SMN2 genes based on DHPLC: a reliable method fro detection of non-homozygous patients with spinal muscular atrophy. Natl Med J China. 2008, 88(8): 1259-1263

[89] Li Xiaoqiao, Yao Fengxia, Su Liang, et al. A simplified approach for detecting homologous deletion of *SMN1* gene in spinal muaeular atrophy. J Med Res 2009, 38(5):29-32

11

Fetal Therapy: Where Do We Stand

Sebastian Illanes and Javier Caradeux
Fetal Medicine Unit, Department of Obstetrics & Gynaecology and Laboratory of Reproductive Biology, Universidad de los Andes Chile

1. Introduction

The last three decades have seen enormous scientific and technological advances, which have allowed the emergence of fetal medicine as a discipline and the possibility of fetal therapy. The development of different tools such as ultrasound, allows inspection and examination of the fetus, and a wide range of invasive procedures can be used for diagnostic and therapeutic purposes.

The value of a fetal therapy relates to the balance between benefits and risks of the in-uterus intervention, contrasted with the natural history and prognosis of each pathological condition. Several studies have shown that any problem diagnosed prenatally, usually has a worse prognosis than when the diagnosis is made postnatally. This improvement of prognosis with time relates to the gestational age at diagnosis, because of early detection of the most severe cases. It also relates to complications occurring during the pregnancy such as the emergence of associated genetic syndromes resulting in the worst prognosis cases being excluded by for example miscarriage. Therefore we should be very cautious about counselling a pregnant woman based on neonatal data and we need to adjust the prognosis given depending on the gestational age of the pregnancy.

We have classified the possible antenatal therapeutic interventions as transplacental treatment, invasive procedures, including transfusion and fetal surgery and future perspectives which we consider in an experimental stage but with clear possibilities of success.

2. Transplacental therapy: Fetal pharmacotherapy

Pharmacological therapy can be used to treat fetal disorders or improve the ability of the fetus to adapt to extra-uterine life. The transplacental route is the most commonly used way to administer drugs. However, transfer can be poor either because of the nature of the drug itself (e.g. digoxin) or if the condition requiring treatment reduces placental function (e.g. a hydropic placenta). Other approaches to drug therapy include direct fetal administration by the intra-amniotic route but these have a very limited role at present because of the invasive nature of the procedures and because very little is known regarding the effects of fetal physiology on fetal drug distribution and effects *(Koren G. 2002 - Thein AT. 1998)*.

2.1 Therapies to improve the ability of the fetus to adapt to extra-uterine life

Several methods have been used to accelerate fetal maturation in fetuses at risk of preterm delivery, and the example most extensively studied and used is corticosteroids for lung maturity. Liggins was the first to describe this effect in 1969 *(Liggins GC. 1969)*, and 40 years later the administration of these drugs remain the most important step to prevent respiratory distress syndrome and intraventricular haemorrhage in preterm infants *(Crowley P. 2004 – Onland W 2011)*. The effect of treatment is optimal if the baby is delivered more than 24 hours and less than seven days after the start of treatment *(Crowley. 2004 – Bronwnfoot FC. 2008)*. Use of repeat corticosteroid courses is at the moment under review. Some studies have shown a potential benefit of weekly repeat courses of antenatal corticosteroids in the occurrence and severity of neonatal respiratory disease but the short-term benefits are associated with a reduction in weight and head circumference, by the moment weekly repeated courses of steroids are not recommended *(Bevilacqua E. 2010 - ACOG Committee Opinion. No. 402 – RCOG Guideline No. 7)*. More studies are needed to assess the long term effect of repeated steroid exposure on the developing human brain *(Bevilacqua E. 2010 - ACOG Committee Opinion. No. 402 – RCOG Guideline No. 7 – Lamer P. 2002 – Crowther CA. 2004)*. Some authors have suggested a role for corticosteroids in elective term cesarean in order to reduce the higher incidence of respiratory distress presented by this group compared with vaginal term deliveries; however more studies are needed to recommend this approach *(Sotiriadis A. 2009)*.

2.2 Preventative therapies

A number of modalities have been studied over the years to try to prevent fetal serious disease that can lead to fetal death or serious long-term sequel in the child. An example of this strategy is the prevention of neural tube defects (NTDs). These conditions include open spina bifida, anencephaly and encephalocele, and complicate 1 or 2 every 1000 pregnancies in the UK *(Abramsky L. 1999)*, and can be prevented by the administration of folic acid during pregnancy *(MRC. 1991 - Czeizel AE. 1992)*. This is the first congenital malformation to be primarily prevented by pharmacological fetal therapy *(RCOG 2003)*. In 1996, the US Food and Drug Administration, initiated folic acid fortification of flour and mean folate levels in the population improved with substantial decrease in the risk of NTDs *(Koren G. 2002)*, this policy have been implemented in many countries *(RCOG 2003)*. Recent studies demonstrate this protective role of folate for NTDs, showing a protective effect of daily folic acid supplementation in preventing the disease (RR 0.28, 95% CI 0.15 to 0.52), with a significant protective effect for recurrence (RR 0.32, 95% CI 0.17 to 0.60) *(De-Regil LM. 2010)*.

Another successful strategy is the maternal administration of IVIg and/or corticosteroids to the mother to prevent severe fetomaternal alloimmune thrombocytopenia (FMAIT). This pathology occurs when a woman becomes alloimmunised against fetal platelet antigens inherited from the father of the baby which are absent from the maternal platelets. The most common of them is anti-HPA-1 *(Kaplan C. 2002)*. This condition is more frequent than is often realised since it occurs in about 1 in 1200 births *(Mueller EC. 1985 - Blanchette VS 1990 – Kaplan C. 1994)*. The main complication of this disease is bleeding which may have severe consequences such as fetal intracranial haemorrhage (ICH) resulting in death or long-term disability *(Montemagno R. 1994)*. Unlike red cell alloimmunisation, this disease often affects the first pregnancy, possibly due to the presence of the antigens in the trophoblast. The risk of recurrence in subsequent pregnancies with increasing severity is very high being 50-100% depending on the zygocity of the father for the relevant antigen *(Murphy MF. 2000)*. Bussel *(Bussel JB. 1996)* demonstrated that treatment with IVIg produced an increase in the platelet count of fetuses with alloimmune thrombocytopenia and observational studies have suggested an improvement in clinical outcome and reduction in the risk for intracranial haemorrhage when IVIg is administered to the mother throughout pregnancy *(Rayment R. 2005)*. Maternal therapy with IVIg may result in a fetal platelet count exceeding 50 x 10^9/l in 67% of pregnancies with a history of sibling affected by FMAIT *(Birchall JE. 2003)*, reducing the need of FBS and transfusions avoiding the complications of this technique. Although, the optimal management of FMAIT remains unclear and further trials would be required to determine optimal treatment for this condition. *(Rayment R.2011)*

In recent years, observational studies have indicated a relationship between antenatal treatment with magnesium sulfate in preeclampsia and preterm deliveries, and a consequent decrease in cerebral palsy in preterm infants with low birth weight *(Nelson KB. 1995 – Hirtz DG. 1998)*. Many randomized controlled trials have been conducted to examine this association. Recent meta-analysis conclude that the use of magnesium sulfate administered to patients at risk of preterm delivery before 34 weeks reduces the risk of cerebral palsy and gross motor dysfunction, without increase in pediatric mortality *(Costantine M. 2009 - Conde-Agudelo A. 2009 - Doyle LW. 2009)*.

2.3 Therapy for fetal disease

Fetal arrhythmias are good examples of pathologies which can be treated by therapeutic fetal drug administration. Although tachycardia (fetal ventricular heart rate faster than 180 bpm.) is sometimes intermittent, the chance of hemodynamic complications and development of fetal hydrops remains high *(Yasuki M. 2009)*. The indications for therapy may depend on its etiology, fetal age and disease severity *(McElhinney DB. 2010 - Strasburger JF 2010)*. For intermittent tachycardia, treatment is generally unnecessary, unless hydrops or cardiac dysfunction is evident. In preterm fetuses, sustained tachycardia should probably be treated regardless of cardiac dysfunction or hydrops, because these sequelae can develop rapidly *(McElhinney DB. 2010)*. When the patient presents with hydrops most arrhythmias can often be controlled with transplacental treatment, but the mortality in this group remains quite high *(Conde-Agudelo A. 2009)*.

Over the years, most antiarrhythmic agents have been used to treat fetal supraventricular tachycardia *(McElhinney DB. 2010)* and most fetuses are successfully treated in utero by transplacental administration of antiarrhythmic drugs *(Yasuki M. 2009)*. Digoxin is widely accepted as a first-line antiarrhythmic drug. Sotalol, flecainide and amiodarone are used as second-line drugs when digoxin fails to achieve conversion to sinus rhythm *(Yasuki M. 2009 - McElhinney DB. 2010)*. For fetuses with hydrops, digoxin is rarely effective *(Yasuki M. 2009 - McElhinney DB. 2010 - Strasburger JF 2010)* because the placental transfer of the digoxin is limited. Hence, sotalol or flecainide, which have good placental transfer ability, should be used from the beginning of fetal treatment for hydrops. *(Yasuki M. 2009 - McElhinney DB. 2010 - Strasburger JF 2010)*

The safety of the mother is of great concern when managing fetal tachycardia, even after some studies did´nt find any serious effects in the mother *(Simpson JM. 1998)*.

Administration of antiarrhythmic drugs for intrauterine treatment may cause pro-arrhythmia and threaten the mother. So ECG monitoring is recommended during dosage increase *(Yasuki M. 2009)*. However, these complications are generally tolerable and reversible *(Strasburger JF 2010)*.

Although intrauterine treatment is very effective in fetuses with tachycardia, treatment after delivery is also very effective. Hence, decisions for which cases are treated in utero or postnatally is often difficult. So, it is important not to select postnatal treatment too quickly in premature gestation, even when the fetus has already developed hydrops *(Yasuki M. 2009)*. Once the tachycardia is converted to sinus rhythm, the hydrops will recover and the fetus can be delivered at term by vaginal birth. However, when the hydrops continues for more than 2 weeks without conversion of tachycardia, postnatal treatment is recommended *(Yasuki M. 2009)*.

The efficacy of prenatal treatment for fetal bradicardia (fetal ventricular heart rate is less than 100 bpm) is limited compared with treatment for fetal tachycardia. Approximately half of all cases are caused by associated congenital heart disease, and the remaining cases that have normal cardiac structure are often caused by maternal SS-A antibody *(Yasuki M. 2009)*. Beta stimulants and steroids have been reported as effective transplacental treatments for fetal AV block *(Yasuki M. 2009)*. But the utility of these drugs still controversial (*McElhinney DB. 2010 - Strasburger JF 2010)*. Work is being done to develop leads and devices to improve fetal pacing *(Strasburger JF 2010)*.

3. Invasive procedure

3.1 Transfusion therapy

3.1.1 Red cell isoimmunisation

Haemolytic disease of the fetus and newborn (HDFN) is due to maternal alloantibodies directed against paternally inherited antigens on fetal red cells and was a significant cause of fetal and neonatal morbidity and mortality until the introduction of anti- D immunoglobulin during pregnancy and shortly after delivery. However, it is still a major problem in affected pregnancies *(Illanes S. 2008)*.

Intrauterine blood transfusion of anaemic fetuses represents one of the great successes of fetal therapy. The first approach was intraperitoneal blood transfusion introduced in 1963 by Liley *(Liley AW. 1963)*. Subsequently Rodeck *(Rodeck CH. 1981)* described intravascular fetal blood transfusion (IVT) by needling of the chorionic plate or umbilical cord vessels under direct vision by fetoscopy. In 1982 Bang in Denmark *(Bang J. 1982)* started IVT by umbilical cord puncture under ultrasound guidance which is now widely used by an increasingly large number of centres. IVT has produced a marked improvement in survival of the anaemic hydropic fetus and can also prevent this complication from developing by treating anaemic non-hydropic fetuses where moderate or severe anaemia is detected noninvasively by Doppler ultrasonography on the basis of an increase in the peak velocity of systolic blood flow or time-averaged mean velocity in the middle cerebral artery *(Mari G. 2000 - Abdel-Fattah SA. 2002)*.

The emphasis of current clinical management of HDFN is a non-invasive approach. This applies to the detection of fetuses at risk of HDFN with the use of cell-free fetal DNA in the plasma of pregnant women for the determination of fetal RhD genotype which is now available as a service world-wide. In addition when a fetus is antigen positive, the follow-up of these fetuses is for the detection of moderate or severe anaemia non-invasively by Doppler ultrasonography. When anaemia is suspected, an invasive approach is required in order to perform an IVT which should only be attempted when the fetus needs transfusion. This approach reduces the iatrogenic conversion of mild to severe disease which occurred as a result of the previous management approaches and this change represents one of the genuine successes of fetal therapy *(Illanes S. 2008)*.

3.1.2 Transient aplastic anaemia (parvovirus)

Parvovirus B19 accounts for about 25% of cases of nonimmune hydrops fetalis in anatomically normal fetuses *(Hall J. 1994)* as a result of fetal anaemia following tropism of B19 virus for erythroid precursor cells and the massive destruction of the infected erythroid cells and possibly myocarditis resulting in cardiac failure *(Yaegashi N. 1999 - Von Kaisenberg CS. 2001)*. The mean gestational age of presentation of hydrops is 22 weeks but there are some reports of earlier presentation which might often be undiagnosed *(Yaegashi N. 1998 - Sohan K. 2000)*.

Also some have suggested it may be a cause of apparently unexplained late still birth *(Norbeck O. 2002)*. The highest risk for a fetus developing hydrops is when maternal infection is before 20 weeks gestation probably due to the rapidly increasing red cell mass and short half-life of fetal red cells *(Thein AT. 1998)*. Diagnostic techniques aim at detecting maternal antibodies or either viral particles or DNA by PCR in maternal serum, amniotic fluid or fetal blood *(Von Kaisenberg CS. 2001)*.

The fetal loss rate following maternal parvovirus infection is about 10% *(PHLS. 1990)* but this is much higher when hydrops develops, so management is by FBS for diagnosis of anaemia followed by transfusion if necessary *(Soothill P. 1990)*. In fact, the rates of death among those who receive an intrauterine transfusion are significantly lower than among those who did not *(Von Kaisenberg CS. 2001 - Fairley CK. 1995)*. However, consideration should be given to the high fetal loss rate in cases of hydrops after fetal blood sampling *(Maxwell DJ. 1991)*. Fetal blood results in these cases show a negative Coomb's test, anaemia, thrombocytopenia, and low reticulocyte count *(Thein AT. 1998)*. If the reticulocyte count is high at the first transfusion this may indicate recovery already occurring and so a second transfusion may not be necessary. Usually FBS is repeated if hydrops returns or more recently when Doppler studies suggest worsening anaemia.

In spite of some reports of hydrops due to fetal parvovirus infection resolving without treatment *(Pryde PG. 1992 - Rodis JF. 1998)*, in our view if non-immune hydrops presents without obvious fetal malformations and anaemia is expected from the Doppler results, even if the mother does not give a clear history of parvovirus exposure, FBS should still be done urgently without waiting for maternal confirmatory tests and intra-uterine transfusion be done if there is evidence of severe fetal anaemia.

In contrast with other causes of fetal anaemia and hydrops, fetal complications caused by hPV B19 have the potential to resolve as the fetus mounts its own immune response *(Lamont R. 2011)*. So if other signs of fetal well-being are present, it might be possible to continue with conservative measurements *(Lamont R. 2011)*.

3.2 Amniotic fluid management

Amniotic fluid surrounds the fetus in intrauterine life providing a protected, low-resistance space suitable for fetal movements, growth and development. Disturbance of the balance between amniotic fluid production and consumption leads to oligo- or polyhydramnios, both of which are associated with poor perinatal outcome related to the degree of fluid volume change (Chamberlain PF. 1984).

Severe polyhydroamnios can cause maternal abdominal discomfort, respiratory embarrassment and preterm delivery *(Kyle PM. 1997 – Phelan JP. 1990)*. Amniotic fluid reduction can relieve maternal symptoms with severe polyhydramnios and prolong the gestation in both singleton and multiple pregnancies and is one of the possible treatments for TTTS *(Kyle PM. 1997 - Wee LY. 2002)*. Abruption can be a complication of removal of large volumes of amniotic fluid and this risk has been estimated at about 3-4% *(Leung WC. 2004)*. Common criteria for amniotic fluid drainage are AFI > 40 cm or the deepest single pool of >12 cm but many prefer to make the decision mostly on maternal discomfort *(Thein AT. 1998)*. Removal of a small volume can rapidly reduce amniotic fluid pressure but it usually re-accumulates quickly and approximately 1 litre needs to be removed for every 10cm the AFI is elevated *(Kyle PM. 1997 - Abdel-Fattah SA. 1999)*. The procedure often has to be repeated in order to prolong gestational age until maturity allows delivery. The insertion of a tube to achieve chronic long-term drainage has been tried in the past but there is a high risk of infection and no evidence supporting this approach.

Oligohydramnios is found in 3-5% of pregnancies in the third trimester, but severe cases relating to impaired outcome are less common *(Kyle PM. 1997)*. The significance of this finding relates mostly to the underlying cause, so the prognosis and the possibility of treatment depends on the aetiology. Attempts at therapy focus on restoring the amniotic fluid to allow continue development of the lungs during the canalicular phase. Quintero et al *(Quintero RA. 1999)* described effective resealing in cases of iatrogenic previable PPROM by intra-amniotic injection of platelets and cryoprecipitate although this approach has not been reported to work after spontaneous membrane rupture. Some reports have also shown that in pregnancies with preterm premature rupture of membranes (PPROM) with oligohydramnios at <26 weeks' gestation, serial amnioinfusions improve the perinatal outcome when compared to those with persistent oligohydramnios *(Locatelli A. 2000 - De Santis M. 2003)*. Fisk et al have recently described an amnioinfusion test procedure to try and pre-select cases of midtrimester PPROM which may benefit from serial amnioinfusion. A quarter of patients who retained infused fluid went on to subsequent serial amnioinfusion and prolongation of pregnancy with decrease in the risk of pulmonary hypoplasia *(Tan LK. 2003)*. However, there are risks of procedure related complications such as chorioamnionitis, placental abruption and extreme prematurity, so ideally a large series in a prospectively randomised trial would be needed to assess the benefits.

Amnioinfusion has also been used to prevent or relieve variable decelerations from umbilical cord compression in cases of rupture of membranes and to dilute meconium when present in the amniotic fluid and so reduce the risk of meconium aspiration during labour. A Cochrane review found that amnioinfusion for oligohydramnios helps when the baby shows signs of distress. If the baby shows no signs of distress from oligohydramnios, then amnioinfusion is not helpful. So there is no role for prophylactic amnioinfusion *(Novikova N. 1996)*. Another studies shows improvements in perinatal outcome when it is used to dilute meconium, only in settings where facilities for perinatal surveillance are limited *(Xu H. 2007 - Hofmeyr GJ. 2010)*.

3.3 Shunting

3.3.1 Pleuro-amniotic shunting

A pleural effusion may be an isolated finding or may occur in association with hydrops fetalis. When severe, this condition can produce hydrops, pulmonary hypoplasia by lung compression and polyhydramnios with secondary risks of preterm delivery *(Phelan JP. 1990)*. When due to a reversible cause such as chylothorax, the treatment of this condition by pleuro-amniotic shunting can be a very effective method *(Sohan K. 2001)* and can reverse the complications and prevent death. However, drainage does not help cases in which the pleural effusion is caused by an underlying progressive disease, or when the effusions are mild and so will not produce secondary effects or when the problem is diagnosed so late that pulmonary hypoplasia has already occurred and is irreversible.

When making the difficult decision of whether or not to shunt, the risks of thoracoamniotic shunting must be considered. The recommendation is that large pleural effusions, especially those with hydropic changes, should be seen urgently in a center that can offer tertiary level ultrasound examination, aspiration and shunting because, with appropriate treatment, 50% of fetuses survive *(Smith RP. 2005)*. Recently Yinon et al. conducted a retrospective study of 88 fetuses with large pleural effusions who underwent pleuroamniotic shunting, to evaluate perinatal outcome associated to the procedure. They concluded that carefully selected fetuses with primary pleural effusions can benefit from pleuroamniotic shunting, allowing hydrops to resolve with a survival rate of almost 60% *(Yinon Y. 2010)*.

Another approach for management of fetal chylothorax that is under evaluation is the use of pleurodesis with OK-432. First case-reports about its utility where published in 2001 revealing rapid and effective control of pleural effusion *(Tanemura M. 2001 - Okawa T 2001)*. A posterior review conducted by Chen et al. pooled a total of 9 cases, concluding that the success of the procedure depends on the complete aspiration of the pleural cavity and the demonstration of adhesions by ultrasonography following the procedure *(Chen M. 2005)*. A recent report published last year, that included a total of 45 cases show that this treatment is only useful in those cases without hydrops, converting the use of OK-432 pleurodesis in a plausible alternative to the classic management with thoracoamniotic shunting *(Yang YS. 2011)*.

3.3.2 Vesico-amniotic shunting

Lower urinary tract obstruction has a significant impact on perinatal morbidity and mortality, related principally to pulmonary hypoplasia and renal impairment that produce at least a 40% of mortality *(Nakayama DK. 1986 - Freedman AL. 1996)*. Animal models of releasing obstruction have been very successful but these models are often different from human congenital urinary tract obstruction *(Agarwal SK. 2001)*. The insertion of a double pig-tailed vesico-amniotic catheter is the most commonly used method to relieve this obstruction in vivo but complications are quite common, including failure of drainage or migration of the shunt, premature labour, urinary ascites, chorioamnionitis and iatrogenic gastroschisis *(Coplen DE. 1997)*. The main concern about vesico-amniotic shunting is that by the time severe obstructive uropathy is detected, renal function may be already severely and irreversibly damaged *(Freedman AL. 1996)*. Needle drainage has been used to obtain an assessment of renal function and helping to identifying fetuses with potential to benefit from in uterus surgical intervention *(Agarwal SK. 2001)*. Sometimes needle aspiration can appear to be therapeutic for megacystis in very early in the second trimester perhaps as a result of releasing urethral oedema secondary to pressure *(Carroll SG. 2001)*.

Recent data about antenatal bladder drainage appears to improve perinatal survival in cases of congenital lower urinary tract obstruction, but may confer a high residual risk of poor postnatal renal function, based on observational studies *(Morris RK. 2010)*. Currently, a clinical trial (PLUTO trial) comparing conservative management to vesicoamniotic shunting in singleton fetuses below 28 weeks gestation with isolated bladder outflow obstruction is at development *(PLUTO trial. 2007)*.

3.4 Laser treatment

Monochorionic (MC) twins account for 20% of spontaneous twin pregnancies and almost 5% occur as a result of medically assisted reproduction *(Chalouhi GE. 2011)*. Twin-twin transfusion syndrome (TTTS) affects 10% to 15% of monozygous twin pregnancies with monochorionic placentation *(Chalouhi GE. 2011 - Sebire NJ. 1997 - Carroll SG. 2002)*.

Without treatment, there is a very high risk of perinatal mortality and perinatal morbidity due to preterm delivery but also as a result of acquired brain injury in utero *(Denbow ML. 1998)*. When TTTS is of early onset, the prognosis is even worse and interruption of the vascular anastomosis by fetoscopic laser ablation is a sensible treatment that has been used since the beginning of the 1990s *(De Lia JE 1990)*. TTTS management has encompassed non-specific, sometimes symptomatic, treatments including amnioreduction, septostomy and even expectant management. To date, the only treatment addressing the pathophysiology of the syndrome is fetoscopic selective laser coagulation of placental vessels (SLCPV) *(Chalouhi GE. 2011)*.

With this treatment, in a third of pregnancies both twins survive, in another third one twin survives and in the remaining third both twins die *(Ville Y. 1995)*. The recently published Eurofetus study showed that laser therapy is associated with improved perinatal outcome compared with amnioreduction in women presenting with TTTS before 26 weeks' gestation *(Senat MV. 2004)*. To improve these results we need better ways of identifying all arterial-venous (A-V) anastomoses before ablation, which will enable a true rendering into a DC placenta with minimal destruction of viable placental territory. There have been some attempts of delineating placental vascular anatomy in utero with contrast agents and power Doppler but without clear success *(Denbow ML. 2000)*.

Laser ablation has also been used successfully to treat acardiac twin pregnancies that complicate 1% of monozygous twin pregnancies with monochorionic placentation *(Moore TR. 1990)* and are associated with congestive cardiac failure in the pump twin leading to polyhydramnios and preterm delivery with a reported perinatal mortality in untreated cases as high as 55% *(Tan TY. 2003)*. Laser or diathermy ablation is used to occlude the cord or the pelvic vessels within the abdomen of the acardiac twin *(Rodeck C. 1998 - Soothill P. 2002)*. A recent review suggests that intrafetal ablation is the treatment of choice for acardiac twins because it is simpler, safer and more effective when compared with the cord occlusion techniques *(Soothill P. 2002)*.

3.5 Fetoscopic / Open fetal surgery

Although most malformations diagnosed prenatally are best managed after birth, a few severe ones may be better treated before birth. The fetal malformations that warrant consideration for open surgical correction in uterus are those that interfere with normal growth, development and are life-threatening, so that correction of the defect may prevent these effects. At present, only a few malformations have been successfully corrected, including fetal myelomeningocele (MMC) and congenital diaphragmatic hernia (CDH).

3.5.1 Hydrocephaly and neural tube defects

Fetal MMC can produce *(Johnson MP. 2003)* obstructive hydrocephalus in up to 85% of cases requiring ventriculoperitoneal shunting. MMC can have other long term sequelae such as motor impairment of the legs and loss of bowel and bladder control. The damage may be due to the defect in the bony spinal column exposing the spinal cord to the trauma from the amniotic fluid and the uterine environment *(Evans MI. 2002)* raising the possibility of covering the spinal cord in the uterus to avoid the damage. The accumulated experience with fetal MMC repair has been encouraging and suggests a decreased need for ventriculoperitoneal shunting, arrest or slowing of progressive ventriculomegaly, and consistent resolution of hindbrain herniation in the short term follow up *(Johnson MP. 2003)*. However, further long-term follow-up is needed to evaluate neurodevelopment and bladder and bowel function. Since 2003 the *MOMS trial* is recruiting patients to assess the better management for these cases. So most centres still await for result before recommend the clinical intervention *(Luks FI. 2011)*.

3.5.2 Congenital diaphragmatic hernia

Congenital diaphragmatic hernia has a high mortality rate, and many clinical and experimental efforts have been made in order to reduce it. Open fetal repair of the diaphragmatic defect was attempted but with an unacceptable high mortality rate and so has been abandoned *(Evans MI. 2002)*. Fetoscopic temporary tracheal occlusion, have emerge as an alternative to open fetal surgery on the basis that the accumulation of lung fluid secretions can expand the lungs and so reduce the herniated viscera and avoid pulmonary hypoplasia. This approach may improve lung growth and development *(Sydorak RM. 2003)*; however, complications related to tracheal dissection, premature delivery and late morbidity are significant *(Deprest J. 2004)*. New techniques have been proven in experimental stage with less invasive approach but most studies have felt to prove any improvement of survival or morbidity rates when compared intrauterine fetal endoscopic tracheal occlusion approach with optimal postnatal care. However, there is a small group of extremely severe cases that could benefit from prenatal intervention *(Luks FI. 2011)*.

The exact definition of this subgroup of patients is still being debated. In 2003 *Harrison et al.* Correlated survival rates with lung-to-head ratio (LHR). Using this ratio good prognosis (100% survival) was associated with an LHR > 1.4. Poor prognosis (less than 30% survival) was associated with an LHR < 1.0 *(Harrison MR. 2003)*.

Actually, a RCT of *Luks et al.* is recruiting patients to evaluate the benefits of fetal tracheal occlusion with a detachable balloon for an LHR < 0.9 *(Luks FI. 2008)*.

4. Interventions in experimental stages

4.1 Ablation of tumours

Some tumours may growth to massive proportion in uterus, inducing high-output failure leading to fetal hydrops that end most uniformly in fetal demise. Fetal sacrococcygeal teratoma is a good example of this and surgery may have a role before the onset of hydrops in order to avoid this complication or after in order to resolve it *(Luks FI. 2011)*. Ablation of the majority of the tumour tissue is not usually necessary and perhaps only ligation or coagulation of the vascular steal can reverse or avoid the high-output fetal heart failure *(Paek BW. 2001)*. Open fetal surgery with a high incidence of technique related complications has been moving to less invasive approach such as radiofrequency ablation and fetoscopic resection *(Hirose S. 2003)* but more studies are needed to assess the impact of these types of managements and what groups of fetus benefit from them. With cervical teratomas another possibility for tracheal obstruction can be the EXIT procedure where the fetus is partially delivered, maintaining the uteroplacental circulation in order to perform the surgery and achieve adequate ventilation *(Murphy DJ. 2001)*.

4.2 Stem cell transplantation

At the present time, the most likely and eminent application of stem cell therapy to the fetus is in utero hematopoietic stem cell transplantation *(Matthew T. 2009)*. Bone marrow transplantation of normal haematopoietic stem cells can sustain normal haemopoeisis and be an alternative in treatment of lethal haematological disease. In the case of congenital disease like haemoglobinopathies, immunodeficiency disorders and inborn errors of metabolism that can be diagnosed prenatally and cured or improved by the engraftment of normal stem cells are theoretically an attractive alternative for the in utero transplantation of stem cells *(Evans MI. 2002)*. The unique characteristic of the hematologic and inmunologic system in the human fetus, could circumvent the postnatal problems of transplantation, such as graft-verus-host disease, and the remarkable ability of stem cells to proliferate, differentiate and become tolerant to host antigens are encouraging. However, most research on stem cell therapy to date has focused on disorders of old age that are not genetic. So, very little is known about the disorders that can occur in utero and how stem cells might be of benefit *(Mummery C. 2011)*. Finally, there is a small amount of evidence about safety and effectiveness in animals for transfer of treatment to fetuses at the present time *(Mummery C. 2011)*.

4.3 Gene therapy

The goal of gene therapy is to treat disease before damage secondary to the gene pathology is produce. Fetal gene therapy for many disorders already has been demonstrated in rodent and large animal models *(Matthew T. 2009)*. Some reports show that using a percutaneous ultrasound-guided injection of gene transfers in the airway or in the amniotic cavity in animal, provided levels of gene expression in lung and intestine that could be relevant for a therapeutic application *(David A. 2003 - Garrett DJ. 2003)*. In spite of the large amount of experimentation already made in this field, today we are still unsure whether or not this technique will provide the desired therapeutic effect and whether expression of the transferred genes will provide real clinical benefit *(Matthew T. 2009)*. Safety concerns need to be investigated extensively in appropriate preclinical animal models before application in humans. The ethics of fetal gene therapy also need to be considered.

5. Conclusions

Much has been achieved in the prevention, diagnosis and management of fetal pathology. This has allowed the development of interventions that have proven to be beneficial and safe for both fetus and mother. However, much remains to be investigated. The rapid progress in molecular and genetic research continues to be promising. However, the ethical and moral implications associated constitute a very important point that should not be omitted.

This article is a review of the evidence available at the time of publication and at no stage intended to be the basis for decision making and behaviours in particular cases, were different variables have to be pondered that exceed the scope of this chapter. It is the duty of the specialists to inform their patients and taking into account all the edges and risk for each management.

6. References

Abdel-Fattah SA, Carroll SG, Kyle PM, Soothill PW. *Amnioreduction: how much to drain?* Fetal Diagn Ther. 1999 Sep-Oct; 14(5): 279-82

Abdel-Fattah SA, Soothill PW, Carroll SG, Kyle PM. Middle cerebral artery Doppler for the prediction of fetal anaemia in cases without hydrops: a practical approach.Br J Radiol. 2002 Sep; 75 (897):726-30.

Abramsky L, Botting B, Chapple J, Stone D. *Has advice on periconceptional folate supplementation reduced neural-tube defects? Lancet* 1999;354:998-9.

Agarwal SK, Fisk NM. *In utero therapy for lower urinary tract obstruction.* Prenat Diagn. 2001 Nov;21(11):970-6.

Agustín Conde-Agudelo, MD, MPH; Roberto Romero, MD. *Antenatal magnesium sulfate for the prevention of cerebral palsy in preterm infants less than 34 weeks' gestation: a systematic review and metaanalysis.* American Journal of Obstetrics & Gynecology 2009 JUNE; 595-609

American College of Obstetricians and Gynecologists. Committee on Obstetric Practice. *ACOG Committee Opinion. No. 402: Antenatal corticosteroid therapy for fetal maturation.* Obstet Gynecol 2008;111:805–7.

Bang J, Bock JE, Trolle D Ultrasound guided fetal intravenous transfusion for severe rehus haemolytic disease. BMJ 1982; 284: 373–374.

Bevilacqua E, Brunelli R, Anceschi MM. *Review and meta-analysis: Benefits and risks of multiple courses of antenatal corticosteroids.* J Matern Fetal Neonatal Med. 2010 Apr;23(4):244-60

Birchall JE, Murphy MF, Kaplan C, Kroll H; European Fetomaternal Alloimmune Thrombocytopenia Study Group. *European collaborative study of the antenatal management of feto-maternal alloimmune thrombocytopenia.* Br J Haematol. 2003 Jul; 122(2): 275-88.

Blanchette VS, Chen L, de Friedberg ZS, Hogan VA, Trudel E, Decary F. *Alloimmunization to the PLA1 platelet antigen: results of a prospective study*. British Journal of Haematology 1990; 74:209-15.

Brownfoot FC, Crowther CA, Middleton P. *Different corticosteroids and regimens for accelerating fetal lung maturation for women at risk of preterm birth.* Cochrane Database Syst Rev. 2008 Oct 8;(4):CD006764.

J. B. Bussel, R. L. Berkowitz, L. Lynch, M. L. Lesser, M. J. Paidas, C. L. Huang and J. G. McFarland. *Antenatal management of alloimmune thrombocytopenia with intravenous gamma-globulin: a randomized trial of the addition of low-dose steroid to intravenous gamma-globulin. Am J Obstet Gynecol* 174 1996, pp. 1414–1423.

Carroll SG, Soothill PW, Abdel-Fattah SA, Porter H, Montague I, Kyle PM. *Prediction of chorionicity in twin pregnancies at 10-14 weeks of gestation*. BJOG. 2002 Feb; 109(2):182-6.

Carroll SG, Soothill PW, Tizard J, Kyle PM. *Vesicocentesis at 10-14 weeks of gestation for treatment of fetal megacystis.* Ultrasound Obstet Gynecol. 2001 Oct;18(4):366-70.

Chamberlain PF, Manning FA, Morrison I, Harman CR, Lange IR. *Ultrasound evaluation of amniotic fluid volume. I. The relationship of marginal and decreased amniotic fluid volumes to perinatal outcome*. Am J Obstet Gynecol. 1984 Oct 1; 150(3): 245-9.

Chamberlain PF, Manning FA, Morrison I, Harman CR, Lange IR. *Ultrasound evaluation of amniotic fluid volume. II. The relationship of increased amniotic fluid volume to perinatal outcome*. Am J Obstet Gynecol. 1984 Oct 1; 150(3): 250-4.

Coplen DE. *Prenatal intervention for hydronephrosis*. J Urol. 1997 Jun; 157(6):2270-7.

Costantine MM, Weiner SJ; Eunice Kennedy Shriver. *Effects of antenatal exposure to magnesium sulfate on neuroprotection and mortality in preterm infants: a meta-analysis*. National Institute of Child Health and Human Development Maternal-Fetal Medicine Units Network. Obstet Gynecol. 2009 Aug;114(2 Pt 1):354-64.

Crowley P. *Prophylactic corticosteroids for preterm birth (Cochrane Review)*. In: *The Cochrane Library*, Issue 1, 2004.

Crowther CA, Alfirevic Z, Haslam RR. *Prenatal thyrotropin-releasing hormone for preterm birth (Cochrane Review)*. In: The Cochrane Library, Issue 1, 2004.

Czeizel AE, Dudas I. *Prevention of the first occurrence of neural-tube defects by periconceptional vitamin supplementation. N Engl J Med* 1992;327:1832-5.

Christine Mummery, Magnus Westgren2 and Karen Sermon. *"Current controversies in prenatal diagnosis 1: is stem cell therapy ready for human fetuses?"* Prenat Diagn 2011; 31: 228–230.

David A, Cook T, Waddington S, Peebles D, Nivsarkar M, Knapton H, Miah M, Dahse T, Noakes D, Schneider H, Rodeck C, Coutelle C, Themis M. *Ultrasound-guided percutaneous delivery of adenoviral vectors encoding the beta-galactosidase and human factor IX genes to early gestation fetal sheep in utero*. Hum Gene Ther. 2003 Mar 1; 14(4):353-64.

De-Regil LM, Fernández-Gaxiola AC, Dowswell T, Peña-Rosas JP. *Effects and safety of periconceptional folate supplementation for preventing birth defects*. Cochrane Database Syst Rev. 2010 Oct 6;(10):CD007950.

Deprest J, Gratacos E, Nicolaides KH; *FETO Task Group Fetoscopic tracheal occlusion (FETO) for severe congenital diaphragmatic hernia: evolution of a technique and preliminary results*. Ultrasound Obstet Gynecol. 2004 Aug; 24(2):121-6

Denbow ML, Eckersley R, Welsh AW, Taylor MJ, Carter RC, Cosgrove DO, Fisk NM. *Ex vivo delineation of placental angioarchitecture with the microbubble contrast agent Levovist.* Am J Obstet Gynecol. 2000 Apr; 182(4):966-71.

Denbow ML, Battin MR, Cowan F, Assopardi D, Edwards AD, Fisk NM. *Neonatal cranial ultrasonographic findings in preterm twins complicated by severe fetofetal transfusion syndrome*. Am Obstet Gynecol 1998; 178:479-83.

De Lia JE, Cruikshank DP, Keye WR (1990) *Fetoscopic neodyminm:YAG laser occlusion of placental vessels in severe twin-twin transfusion syndrome*. Obstet Gynaecol 75:1046–1053.

De Santis M, Scavo M, Noia G, Masini L, Piersigilli F, Romagnoli C, Caruso A. *Transabdominal amnioinfusion treatment of severe oligohydramnios in preterm premature rupture of membranes at less than 26 gestational weeks*. Fetal Diagn Ther. 2003 Nov-Dec; 18(6): 412-7.

Doyle LW, Crowther CA, Middleton P, Marret S. *Antenatal magnesium sulfate and neurologic outcome in preterm infants: a systematic review*. Obstet Gynecol. 2009 Jun;113(6):1327-33

Evans MI, Harrison MR, Flake AW, Johnson MP. *Fetal therapy*. Best Pract Res Clin Obstet Gynaecol. 2002 Oct; 16(5):671-83.

Fairley CK, Smoleniec JS, Caul OE, Miller E. *Observational study of effect of intrauterine transfusions on outcome of fetal hydrops after parvovirus B19 infection*. Lancet. 1995 Nov 18; 346(8986): 1335-7.

Freedman AL, Bukowski TP, Smith CA, Evans MI, Johnson MP, Gonzales R. 1996. *Fetal therapy for obstructive uropathy: specific outcome diagnosis*. J Urol 156: 720.

Garrett DJ, Larson JE, Dunn D, Marrero L, Cohen JC. *In utero recombinant adeno-associated virus gene transfer in mice, rats, and primates*. BMC Biotechnol. 2003 Sep 30; 3(1):16.

G. E. Chalouhi, M. Essaoui, J. Stirnemann, T. Quibel, B. Deloison, L. Salomon and Y. Ville. *Laser therapy for twin-to-twin transfusion syndrome (TTTS) Review*. Prenat Diagn 2011; 31: 637–646.

Hall J. *Parvovirus B19 infection in pregnancy. Arch Dis Child Fetal Neonatal Ed* 1994; 71: F4–5

Harrison MR, Keller RL, Hawgood SB, Kitterman JA, Sandberg PL, Farmer DL, Lee H, Filly RA, Farrell JA, Albanese CT. *A randomized trial of fetal endoscopic tracheal occlusion for severe fetal congenital diaphragmatic hernia*. N Engl J Med. 2003 Nov 13;349(20):1916-24.

Hirose S, Farmer DL. *Fetal surgery for sacrococcygeal teratoma*. Clin Perinatol. 2003 Sep; 30(3):493-506.

Hirtz DG, Nelson KN. *Magnesium sulfate and cerebral palsy in premature infants*. Curr Opin Pediatr 1998;10:131–7.

Hofmeyr GJ, Xu H. *Amnioinfusion for meconium-stained liquor in labour*. Cochrane Database Syst Rev. 2010 Jan 20;(1):CD000014.

S. Illanes, P. Soothill. *Current aspects of the clinical management of haemolytic disease of the newborn and foetus.* Hematology Education: the education program for the annual congress of the European Hematology Association 2008; 2:175-178

Johnson MP, Sutton LN, Rintoul N, Crombleholme TM, Flake AW, Howell LJ, Hedrick HL, Wilson RD, Adzick NS. *Fetal myelomeningocele repair: short-term clinical outcomes*. Am J Obstet Gynecol. 2003 Aug;189(2):482-7

Kaplan C. *Alloimmune thrombocytopenia of the fetus and neonate: prospective antenatal screening.* In: Third European Symposium on Platelet and Granulocyte Immunobiology. Cambridge, UK, 1994.

Kaplan C. *Alloimmune thrombocytopenia of the fetus and the newborn*. Blood Rev. 2002 Mar; 16(1): 69-72.

Koren G, Klinger G, Ohlsson A. *Fetal pharmacotherapy. Drugs.* 2002; 62(5):757-73.

Kyle PM, Fisk NM (1997) *Oligohydramnios and polyhydramnios*. In: Fisk NM, Moise KJ Jr (eds) Fetal therapy, invasive and transplacental. Cambridge University Press, Cambridge, pp 203–217

Lamer P. *Current controversies surrounding the use of repeated courses of antenatal steroids.* Adv Neonatal Care. 2002 Dec;2(6):290-300

Lamont R, Sobel J, Vaisbuch E, Kusanovic J, Mazaki-Tovi S, Kim S, Uldbjerg N, Romero R. *Parvovirus B19 infection in human pregnancy*. BJOG 2011;118:175–186.

Leung WC, Jouannic JM, Hyett J, Rodeck C, Jauniaux E. *Procedure-related complications of rapid amniodrainage in the treatment of polyhydramnios.* Ultrasound Obstet Gynecol. 2004 Feb;23(2):154-8

Liggins GC. *Premature delivery of fetal lambs infused with glucocorticoids.* J Endocrinol 1969; 45: 515-23.

Liley AW Intrauterine transfusion of fetus in haemolytic disease. BMJ II 1963: 1107–1109.

Locatelli A, Vergani P, Di Pirro G, Doria V, Biffi A, Ghidini A. *Role of amnioinfusion in the management of premature rupture of the membranes at <26 weeks' gestation.* Am J Obstet Gynecol. 2000 Oct; 183(4): 878-82.

Luks FI. *New and/or improved aspects of fetal surgery*. Prenat Diagn. 2011 Mar;31(3):252-8. doi: 10.1002/pd.2706. Epub 2011 Feb 4.

Luks FI. 2008. *Fetal tracheal balloon study in diaphragmatic hernia.* http://clinicaltrials.gov/ct2/show/NCT00966823?term=luks&rank=1

Mari G, Deter RL, Carpenter RL, Rahman F, Zimmerman R, Moise KJ Jr, Dorman KF, Ludomirsky A, Gonzalez R, Gomez R, Oz U, Detti L, Copel JA, Bahado-Singh R, Berry S, Martinez-Poyer J, Blackwell SC. Noninvasive diagnosis by Doppler ultrasonography of fetal anemia due to maternal red-cell alloimmunization. Collaborative Group for Doppler Assessment of the Blood Velocity in Anemic Fetuses. N Engl J Med. 2000 Jan 6; 342 (1):9-14.

Matthew T. Santore, Jessica L. Roybal, Alan W. Flake. *Prenatal Stem Cell Transplantation and Gene Therapy*. Clin Perinatol 36 (2009) 451–471

Maxwell DJ, Johnson P, Hurley P, Neales K, Allan L, Knott P. *Fetal blood sampling and pregnancy loss in relation to indication*. Br J Obstet Gynaecol. 1991 Sep; 98(9): 892-7.

McElhinney DB, Tworetzky W, Lock JE. *Current status of fetal cardiac intervention*. Circulation. 2010 Mar 16;121(10):1256-63.

M. Chen, J.C. Schin, B.T. Wang, C.P. Chen and C.L. Yu. *Fetal OK-432 pleurodises: complete or incomplete?*.Letters to the Editor. Ultrasound Obstet Gynecol 2005; 26: 789-796

Montemagno R, Soothill PW, Scarcelli M, O'Brien P, Rodeck CH. *Detection of alloimmune thrombocytopenia as cause of isolated hydrocephalus by fetal blood sampling*. Lancet. 1994 May 21; 343(8908): 1300-1.

Morris RK, Malin GL, Khan KS, Kilby MD. *Systematic review of the effectiveness of antenatal intervention for the treatment of congenital lower urinary tract obstruction*. BJOG. 2010 Mar;117(4):382-90.

MRC, *Prevention of neural tube defects: results of the Medical Research Council Vitamin Study.* MRC Vitamin Study Research Group. *Lancet* 1991;338:131-7.

Mueller Eckhardt C, Mueller Eckhardt G, Willen-Ohff H, Horz A, Kuenzlen E, O'Neill GJ et al. *Immunogenicity of and immune response to the human platelet antigen Zwa is strongly associated with HLAB8 and DR3.* Tissue Antigens 1985;26: 71-6.

Murphy DJ, Kyle PM, Cairns P, Weir P, Cusick E, Soothill PW. *Ex-utero intrapartum treatment for cervical teratoma.* BJOG. 2001 Apr;108(4):429-30

Murphy MF, Williamson LM. *Antenatal screening for fetomaternal alloimmune thrombocytopenia: an evaluation using the criteria of the UK National Screening Committee.* Br J Haematol. 2000 Dec; 111(3):726-32.

Nakayama DK, Harrison MR, de Lorimier AA. 1986. *Prognosis posterior urethral valves presenting at birth.* J Pediatr Surg 43–45.

Nelson KB, Grether JK. *Can magnesium sulfate reduce the risk of cerebral palsy in very low birthweight infants?* Pediatrics 1995;95:263-9.

Norbeck O, Papadogiannakis N, Petersson K, Hirbod T, Broliden K, Tolfvenstam T. *Revised clinical presentation of parvovirus B19-associated intrauterine fetal death.* Clin Infect Dis. 2002 Nov 1;35(9):1032-8.

Novikova N, Hofmeyr GJ, Essilfie-Appiah G. *Prophylactic versus therapeutic amnioinfusion for oligohydramnios in labour.* Cochrane Database of Systematic Reviews 1996, Issue 1. Art. No.: CD000176. DOI: 10.1002/14651858.CD000176.

T. Okawa, Y. Takano, K. Fujimori, K. Yanagida and A. Sato. *A new fetal therapy for chylothorax: pleurodesis with OK-432.* Ultrasound Obstet Gynecol. 2001; 18: 376-377.

Onland W, de Laat MW, Mol BW, Offringa M. *Effects of antenatal corticosteroids given prior to 26 weeks' gestation: a systematic review of randomized controlled trials.* Am J Perinatol. 2011 Jan;28(1):33-44. Epub 2010 Jul 20.

Paek BW, Jennings RW, Harrison MR, Filly RA, Tacy TA, Farmer DL, Albanese CT. *Radiofrequency ablation of human fetal sacrococcygeal teratoma.* Am J Obstet Gynecol. 2001 Feb; 184(3):503-7.

Phelan JP, Park YW, Ahn MO, Rutherford SE. *Polyhydramnios and perinatal outcome.* J Perinatol 1990;10:347-50.

Pluto Collaborative Study Group. *"PLUTO trial protocol: percutaneous shunting for lower urinary tract obstruction randomised controlled trial"*. BJOG. 2007;114(7):904.

Pryde PG, Nugent CE, Pridjian G, Barr M, Faix RG. *Spontaneous resolution of nonimmunne hydrops fetalis secondary to human parvovirus B19 infection.* Obstet Gynaecol 1992; 79:859–861

Prospective study of human parvovirus (B19) infection in pregnancy. Public Health Laboratory Service Working Party on Fifth Disease. BMJ. 1990 May 5; 300(6733): 1166-70.

Quintero RA, Morales WJ, Allen M, Bornick PW, Arroyo J, LeParc G: *Treatment of iatrogenic previable premature rupture of membranes with intra-amniotic injection of platelets and cryoprecipitate (amniopatch): preliminary experience.* Am J Obstet Gynecol 1999; 181:744–749.

Rayment R, Brunskill SJ, Stanworth S, Soothill PW, Roberts DJ, Murphy MF. *Antenatal interventions for fetomaternal alloimmune thrombocytopenia.* Cochrane Database Syst Rev. 2005 Jan 25;(1):CD004226

Rayment R, Brunskill SJ, Soothill PW, Roberts DJ, Bussel JB, Murphy MF *Antenatal interventions for fetomaternal alloimmune thrombocytopenia..* Cochrane Database Syst Rev. 2011 May 11;5: CD004226.

Rodeck C, Deans A, Jauniaux E. *Thermocoagulation for the early treatment of pregnancy with an acardiac twin.* N Engl J Med. 1998 Oct 29; 339(18):1293-5.

Rodeck CH, Kemp JR, Holman CA, Whitmore CA, Karnicki J,Austin MA. Direct intravascular fetal blood transfusion by fetoscopy in severe Rhesus isoimmunisation. Lancet I 1981:625– 627.

Rodis JF, Borgida AF, Wilson M, Egan JF, Leo MV, Odibo AO, Campbell WA. *Management of parvovirus infection in pregnancy and outcomes of hydrops: a survey of members of the Society of Perinatal Obstetricians.* Am J Obstet Gynecol. 1998 Oct; 179(4): 985-8.

Royal College of Obstetrician and Gynaecologist (RCOG). *Antenatal Corticosteroids to Reduce Neonatal Morbidity and Mortality.* Guideline No. 7; Oct. 2010

Royal College of Obstetrician and Gynaecologist. *Periconceptional Folic Acid and Food Fortification in the Prevention of Neural Tube Defects.* Scientific Advisory Committee Opinion Paper 4 . April 2003.

Sebire NJ, Snijders RJ, Hughes K, Sepulveda W, Nicolaides KH. *The hidden mortality of monochorionic twin pregnancies.* Br J Obstet Gynaecol 1997; 104:1203-7.

Senat MV, Deprest J, Boulvain M, Paupe A, Winer N, Ville Y. *Endoscopic laser surgery versus serial amnioreduction for severe twin-to-twin transfusion syndrome. N Engl J Med* 2004;351:136-44

Simpson JM, Sharland GK. *Fetal tachycardias: management and outcome of 127 consecutive cases.* Heart. 1998 Jun; 79(6):576-81.

Smith RP, Illanes S, Denbow ML, Soothill PW. *Outcome of fetal pleural effusions treated by thoracoamniotic shunting.* Ultrasound Obstet Gynecol. 2005 Jul;26(1):63-6

Sohan K, Carroll S, Byrne D, Ashworth M, Soothill P. *Parvovirus as a differential diagnosis of hydrops fetalis in the first trimester.* Fetal Diagn Ther. 2000 Jul-Aug; 15 (4): 234-6.

Sohan K, Carroll SG, De La Fuente S, Soothill P, Kyle P. *Analysis of outcome in hydrops fetalis in relation to gestational age at diagnosis, cause and treatment.* Acta Obstet Gynecol Scand. 2001 Aug; 80(8):726-30.

Soothill P. *Intrauterine blood transfusion for non-immune hydrops fetalis due to parvovirus B19 infection.* Lancet. 1990 Jul 14; 336(8707): 121-2.

Soothill P, Sohan K, Carroll S, Kyle P. *Ultrasound-guided, intra-abdominal laser to treat acardiac pregnancies.* BJOG. 2002 Mar;109(3):352-4

Sotiriadis A, Makrydimas G, Papatheodorou S, Ioannidis JP. *Corticosteroids for preventing neonatal respiratory morbidity after elective caesarean section at term.* Cochrane Database Syst Rev. 2009 Oct 7;(4):CD006614.

Strasburger JF, Wakai RT. *Fetal cardiac arrhythmia detection and in utero therapy.* Nat Rev Cardiol. 2010 May;7(5):277-90.

Sydorak RM, Harrison MR. *Congenital diaphragmatic hernia: advances in prenatal therapy.* Clin Perinatol. 2003 Sep; 30(3):465-79.

Tan LK, Kumar S, Jolly M, Gleeson C, Johnson P, Fisk NM. *Test amnioinfusion to determine suitability for serial therapeutic amnioinfusion in midtrimester premature rupture of membranes.* Fetal Diagn Ther. 2003 May-Jun; 18(3): 183-9.

Tan TY, Sepulveda W. *Acardiac twin: a systematic review of minimally invasive treatment modalities.* Ultrasound Obstet Gynecol. 2003 Oct; 22(4):409-19.

M. Tanemura, N. Nishikawa, K. Kojima, Y. Suzuki and K. Suzumori. *A case of successful fetal therapy for congenital chylothorax by intrapleural injection of OK-432.* Ultrasound Obstet Gynecol. 2001; 18: 371-375.

Thein AT, Soothill P. *Antenatal invasive therapy.* Eur J Pediatr. 1998 Jan; 157 Suppl 1: S2-6.

TR Moore, S Gale and K Benirschke. *Perinatal outcome of forty-nine pregnancies complicated by acardiac twinning. Am J Obstet Gynecol* 163 1990, pp. 907–912

Ville Y, Hyett J, Hecher K, Nicolaides KH (1995) *Preliminary experience with endoscopic laser surgery for severe twin-twin transfusion syndrome.* N Engl J Med 332:224–227.

Von Kaisenberg CS, Jonat W. *Fetal parvovirus B19 infection.* Ultrasound Obstet Gynecol. 2001 Sep; 18(3): 280-8.

Wee LY, Fisk NM. *The twin-twin transfusion syndrome.* Semin Neonatol. 2002 Jun; 7(3): 187-202.

Xu H, Hofmeyr J, Roy C, Fraser W D. *Intrapartum amnioinfusion for meconium-stained amniotic fluid: a systematic review of randomised controlled trials.* BJOG. An International Journal of Obstetrics and Gynaecology 2007 114(4):383-390

Yaegashi N, Niinuma T, Chisaka H, Uehara S, Moffatt S, Tada K, Iwabuchi M, Matsunaga Y, Nakayama M, Yutani C, Osamura Y, Hirayama E, Okamura K, Sugamura K, Yajima A. *Parvovirus B19 infection induces apoptosis of erythroid cells in vitro and in vivo.* J Infect. 1999 Jul; 39(1): 68-76

Yaegashi N, Niinuma T, Chisaka H, Watanabe T, Uehara S, Okamura K, Moffatt S, Sugamura K, Yajima A. *The incidence of, and factors leading to, parvovirus B19-related hydrops fetalis following maternal infection; report of 10 cases and meta-analysis.* J Infect. 1998 Jul; 37(1): 28-35.

Yang YS, Ma GC, Shih JC, Chen CP, Chou CH, Yeh KT, Kuo SJ, Chen TH, Hwu WL, Lee TH, Chen M. *Experimental treatment of bilateral fetal chylothorax using in utero pleurodesis.* Ultrasound Obstet Gynecol. 2011 May 16.

Yasuki Maeno1, Akiko Hirose1, Taro Kanbe1 and Daizo Hori. *"Fetal arrhythmia: Prenatal diagnosis and perinatal management"*. J. Obstet. Gynaecol. Res. Vol. 35, No. 4: 623–629, August 2009.

Yinon Y, Grisaru-Granovsky S, Chaddha V, Windrim R, Seaward PG, Kelly EN, Beresovska O, Ryan G *Perinatal outcome following fetal chest shunt insertion for pleural effusion.* Ultrasound Obstet Gynecol. 2010 Jul;36(1):58-64.